Spiritual Management

— And —

Road to Eternity

Secrets of Beauty, Health, Youth and Liberation

Dr. Chan Baidjnath Misier

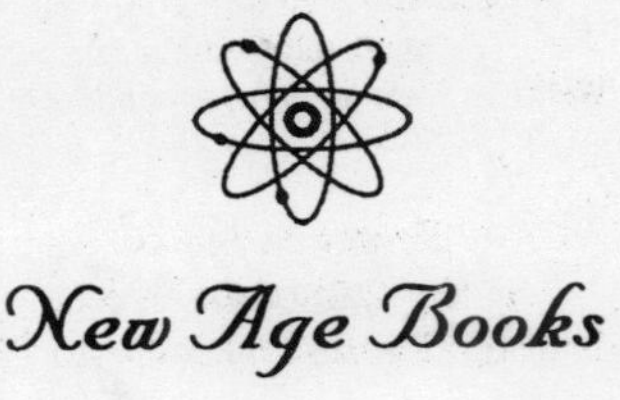

New Age Books

ISBN: 81-7822-278-7

First Indian Edition: Delhi, 2007

Published by
NEW AGE BOOKS
A-44, Naraina Industrial Area, Phase-I
New Delhi 110 028 (INDIA)
Email: nab@vsnl.in
Website: www.newagebooksindia.com

Printed in India
at Shri Jainendra Press
A-45, Naraina Phase-I, New Delhi 110 028

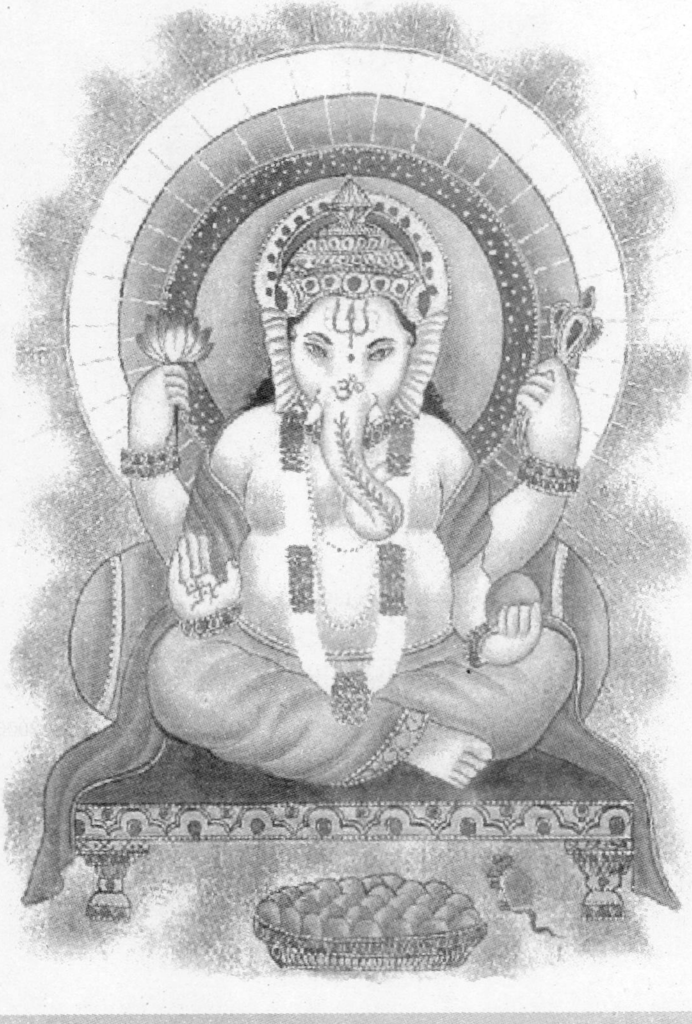

Śrī Gaṇeśāye Namaḥ

Śrī Guruve Namaḥ

Worship to Viśvanātham

gangā taranga
ramaṇya jatā kalāpam gaurī
nirantara vibhūśita vāma bhāgam
nārāyaṇā priya managa madāpahāram
vārāṇasi pura patim bhaja viśvanātham

CONTENTS

ABBREVIATIONS

AV	Atharva Veda
RV	Rig Veda
YV	Yajur Veda
SV	Sāma Veda
Bh.G.	Bhagvad Gītā
BhT.	Śrīmad Bhāgvatam
PYS	Patāñjali Yoga Sūtras
Mnd. Up	Muṇḍaka Upaniṣad
Ch. Up.	Chāṇdogya Upaniṣad
Kath. Up.	Kaṭha Upaniṣad
Ai.Up.	Aitareya Upaniśad
Brhd. Up.	Bṛhadāraṇyaka Upaniṣad
Sv. Up.	Śvetāṣvatara Upaniṣad
Mdk. Up	Māṇḍukya Upaniṣad
Ken. Up.	Kenopaniṣad
Is. Up.	Īṣopaniṣad
Pr. Up.	Praśna Upaniṣad
MS	Manu Smṛti
BS	Brahm Sūtra
Asht.G.	Aṣṭavakra gītā
VCM.	Vivekacūḍamaṇī

ACKNOWLEDGEMENT

I like to acknowledge my debt to numerous good spiritual advisors in Suriname, The Netherlands and India, who through their comments, corrections, encouragement and sometimes gentle prodding, have made this publication possible. I would like to express my gratitude and appreciation to Sudesh K. Hira, M.Sc. for his guidance and editing and to complete this work in time for publication.

Special thanks go to Dr. Premāchārya Shāstrī Jī for his incisive observations and clarification of crucial points of doctrine, and his continuous moral support; all Vedic and Yogic global teachers for their patient and thorough explanation of many difficult passages; and New Age Books without whose timely follow-up this book could never have achieved the worldwide dissemination it now enjoys.

This Veda Cosmic Science was made possible by a grant from the Foundation Āshrama The Netherlands, and the support of many global spiritual masters. The research has been jointly supervised by Professor G. Neeran, India and Professor M.K. Gautam, The Netherlands.

Dr. Chan Baidjnath Misier

FOREWORD

We need to educate the youth today about the sacred responsibility of preserving life and sharing the wealth of our global resources. This requires a new coalition of cooperation among the world's religions. A better understanding of the universe, about our lives, our own faith and religion is necessary because a comparison of different religions will bring out some common factors as well as some differences, both of which are essential. The common points help us to come to a better, a deeper understanding about our own religion. The differences bring out the borders of our religion and comparisons of the capacity of our own religion vis-ē-vis the others. Difference keeps our interests. Differences are complementary, they make us complete. It means that we have something to learn from those who are different from ourselves. People of all nationalities need to go beyond the external, and into the inner self to discover and establish everlasting peace based on a complete and holistic knowledge of spirituality.

This book *Spiritual Management and Road to Eternity* explores alternate secrets of Cosmic Science. We find discussions on the field of Jñāna Yoga or wisdom, the beauty of our nature and creation, sacrifice, physiology of breathing and its effect on the mind and emotions. It further goes to evaluate, on the bases of authoritative Sanskrit texts (the Vedas); the Ocean of Science, the creation, dissolution and salvation of the universe. It suggests many practical methods that help in harmonising the two kinds of energies in our body and in the cosmos in the achievement of mental and physical balance. There are chapters which deal with Yogic and Tantric meditations guiding the way to good health, a calm mind and controlling emotions. The roads to perfection are via concentration and meditation. These are paths for learning and teaching too. Concentration is the key factor for the student. Fix the mind on one object either within or outside the body. Steadily keep it there for some time. Purify the mind first through the practice of right conduct and then take to the practice of concentration. Concentration without purity of mind is of no avail. There are some occultists who have acquired the art of concentration but lack good character. That is the reason why they do not make any progress in the spirituality.

Ethical perfection is a matter of paramount importance. A scientist concentrates his mind on making new inventions. Through concentration he opens the layers of the gross mind and penetrates deep into the higher regions of the mind to gain deeper understanding. He concentrates all the energies of his mind into one field and focuses on the materials he is analysing to gain insight of their potentials. One has to tread on the spiritual path step by step, stage by stage. There are no shortcuts. Lay the foundation of right conduct, postures, regulation of breath and abstraction to start with. Only then will the superstructure of concentration and meditation be successful. It is very difficult to practise concentration when one is hungry or when one is suffering. We need to work and solve problems on several fields in several parts of the world.

Today, we possess sufficient economic, cultural and spiritual resources to introduce better global order, but old and new ethnic, national, social, economic, and religious tensions threaten and inhibit the peaceful building of a better world.

We have experienced greater technological progress than ever before, yet we see that worldwide poverty, hunger, death of children, unemployment, misery, and the destruction of nature are on the increase. Many peoples are threatened with economic ruin, social disarray, political marginalisation, ecological catastrophe and moral collapse. A decade later, the situation has grown worse.

Holy sacrifice or Pūjā and meditation (Yoga) are royal roads to the attainment of salvation or Mokṣa. Besides this, it's maintaining of the entire universe. These methods are so-called 'aircrafts' that help the aspirant to soar high in the realms of eternal bliss and everlasting peace. It is a mysterious ladder that connects earth and heaven and takes the aspirant to the immortal abode of Brahma. Meditation is the continuous flow of one thought of God or Ātmā, like the continuous flow of oil from one vessel to another. Meditation follows concentration.

If you have contentment, cheerfulness, patience, unruffled state of mind, sweet voice, one-pointedness of mind, light body, fearlessness, desirelessness, disgust for worldly things, consider it that you are advancing in the spiritual path and that you are nearing God. All desires and cravings slowly melt away. The intellect ceases to function.

You will be very close to the source, Ātmā or Soul. You will enjoy the waves of bliss and peace. All sensual objects will have no attraction for you now. The world will appear to you as a long dream. Jñāna will dawn in you by constant and deep meditation. The body-idea will vanish. You will realise the significance of the Mahavakya, 'Tat Tvam Asi."

Finally we can proclaim that the Saṃpūrnānandā Sanskrit University (Varanasi, India) and the European University of West and East (The Netherlands) highly praised the author,

Dr. C. Baidjnath Misier, and can declare this as a well-received book. We find here a clear sample of the core part of the identity which is the fruit in this book, even the author is a Non-Resident Indian (NRI). It is not important how a tree grows; the taste of the fruit is the character of the heritage. The deeper you search the roots the more you find and disclose the secrets of a culture. People are born and die in a culture.

Each chapter contains profound teachings clearly described with many Vedic mantras and other holy scriptures. Amenability to living ideas concerning spirituality is certainly needed in a society where modern science is developing very fast. The author places special accent on the pertinence of the teachings in Hinduism, viz. civilisation, culture and rituals in modern time. This work also describes the possibilities of operating more efficiently in this scientific world and has potentials to do the right things in the right manner. Thus, the book answers ideally the need for a lucid, succinct presentation of the principal aspects of Hinduism and its relevance to the apparent spiritual poverty of contemporary society.

Prof. M.K. Gautam
Vice-Chancellor of the
European University of West and East

PREFACE

The Hindu way of life is robust, joyful communion, amazingly in step with the most advanced ideology of modern times, in love with life, deeply human, as well as humane, delightfully aware of the individual's personal life needs compiled into a religion. This way of life deepens our understanding and appreciation of the Hindu religion. Besides that it also stimulates and increases our awareness to include and appreciate the truth in all religions. The chapter *Understanding the Spiritual World* (Ch. 2) gives an idea of the spirituality in Hinduism and its components.

The source of Hinduism is based on the knowledge of the Vedas, which are the highest authority in religious, ceremonial, and social matters. The Veda or knowledge is Cosmic Science. It contains knowledge of the cosmic universe, of all the creatures and God. It describes two paths to achieve the ultimate reality. The primarily technique that unites the seeker with the ultimate reality is pūjā or sacrifice (karma kanḍa). This is a visible interactive technique of divine ritual to purify the heart and to achieve union with God. Holy scriptures express the divine ritual as a method to keep the Lord in your heart. "As chaste women bring their gentle husbands under control by service, the pure devotees, who are equal to everyone and completely attached to the Supreme in the core of the heart, bring Him under their full control" (BhT. 9.4.66).

Man does not live by bread alone. Beauty and happiness are essential in life. Happiness is always present in anyone. Meditation makes one experience the happiness, whatever the circumstances. It is up to a person to draw from the source of Ānanda (happiness). Mantra or hymn is also a way to become aware of that source of Ānanda in oneself. That source is also called Paramātmā or unconditional consciousness, the kingdom of God. The Bhāgavatam provides an impression of unity and how to liberate the human being from bondage. "For one who has accepted the boat of the lotus feet of the Lord, who is the shelter of the cosmic manifestation and is famous as Mukunda, or the giver of mukti, the ocean of the material world is like the water contained in a calf's footprint (Parampadam), or the place where there are no material miseries, or Vaikuṇṭha, is his goal, not the place where there is danger in every step of life." (BhT. 10.14.58).

The second technique is the philosophy of Brahman (jñāna kaṇḍa). This knowledge or wisdom is related with yoga, jñāna yoga, this borderless path requiring tremendous strength of will and intellect. The practitioner of this yoga is training his mind to search for its own nature. Jñāna yoga explains the relationship between the Soul (Ātmā) and the Super Soul (Paramātmā). The Supreme Lord is so kind upon the living entity that He always accompanies, as two friends, the individual soul and in all circumstances is present as the Supersoul, or Paramātmā (Mnd. Up. 3.1.1). However, Yoga's, our doctor for health, beauty, pleasure, rust, peace, harmony, is the importance of awakening of the Kuṇḍalini a potent occult energy symbolized by a serpent having three and a half coils, and sleeping with its tail in its mouth. Jñāna yoga's, the wisdom that explains the technique to achieve salvation from rebirth. This book decodes the secrets of how to enter into the world of Goddess. The four stages in liberation are Sālokya, Sārūpya, Sāmīpya and Sāyujya. The destiny of the beginning (Sa) or to enter the place of the demigods (loka). To be involved in the general society of the spirits or Angels and to participate in cosmic decisions. The upturn to a new identity (rūpa)! A true God's world in which we want to develop a solid relationship with Him (mīpa). The last stage is in spirituality, the merge of the soul with the Super Soul (yuja) which means Mukti or salvation, the end of the birth- and death cycle. Yuja is the pipeline or light tunnel. As long we are not completely grown in spirituality, we will wander around within the creation, and will never find the way to God. Intermixing is only possible with capable management and action in the process of dissolving (body) and resolving of the soul in the Super Soul. Jñāna yoga, gives the facets of this technique in cosmic outlook. This chapter explains this path, which contains everything concerning knowledge: know how, insight and wisdom. It also regards the total process of pūjā, yoga, language, manners, behaviours and (greeting) sign (in theory and practice). Within the process it gives techniques how to achieve self-realization through the several paths of yoga.

This book points to that essence of eternal truth that animates every great religion in the world for the sake of well-being and for the benefit of future generations. It is written in harmony with the findings of modern science, yet it provides them with deeper meaning according to the Vedas and other relevant scriptures of Hinduism. It also provides an understanding of Hinduism as the inner way that all souls tread, characterised by profound wisdom, discipline and devotion, and with a genuine toleration and appreciation of religious diversity that is so much needed in our world. In clear and accessible language, Jñāna yoga topics covered include: important reading which is prepared to take on a new view of reality and your own nature. This is the inner beauty which is sweet like honey for every creature in nature, the spiritual universe.

Dr. Chan Baidjnath Misier
Pro. Vice Chanceller of the
European University of West and East

Introduction

Jñāna yoga in cosmic perspective

We must often check the oil meter of a car to ensure it's smooth functioning. Similarly we must often think in which direction the material and immaterial world develop within the current situation. We know that we are damaging the environment; the hole in the ozone is visible proof. Sometimes more destruction falls upon a particular area on the globe than raindrops. People present themselves with masks instead of their true face. *Quo Vadis?* Did science make more progress than necessary? How do we treat each other and our surroundings? This is a question we must answer now to make a plan toward attaining rest, peace, love and harmony in our society. The quotation: "make a better world, but start with yourself" says enough. People today, live with too many anxieties leading to tension, stress etc. In short, the world is in a state of Śirāsana: on the head (upside down)!

What is yoga? Which science should we use to solve environmental, societal and spiritual problems? This is the crucial question for everybody. We can ask ourselves: who are we and what is our task? Jñāna yoga offers perspectives in this impenetrable issue. But, what is Jñāna yoga?

Back to the sources

The Supreme Lord Śiva said in the Atharva Veda, one of the four books of the cosmic science, about yoga: "Through yoga I rise higher from physical force to mental force; from mental force to spiritual force, from spiritual force to God, the Blissful light" (AV 695). This threefold stage is based on practical cosmic knowledge and elevated conditions of yoga. Śiva confirms that the aim of yoga is to rise from a physical to a spiritual force and eventually eternal light.

The significance of 'force' is explained in the Rig Veda with a comparison of Indra Deva. "All our praises magnify Indra, spreading or pervading like the ocean (expansive), the most valiant of warriors who fight in chariots, the Lord of food, the protector of the virtues as the firmament" (RV 1.11.1; YV 17.61, 911). Indra is the preserver of food. Food indicates *physical power.* Courage or bravery points to *mental power* and the grateful homage to God, in words or song. The aim is to generate all aspects of knowledge: in the hymn it is called protection of virtues. This cumulative effect is comparable to the fire sacrifice or spiritual power—Sacrificial fire delivers the quintessence of the gross food (elements) in astral form to the gods, as amṛita or nectar of life (RV 1.12.1; SV 790).

The Atharva Veda explains sacrifice and denotes the method of protection and the continuation of yoga and pūjā. "Whosoever there are among the learned, the performers of seasonal sacrifices, the respectable at sacrifices, the performers of mental sacrifice in the form of yoga, the immortal, the expert in Vedic learning, may they all deliver unto us a vast sermon about Vedic lore today. O the learned people, may you ever protect us with peace-giving means" (AV 19.7.5, 4595). Regarding to the rising forces, we have to go back to the original source. This means that we have to attempt to an integration of the human soul with the Super soul; the Jīva with Śiva. The merging process happens through bliss and glitter!

The above mentioned three hymns of wisdom mention the stages of this particular path to blissfulness (Jīva up to Śiva). In the beginning of life, we find this bliss in our heart as true love, rest and peace. However, the heart is the rest place of our soul. Mainly, this process becomes the first success in life, the moment the sun lights our physical body. The next step in the immaterialistic way of life is connecting our heart with the heart of the cosmos, the heaven. The King of the heaven is lord Indra. He encourages the mental power for grateful homage to God. The next growth in our mental power which brings us in contact with lightning (SV 1420: RV 9.93.3). This is another form of God which is visible but too fast for our physical eyes to see a clear picture. The third stage in the spiritual growth is to achieve the highest region of God (YV 3.25; SV 1108). The Rising forces and the increasing growth circulates in our three bodies.

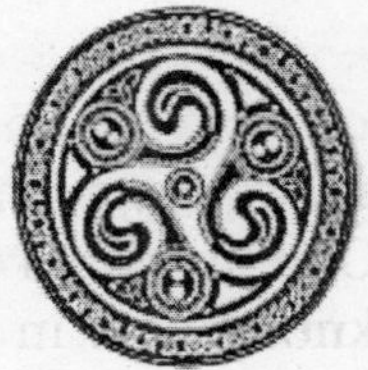

Figure 1: The three forces and bodies

The three bodies correspond with the three in the gāyatrī mantra, known as Bhūh, Bhuvah and Svah; the physic, potential and static energy in every being. The final destination through the human body is to reach Śiva Loka. With the astral part of and in this body we travel to this region and the process of liberation (comparable with 'death') starts from here. In this stage wordly love is characterised by striving toward spiritual love. Love here becomes purely spiritual and free from sensual desire. In this state have the mind totally under control. This is known as the harmony between the inner and the outer source. This is the Sārūpya state, the physical similarity with God, the Jīva and Śiva.

The medium between the soul (sound) and the Super soul (Super sound) is the Sāmanya or the Sāma Veda (Bh.G. 10.22: *Vedānām Sāmavedo-asmi*). The eleven kind of Śāntis or rest and peace, is merging the density of the inner sound with the outer sound: the eternal symphony welcomes us.

Above we have described the three stages of spiritual growth and development in our life in order to reach our final destination. Human beings should strive toward the acquirement of knowledge or wisdom called Jñāna yoga: the peace-giving means.

Jñāna yoga or Cosmic Science

Jñāna yoga is the most difficult path requiring tremendous strength of will and intellect. Hindu philosophy assumes that this entity as pure intelligence remains ever in its purity and only through a transcendent beginningless illusion. It appears to take part in or become associated with our experience. True knowledge or emancipation consists in the inborn or natural understanding of the Self as pure intelligence because everything comes into being by the Soul.

The aim of Jñāna yoga is to optimise the intellect by knowledge and wisdom. This path contains everything concerning knowledge, know-how, insight and wisdom. It regards also the total process of pūjā, yoga, language, manners, behaviour and (greeting) sign (in theory and practice). Within the process it gives off techniques how to achieve self-realization through the several paths of yoga. Jñāna yoga is searching for self-realization in practical life.

An aspirant who practices Jñāna yoga needs to have integrated the lessons of Hinduism or (macro) cosmic science and other yoga paths. This has to be done with selflessness in thoughts and activities, with love for all creation and God, with physical strength and a bright mind. A bright vision means that the aspirant understands that a human being is a microcosmic creature.

The aspirant should study the Vedas concerning the integration of the lessons of Hinduism with (macro) cosmic science. The Vedas contains the source of Hinduism, the basis of the social fabric of Indian lifestyle, the highest authority in religious, ceremonial, and social matters. These are believed to be, not the work of man, but of the Supreme Being Himself, and are therefore eternal. Vedas contain knowledge of God, the cosmic universe and all creatures. It gives two paths and or techniques to achieve ultimate reality.

The first technique is pūjā or sacrifice that unites the seeker with the ultimate reality. This is a visible interaction technique of divine ritual services performed at home or in a temple to purify the heart and to achieve union with God. The establishment of sacrificial knowledge and wisdom you will find in the Rig Veda, started already with the first mantra.

The second technique is spiritual, with physical discipline intended to bring direct insight into ultimate reality. With the philosophy of Vedānta the Jñāna yogi uses his mind to inquire into its own nature. Vedānta literally means "end of the Vedas" but it is interpreted as 'climax of the Vedas'. This philosophy has been fully integrated into Hinduism. Rituals and scriptural knowledge are only a means, not the end. The aim is ultimate unity with God (Mnd. Up. 3.2.4; BhG. 8: 21, 22).

Jñāna yoga leads the devotee to experience his unity with God, just as we perceive the space inside and outside a glass. In the same way we see ourselves as separate from God. Pūjā and yoga teach and provide physical and mental control, a divine love necessary for the "union of a human soul with a divine soul", directly by breaking the 'glass' around the soul; dissolving the veils of ignorance. The Yajur Veda clarifies this with the hymn: "Verily, the unborn soul, receives knowledge from the light of God. It beholds the Primordial God who's existing at or from the very beginning. Through His grace the learned at first attain spirituality. Through His grace the pure souls attain exalted positions. O learned persons, taking your spiritual knowledge, endowed with the lustre of God, to attain supreme happiness. Having reached the stage of final beatitude, and realising that Excellent light, mixed with the emancipated souls, and live in merriment (See also AV 4.14.1 en 2: 693 en 694). The hymn explains also that even after death only wisdom goes along with the soul. Spiritual knowledge is the vehicle to reach the destiny of supreme happiness (SV 3.7.2). We can emphasize that wisdom is the most important aspect of our life here and after. Both techniques are strongly connected with our state of consciousness, in which wisdom is meant to reach the higher consciousness. The figure below shows the connection of the two tehniques and the two-in-one principle's.

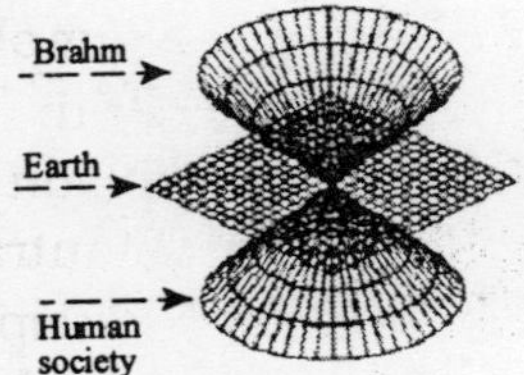

The upper aerial is God or Brahm. Brahm focuses to the complete creation, the universe with all natural characteristics. The square, plateau, states the earth space within all energies for growth and development; the bio data. The connection between the upper and bottom part is called the Ardhanārīprinciple, the two-in-one, which is necessary for love, peace and harmony.

Figure 2: Model of the flowing of cosmic sounds

The process of higher consciousness that takes place in our mind (internal) and in the 'cosmic mind' (universal). This part in our inner body has a variable to measure the distance between two celestial bodies. It is a transitional or intermediate route between two elements, which do not touch each other literally. This is a cosmic transmitting route, the same route of an email or the process of downloading. Practising the yoga system in this regard is just like connecting two-branch networks. This includes a measuring device in which the unknown resistance, capacitance, inductance, or impedance of one component can be measured by balancing the densities in each branch. Also computing the unknown value from the known values of the other components. This so-called celestial bridge circuit is located in the forehead (Ajñā cakra) where the concentration takes place. We describe this process of a cosmic structure as the space within two lines or three or more planes, known as Śiva Tilaka, diverging from a common zero-point with a celestial attendant of Goddess in microform.

The second technique, of spiritual with physical discipline is also used to realize a balance of the body and spirit. Figure 2 also pictures the balance and the biorhythm, which is coordinated by cosmic energies. The practitioner should intend to reach the inner movement, the correct speed and the desired density.

The figure shows a central point, the so-called 0-point, which is the Supreme Being or Brahmā (YV. 40.17: Om Kham Brahmā; BhG. 7.8; Sabdah Khe; Kha means Zero, infinite). Moving above point - zero is tuned to the cosmos (zero means round in shape). The downward radar shows the energy from point-zero forwards human society. A balance can be reached through the mind vibrations or radar . The result of this action is that the inner nature is linked with the cosmic nature. Both positions can be considered as two radars aimed at each other. Just as a radar sends waves and echo powers to determine the presence and location of an object, measuring time and space, in the same way the mind receives waves and echo powers from the cosmos. Receiving in spirituality terms means perception becomes awareness. This is the start of awakening higher consciousness. The last stage of awareness is also called *ex nihilo nihil fit*, out of nothing, comes nothing. Jñāna yoga is the technique to enlarge the mind. This is vital to understand our inner body and the secrets or icons in the cosmos, to experience and enjoy cosmic energy in the form of wisdom.

In the Middle Ages angelology, angels constituted the lowest of the nine celestial orders. These nine orders are compared in Hinduism with the nine powers in female forms, called Durgās. In compassion with the flowing cosmic sounds, the modern radar shows one of the Durgās, Mā Kālarātri, or female power for destruction of the negative demon powers. Because of Kālarātri time (Kāla) comes into existence.

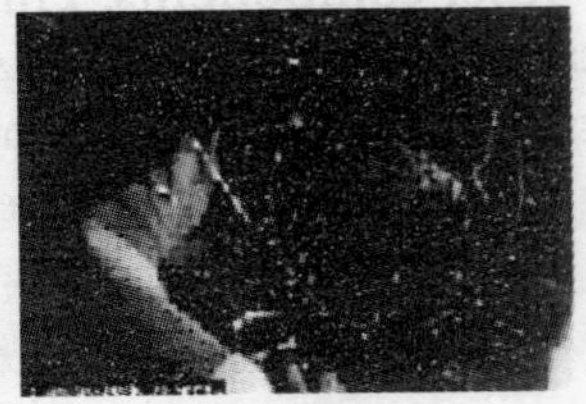

Figure 3: Radar

The comparison with radar means that the radar displays indicate the presence and movement of objects beyond sight. The waves, which do not encounter anything, simply disperse and waves bounced back reveal the shape and position of all objects in the region. The use of energy sources in the cosmos through yoga reduces time and space (distance). According to Jñāna yoga the element space is located in our throat, called the Viśuddha cakra. This is the unlimited or incalculably great three-dimensional realm or expanses in which all material objects are located in microform and all events occur. This microform is recognized in Hindu religious philosophy (Brhd. Up. 2:19) which says that man (microcosm) is a prototype of the universe (macrocosm). Universe is not just a matter. It consists of 'Rata and 'Prāṇa' (matter and spirit). Just as there is consciousness or spirit (Ātmā) behind the physical body (matter) of man, there is Consciousness or spirit behind the physical body of the universe (Sv. Up. 6:17), which is understood as God or Brahmā (Kath. Up. 6: 7,8). Additionally, space and time are connected with sounds in our alphabet.

The Sanskrit character 'Nga' indicates the space in the throat. And in the forehead (ajñā cakra) where time takes place is indicated with the character Ha which means expand or multiply constantly. This Ha-sound is a Devi or energy (angel) which promotes cosmic growth and development. This is a matching principle between the macro and the micro, the cosmic and the human body. The Rig Veda confirms this in the following hymn: "His two nostrils are the generating centers of our breathing and of all other airs, His smelling powers generate the Aśvinī Kumārs demigods (space and time)and all kinds of medicinal herbs, and His breathing energies produce different kinds of fragrance. His eyes are the generating centers of all kinds of forms, which glitter and illuminate. His eyeballs are like the sun and the heavenly planets. His ears hear from all sides and are receptacles for all the Vedas, and His sense of hearing is the generating center of the sky and of all kinds of sound. The air is the moving agent of all the planets, and as such the generating centers for promotion to the deserving planets, the sacrifices, are His bodily surface and are naturally the origin of all auspicious opportunities" (RV 10.90.2-4).

A generating center is defined as a form, type, class, etc. of objects existing at the same time and having many similarities or developed from a common model or ancestor. The ancestor in this matter is the Super Soul or the Supreme Lord. A common model can be compared with a small computer (compare human as a small cosmos) which has similarities with the bigger computer in the macro cosmos. This comparison is not unusual because even computer science uses the above-mentioned Sanskrit alphabet as characters to develop computer programmes such as Internet, email etc.

The Jñāna yoga technique has been a great improvement for computer science. Take for instance the sense becomes sensor, vibration in radar system, sound into echo power expanded or multiplied translates into waves. Internet Technology (IT) is a semi-product of cosmic science or the Veda's. Another example of a Sanskrit character 'Jha' Aśvinī means 'in touch' or contact point. This contact becomes a compassion on a higher or emotional level. It means action and reaction, an Ardhanāri or a two-in-one-principle. Ardha means the Ultimate Reality conceived as the Divine Unity of Śakti (the Divine Feminine) and Śiva (the Divine Masculine). They are One, They are All, They are God. Consider the name most frequently applied to this "Divine Androgyne." This is a being of ambiguous sexual identity; one that combines major aspects of both the male and the female. Śiva represented as a half male and half female, the incarnation as the male and the female principles of the world as the bisexual image of the lunar and solar power. These powers are the bases to create the universe and all creatures, symbolizing his dual nature. This Divine Androgyne or Ardha-nārīśvara is the concept for creation of all creatures in the (human) cosmic world. Lord Brahmā has the same Androgyne status by creating the demigods. The difference between the human and the angel (demigods) is that the human has three bodies (physic, astral and carnal; a three-in-one) and the angel has no physical body. This difference has many influences on the densities of sounds in those bodies. In the cosmos this particular kind of action or contact is made with the energy, which is hidden behind this character Jha. Spirituality decodes and gives insight of icons. This is the energy that the yogi accomplishes when he comes in contact with icons.

Jñāna yoga is indispensable for the development of nature, people and the inner nature of people. Knowledge and wisdom are the power behind the total development of humanity. Veda formulates that attainment to salvation by knowledge the highest stage of spiritual development and to attain the loftiest light of God. The benefactors of humanity and the exhibitors of the path of righteousness have been worshipped. The yogi or practitioner of Jñāna yoga makes a concentrated link between its own energy source with the energy sources in the universe to achieve balance between inner peace and peace in society. The practical method can be compared with the door of a lift, which opens as soon as a laser beam contacts the contra pool. The Rig Veda mentions this in the first chapter as follows: "I solicit understanding from Agni or Sadasaspati. The wonderful, the friend of Indra, the desirable, liberal in bestowing gifts (bountiful). I am drawn nearer in prayer to the wondrous Lord or Guardian who's assembly of priests and worshippers are brought together." This hymn formulates a state, process, or instance of a chemical combination in which materials are heated intensely and combined with oxygen. This process produces light, heat and flame, called Agni. Further it defines a loud, explosive, resounding noise produced by the explosive expansion of air heated by a lightning discharge, named Indra, the King of Heaven. Lightning appears as the renderer of forts, young, the thunderer, unmeasured in strength, the sustainer of all acts, armed with power, and highly spoken of in the Vedas (RV 1.2.4; SV 1250). Friendship means a contact between Agni (fire) and Indra (lightning) and on equal level of energies. This contact produces male and female aspects, a dual nature. The male part of Agni is guarding and protecting, and the female part is a burning passion for enthusiasm and intense devotion (desirable). Agni also means growth in values (gifts), independency (liberal), the total development of humanity (wondrous Lord) and spiritual development (priests and worshippers). The final core of Jñāna yoga is to generate contact, love, peace, religious worship, bliss and wisdom.

Heritage

In chapter 10 of the Rig Veda we find the explanation of the process and the purpose of creation (RV 72.4 and 5). The unmanifested Lord or Brahm, first expanded Himself in the universal form of the Puruṣa (Man) incarnation. This Super form is known as Virāṭ. He in this form manifested all the ingredients for material creation. Then He changes His energy in several forms, with names as passwords, according to the plan of action: to organize, to create and to manage the whole process of creation. This plan is similar to that of a company wherein several people work in each branch based on which they have a designation or (profession) and a job description.

At first there was the creation of the sixteen principles of material action. This was for the purpose of the first creation, the material universe. The material for this creation He took from water. A part of the Puruṣa lies down within the water of the universe, from the navel of His body sprouts a lotus stem, and from the lotus flower atop this stem, Brahmā, the master of all engineers in the universe, is manifested. A stem of a lotus is the rising and central or principal structure, whether above or below the ground, which ordinarily grows in the opposite direction to the root. It is also called the main body of that portion of a plant. Other meanings of the stem are to dam or to stop the flow of a stream, to make progress against any opposition and to direct one's course. Jñāna yoga functions as the stem of the lotus: going back to the root by wisdom (the main body) and progression to self-realisation.

This foregoing process can be described as the second step in the process of evolution, known as the mundane egg or Hiraṇyagarbha. This egg had two parts, a male and a female. The male form was a small part of Brahmā and He changes a part in Him as the female form or Śakti. Mā (Mother) is known as the female part of Brahm. The merge between Brahm and Mā becomes Brahmā. Hiraṇyagarbha is ordained as the heir or protector and sustainer of all creations from the beginning. At the impregnation process of this egg Puruṣa entered for the first time into the nominative form. Ma-Śakti is the energy source in which change is constantly in movement.

Change is necessary for reforming or modernization. This is similar to the moon in the cosmos (full moon, three quarter etc.). This sort of energy is necessary both in heaven and on earth, for impregnation, growth and delivery in which emotion in and love is distinguished.

Brahmā's duty was to form all the creatures of the air and animals both wild and tame. In the scientific creation it is also known as a cosmic sacrifice referring to the first technique of Jñāna yoga. From that Sacrifice Ṛcas (knowledge) and Sāma hymns (rhythm, sounds and music) were also born and from here spells and charms produced: the Yajus. These are the basic principles for creation (YV 31. 1664). Just as the creation and sounds change, so also the physical forms.

This changing of male and female power in the universe got the name Ādi-Puruṣa (Man) and Ādi-Śakti (Woman), the primeval energies or pertaining to the first age, especially for a world. These are also the primary forms of life. The energy mix of this process animates as its vital soul or divine principle; beauty is divine to the superhuman or surpassing excellence. This same process happens on the earth between man and woman. We call this process of render (the female gamete) capable of development by uniting it with the male gamete: the fertilization process or Garbha, instead of Hiraṇyagarbha. Thus we are a link in the forth going process from heaven and are gods on earth in microform. Our tasks in this process are: to take care of the bio cosmos (the environment) etc. for other creatures and cosmic nature. Therefore we need norms and values.

It has been indicated above that Brahmā must produce sacrifices to maintain creation. This maintenance is necessary for creation as for the creatures in heaven. This principle also applies on earth. Those who create are also obliged to maintain the creatures and the surroundings in which they are living. This is a law of nature. Focusing on the current environmental issues on the earth, one is able to adopt that the occupants of this planet do not comply to their obligations sufficiently. This means in practice that we must recalibrate the standards and values on the basis of the current state in the cosmos. Vedic tradition has ensured this in the past by regular small and large yajñas or sacrifice ceremonies that were kept by people. These sacrificial ceremonies had a positive influence on the environment, for rest, peace, and harmony on earth.

God or Puruṣa

Puruṣa, the Person, Super spirit, or Man personified and regarded as the soul and original source of the universe, the personal and life-giving principle in all animated beings, is said to have a thousand, that is, innumerable, heads, eyes, and feet, as being one with all created life (RV 10.90.1). The first mantra of the Puruṣa Sūkta in the Atharva Veda version; arms have been substituted for heads, to agree, apparently, with the number of eyes and feet. The first mantra of the Puruṣa Sūkta (means been spoken by Him, the Puruṣa) mentions a space ten fingers broad (Dasāṅgulam). This is the region of the heart of man wherein the soul was supposed to reside. Although, as the Universal Soul, Puruṣa pervades the universe, so the Individual Soul is enclosed in a space of narrow dimensions. Puruṣa mounts beyond His own condition for the food of living beings. All creatures are one fourth of Him and three fourths are in heaven. With this three fourths Puruṣa rose up and one fourth became the (visible) universe. Thence He moved forth to every side over animate and inanimate creation, the two classes of created things. The two classes are defined as follows: one, are those who can taste the reward and punishment of good and evil actions such as Gods, men, and lower animals (cetanam or conscious, capable of enjoyment), and two are those who are incapable thereof, such as mountains and rivers (acetanam or unconscious). From Him Virāja was born and again Puruṣa from Virāj. Whén born, He spread to the west and east beyond the boundaries of earth (YV 31. 1662).

Puruṣa was Brahmana (Teacher, Priest and Guru), c.f. code of terms, from His mouth (knowledge) and was made Rājanya (Soldier or Defence) from His arms (Power and Manager). From His thighs, he became the Vaiśya (Industrialist, Producer and Businessman) and from His feet he was produced as the Śūdra (Employer and Server). He was born as the Moon from His mind (female power) and the Sun (male power) from His eyes. As Vāyu (wind) and Prāṇa (life elixir) from His ear, and from His mouth as Agni (fire, sacrificial box Havan Kūṇḍa). From His navel He was mid-space; he was the sky from His head; Earth from His feet, and from His ear the Quarters. The hills are His bones, the sky His skull, the sea His blood, and the clouds His brains. When Gods performed the saṁskara Puruṣa, Spring was the butter, Autumn the oblation, Summer was the wood.

The Devas classified the body of Puruṣa. When the Devas performed the sacrament (saṁskara) of Puruṣa, His enclosing sticks were seven in total and His kindling brands (fire marks) were three times seven. The enclosing sticks are symbolically the seven sacred metres, or as six shallow trenches dug round the fire and an imaginary one round the Sun. The twenty-one kindling fire are the three cosmoses (maṇḍalas) with which the three characters of AUM (OM) are formed (Bh.G. 7.8). In each universe there are seven visible main planets. The cosmoses in OM are half-visible because we see an object entirely only from one side. The U-form in the AUM is the Viṣṇu-sign and stands in connection with the energy Viṣṇu. The Bindu or dot is a microform of complete creation. AUM is a none-character icon of god in which the creation is only a part (BhG. 10.25). This hymn, which is generally called the Puruṣa Sūkta, harmonizes the two ideas of sacrifice and creation. Puruṣa Sūkta (RV 10.90.1-16) is in reality a mathematical formula of the creation and creatures, maintenance, tribute, love, rest, peace, harmony and bliss within the entire creation. This formula contains sixteen components. Such as we cannot (re)move a number or sign in a formula, this formula of the Puruṣa Sūkta also is a total coherency. Move of a digit means that the formula doesn't work or the result becomes incorrect.

Yajur Veda (1675) mentions "I know this mighty Puruṣa whose colour is like the Sun, beyond the reach of darkness." The hymn (1676) continues: "He only who knows Him leaves death behind Him. There is no path safer than this to travel. In the womb moves Prajāpati, the Golden Egg or Hiraṇyagarbha: He, never being born, is born in sundry figures." The wise discerns the womb from which He springs. In Him alone stand all existing creatures (AV 10.8.13). A sundry place means every birth that occurs being in reality a rebirth of the creative power Prajāpati. He is transcendental to all kinds of material leaders (gross elements) and controllers or deva's (Angel's) and is worshipped by all creatures.

The Rig Veda explains in chapter 10 (90.2) that "Puruṣa is this All in truth, what has been and what yet shall be. He is the Lord of immortality or the immortal world of the Gods which grows greater by food, that is, by the sacrificial offerings of men." The term 'food' here is not literally food for eating, but the essence of it, such as heat comes from fire. It is also comparable with the essence that reaches God if we sacrifice fruit. He is the Lord or distributor of immortality because He becomes the visible world in order that living beings may obtain the fruits of their actions and gain final liberation (mokṣa) from their bonds.

The sacrifice of the Devas initiated the Puruṣa into the Vedas and the mantras of the Puruṣa Sūkta were the earliest holy ordinances. Since He spoke with the Gods at first, and began the bright and holy One: The Brahmā. He, who may know you thus shall have the Gods in his control (YV 31.1678). There is no one greater than Him, and He is the supreme cause of all causes. He is All in One and One in All.

God and All Creatures

The Lord whose pure form is pure or not affected by the modes of material nature, can be perceived by pure consciousness. Māyā, or illusion, is the condition of spiritual life made impure by material infection. Liberation from this material infection does not mean destruction of the original eternal position of the living entity. Patañjali[1] used the word Citi-Śakti in chapter 3. This Citi-Śakti or transcendental pleasure is real life. The sūtra says: "The seed of bondage having been destroyed by desirelessness even for that, comes absolute-independence (Kaivalya)" (PYS 3.49).

This sūtra means that the Yogi becomes conscious of what he says is knowledge of discrimination as a characteristic of the Sattva. When he comes to think that the discrimination of the distinctive natures, is after all a manifestation of the quality of Essentiality (Sattva) and that the quality of essentiality has been classed with avoidable pains; and that the Puruṣa is unchangeable, pure and other than the quality of essentiality (Sattva) then he begins to lose his desire for that, and then the afflictions having had their seed burnt, become incapable of sprouting again like burnt seeds of rice.

---

[1] *Patañjali Yoga Sūtras,* Translated by Rama Prasada, Munshiram Manoharlal Publishers Pvt Ltd, Delhi, 1988

Then all the seeds of afflictions pass, together with the mind, into latency. When they have become latent, the Puruṣa does not then suffer from the triad of pain, known as physical, mental and spiritual. The state in which the qualities manifest in the mind as afflictions, actions and fruitions do not, having fulfilled their object, come back to action, is the final separation of consciousness from the qualities. This is the state of absolute independence, when the Puruṣa remains in consciousness alone, as in its own nature. This is confirmed in the Vedāntasūtra (1.1.12) as Ānandamayo-abhyasat. This natural transcendental pleasure is the ultimate goal of yoga and is easily achieved by execution of devotional service. The Anandamaya is the Light tunnel where the transfer process starts from human into God force.

His cosmic form within all creations is actually energy or sound in different forms and densities or rhythms. It depends on the quantity of absorption or evolving Vedic knowledge. As soon as the crowded condition is spiritually comparable to the lowest state of the Lord, absorption or liberation starts. The beat of the heart becomes the rhythm of the cosmos and is compared with the small form of the God Vāmana, the form of vibration or the spirit (also called a bindu or dot). This rhythm has three dimensions or three steps, referring to the three worlds (physic, astral and carnal).

In the Vedānta He is described as being one without a second. Because of His spiritual potency, He is untouched by the contamination of material nature, and because He is not subjected to material vision, He is known as transcendental. He has no material activities, nor has He a material form or name. Only in pure consciousness can one perceive the transcendental form of the Lord, through the third eye or the sixth sense.

When one realises that all the gross and subtle forms originate from the ignorance in the self it is then that he/she becomes one in association with the divine. This process is described as a cosmic understanding; the knowledge and consciousness of the micro and macro cosmos. All energies and their activities are then geared to one or another.

Incarnations

We have mentioned above that the Lord changes his energy in several forms to organize, create and to manage the whole process of creation. Considering the threefold duty He takes a form that fits with the process of that creation or managing. These are icons in the cosmos in astral form, images in the material form for prayers (Bhakti yoga). This is comparable with the bites (two-in-one-principle) of a computer. From the ocean of goodness all manifestations of the Lord are innumerable like the countless streams from thousands of lakes. This is a huge network of database and communications with names as passwords. Human beings are a part within this network and are in contact and in participation with the mass Energy source, because we are all a part of that energy. All the powerful sages, the godly, the Manus and their originates, as well as the Prajāpatis (founding fathers) are aspects of the Lord. Beginning from Brahmā and Bhava (Śiva, the source of the Jivas or souls), all the great sages who were born before, the demigods, the demons, the Nāgas (snakes), the human beings, the birds, the beasts, as well as the reptiles, etc., and all phenomenal manifestations of the universes, namely the planets, stars, asteroids, luminaries, lightning, thunder, and the inhabitants of the different planetary systems, namely the Gandharvas, Apsarās, Yakṣas, Rākṣas, Bhūtagaṇas, Uragas, Paśus, Pitas, Siddhas, Vidyādharas, Caranas, and all other different varieties of living entities, including the birds, beasts, trees and everything that be, are all covered by the universal form of the Lord at all times, namely past, present and future, although He is transcendental to all of them, eternally existing in a form not exceeding nine inches, in Him (BhT. 2.6.13-16).

Lord Śiva, as mentioned above, is Mahādeva or the highest power within the gods. His energy as Bhava (RV 10.90.2) makes Him become the great Manager and Destroyer of all the creatures and creations. He changes His outlook for the intentions that He exploits. He is the source of Motherhood as Bhava and as character Kṣa the Ultimate Power of Śakti of the Female Divine. This character is located in the forehead or the Ajñā cakra. His presence here is the third eye. With this eye He controls the past, present and future. With this Kṣa He becomes Lakṣmī, Lakṣmaṇa, etc. The sun is a small part of the third Eye of the Supreme Lord.

We describe some manifestations of the Lord with their names and disciplines. We refer to Śrīmad Bhāgvatam (Book 1, chapter 3) where the creation of the Lord has been described. At first the sons of Brahmā, the Architect and Creator, (the sons are known as Sanaka, Sanandana, Sanātana and Sanatkumāra) were disciplined in austerity for the realization of continuation. The next incarnation, Vārāha (boar), was for the sake of its welfare. He uplifted our world out of the lower regions. For the sake of evolving Vedic knowledge for service in devotion without further material motives He accepted His presence among the learned ṛiṣis or seers, as Nārada Muni.

In the form Nara-Nārāyaṇa (the twin sons of king Dharma) He underwent severe penances to attain control over the senses. With the name Kapila He exhibits to the Brahmin Asuri on the nature of metaphysics and the elements of creation as through time knowledge was lost. As the son of Atri He lectured the transcendental Science. Yajña, the son of Prajāpati Ruci with the help of the gods, ruled over the change of the period of Svayambhuva Manu. As King Ṛiṣabha He showed the path of perfection that is respected by people of all stages of life. As Prithu He accepted the earth for the sake of its cultivation and produces, which made it beautifully attractive. Like a fish, Matsya, in the water He kept Vaivaśvata Manu after the period of Cākṣuṣa Manu on a boat of protection afloat the waters when the world was deeply inundated. We refer here to the same story of Noach in the Bible. As a tortoise, Kūrma, He sustained the Mandāracala Hill of the theists and atheists, which served as a pivot in the ocean. He appeared as Dhanvantari, Lord of medicine and science. He appeared as Narsiṁha half as a Lion and tore apart the king of the atheists like a carpenter does cane. In His incarnation as Bhṛigupati He acted twenty-one times against the ruling class that negated the intelligentsia with reference to the explanation above about the syllable OM (RV 10.90.15, the mathematical formula of the universe).

Seeing the common people as being less intelligent He incarnated as Vyāsadeva to divide the desire tree of the Veda into several branches and subbranches. The Lord appeared as King Rāma in order to perform some pleasing work for the demigods, He exhibited superhuman powers by controlling the Indian Ocean and then killing the atheist King Rāvaṇa, who was on the other side of the sea. Thereafter in the Age of Kali (this era) His birth as Lord Buddha from Anjana in Gaya took place in order to delude the ones envious with the theists.

Like rivulets flowing from inexhaustible sources of water (energies), all these are part of The supreme Lord or Bhagavān as person who gives protection in all ages and worlds against the enemies. All of the above mentioned incarnations and creators are either plenary portions or portions of the plenary portions of the Lord, but the Supreme Lord is the original personality. All these forms of the Lord are certainly of the one without a form that is transcendental; they came about in the self from the modes of the material energy with its elements.

Due to the duties that have to be done by the Lord, He appeared twenty-four times on this earth. In this way He is the producer, manager and controller of the whole universe.

Accidentally we find some remarkable developments in the present stage of modern science. The Navstar Global Positioning System (NGPS) is a network of 24 satellites in orbit around the earth that provides users with information about their position and movement. A navigation satellite sends continuous radio signals to Earth. These signals contain data that a special radio receiver on Earth translates into information about the satellite's position. To manage and to control this system we need many tools which are assumed to be identical to the above mentioned disciplines. For each sector we have several identities, names, codes, passwords etc.

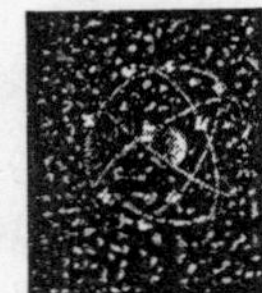

Figure 4: Satellite

Human

The Human Form

Humans are special. In the human race, the mode of passion is very prominent. Humans are always busy in the midst of miserable life, but they think themselves happy in all respects.

Above we explained the process of Hiraṇyagarbha in the paragraph Heritage where male and female energy are necessary for creation. Lord Brahmā explains the importance of human life form: "My dear demigods, the human form of life is of such importance that we also desire to have such life, for in the human form one can attain perfect religious truth and knowledge. If one in this form does not understand the Lord and His abode, it is to be understood that he is very much affected by the influence of external nature. Persons whose bodily features change in ecstasy and who breathe heavily and perspire due to hearing the glories of the Lord are upgraded to the kingdom of God, even though they do not care for meditation and other austerities. The kingdom of God is above the material universe, and this is desired by Brahmā and other demigods" (BhT. 3.13.24 and 25).

Reality and The Imaginary

The conception of the Virāṭ, universal form of the Lord, as appearing in the material world, is imaginary. With the illusory energy (Māyā) subsided there is enrichment with full knowledge of enlightenment, and knowing in the glories of the self. The multifarious forms of the universe are the indestructible source from which all deva's, human beings, animals, etc. originate. This form (the second manifestation of the Puruṣa) is the source and indestructible seed of multifarious incarnations within the universe. From the particles and portions of this form, different living entities, like demigods, men and others, are created.

It is to enable the less intelligent to adjust to the idea of the Lord's having form. But factually the Lord has no material form. To the less intelligent seer they are as clouds in the sky and dust in the air. The air carries clouds and dust, but less intelligent persons say that the sky is cloudy and the air is dirty. Similarly, they also implant material bodily conceptions on the spirit of the self. This unmanifested beyond, which is without a form affected by the modes of nature and is alike that what is unseen and unheard—that is the living being that takes birth repeatedly. Beyond this gross conception of form is another, subtle conception of form which is without formal shape and is unseen, unheard and unmanifested. The living being has his form beyond this subtlety, otherwise he could not have repeated births. More than three-quarters of the body of the Lord is invisible and impenetrable.

Sound as Conditioned Soul

In the Śrīmad Bhāgvatam (5.4.24), another Hindu book, Brahmā mentioned that the Vedas are His eternal transcendental sound incarnation. Therefore the Vedas are Śabda Brahmā. The Yajur Veda (chapter 36.1, 1873) confirms also that Ṛcā is stronghold in *speech*, in the mind as Yajus, in breath as Sāma, also in hearing and in sight. Speech energy is been provided in strength, I breathing in and out. Rhythm or soul is the important part or backbone of music. Our inner soul or atmosphere accepts the soul of the music. This is the way vibrations work.

In chapter 2 (2.1, 2) of the Bhāgvatam sound or soul is explained as follows: "Formerly, prior to the manifestation of the cosmos, Lord Brahmā, by meditating on the Virāṭ R̃ūpa (the Super Puruṣa), regained his lost consciousness by appeasing the Lord. Thus He was able to rebuild creation as it was before. The way of presentation of Vedic sounds is so bewildering that it directs the intelligence of people to meaningless things like heavenly kingdoms. Conditioned souls hover in dreams of such heavenly illusory pleasures, but actually they do not relish any tangible happiness in such places." The Lord of the cosmos is within every living being, but still independent and unaffected by creation, destruction and maintenance. The inactive unborn Lord of the Heart (read beat, sound, vibration or rhythṃ) with His energies and absorptions is also described in the Vedas. Even the Vedic seers are trying to discover His existence in the cosmos along with His true character or activity.

In this world, some Brāhmaṇas thoroughly study all the Vedas, and because they assimilate Vedic conclusions, they are also to be considered the Vedas personified. Brāhmaṇas are situated in the supreme transcendental mode of nature, the sattvaguna. Because of this, they are fixed in mind control (sama), sense control (dama), and truthfulness (satya). They describe the Vedas in their original sense, and out of mercy (anugraha) they preach the purpose of the Vedas to all conditioned souls. They practice penance (tapasya), tolerance (titikṣa), and realise the position of the living entity and the Supreme Lord (anubhava). These are the eight qualifications of the Brāhmaṇas. Therefore among all living entities, no one is superior to the Brāhmaṇas.

Self-realisation and liberation

By self-realisation a person experiences that both the gross and subtle bodies have nothing to do with the pure self. That moment he sees himself as well as the Lord. This is the first step in the process of liberation, which is compared as fruits of our life. One of the well known priest leaders and teachers Dr. Prem Acarya Shastriji explains this matter as fruits namely the four types of liberation: Sālokya, or life in the residence of God; Sārūpya, the acquisition of the likeness with God; Sāmīpya, living near God and Sāyujya, or reunification with God.

Professor R.C. Zaehner,[2] Spalding of Eastern Religions and Ethics at the University of Oxford, refers to this in the book *Hindu Scriptures* that according to the Bṛhadāraṇyaka Upaniṣad (1.23) the process of self-realisation is: "What those (faculties) started in olden times they still do today. So a man should follow but one observance. He should breathe in and breathe out, saying: 'May not the evil one, may not Death take possession of me!' And whatever (observance) he follows, he should want to see it through to the end. Thereby he will

---

[2] *Hindu Scriptures,* R.C. Zaehner, spalding Professor of Eastern Religions and Ethics at the University of Oxford (page 41). J.M. Dent & Sons ltd, 1995.

attain unity (Sāyujya) with that natural phenomenon and will share in its state of being (Sālokata). In this book he also quotes on page 86 (Ch. Up. 3.11.1) about the essence of life 'Thenceforth (the sun), after rising high, will never again rise or set: all alone will it stand in the midst.' Hence the following verse:

There indeed it never sets, Nor does it ever rise at all:
By the truth of this, ye gods, May I never be robbed of Brahmā!

He refers to chapter 3 of this Upaniṣad as follows:

"In chapter 3.1-10, dealing with the sun seen as honey extracted from the Vedas ...are omitted." We find this parallel in the Bhāgvatam: "The sun illuminates both internally and externally by expanding its radiation; similarly, the Lord, by expanding His universal form, maintains everything in the creation both internally and externally" (BhT. 2.5.17). All living entities, including demigods, human beings, animals, birds, insects, reptiles, creepers and trees, depend upon the heat and light given by the sun-god from the sun planet. Furthermore, it is because of the sun's presence that all living entities can see, and therefore he is called Dṛgeśvara, the Supreme Lord presiding over sight.

The above mentioned process of liberation confirms that the term 'yoga' means Yuj. The proof of which we see in the last step of liberation: Sāyujya. Spirituality means love for and to the honey. This process is also described in the sacrifice or pūjā system. To be serviced by the Service.

All the Vedas (for instance 10.90.1-16) and the Bhāgvatam (1.3.1) refer to the pūjā ceremony with its sixteen principles when He starts with His creation. These sixteen steps of devotion are included in the process of purification, in the core part of the ceremony; comparable with the sixteen principles of material action as all ingredients for material creation. After all, Pūjā is a materialized form of yoga; aimed at the purpose of creating the material universe. In connection with the Lord Puruṣa must be preceded just as in the case of the sixteen services. The Gaṇeṣa pūjā as a form of energy or remover of obstacles and cleaning the atmosphere thereby serves as overture while the mother is honoured as creative power by means of the Gaurī pūjā. She permits her son to precede her because of his partnership with Riddhi (luxury) and Siddhi (supernatural properties).

Purpose of life

Our purpose of life as mentioned above is to reunite with the primary source or Energy. The ones with little knowledge cannot know Him in His activities, names and forms by means of speculation and oration. Only he can know of the transcendental glories of the creator who renders unconditional, uninterrupted, favourable service to His fragrant lotus feet: who is all powerful with the wheel of the chariot in His hand. In this world one can be successful if one knows in full about the Supreme Lord who embraces all of His universes and inspires for complete spirit of ecstasy in which one will never find dreaded repetitions of worldly interest. Thus being fixed, one must render service unto the Super soul situated in one's own heart by his infinite power. Because he is the Almighty, eternal and unlimited, He is the ultimate goal of life, and by worshipping Him one can end the course of this conditioned state of existence (BhT. 2.2.6). The Lord's activities in association with His different energies should be described, appreciated and heard in accordance with the teachings of the Supreme Lord. If this is done regularly with devotion and respect, one is sure to get out of the illusory energy of the Lord (BhT. 2.7.53).

People of today do not have enough time. They are all in a hurry. Nevertheless they are aware that they must survive to be able to reach the aim of life. That is why we have analysed yoga and pūjā. Yoga and pūjā are medicines for stress and bring rest, love and peace. The simplest method in this will take less than three minutes per day. For the analysis and method we refer to the chapter Pūjā in this paper. In short we give below an overview and impact of yoga and pūjā.

Table 1: Influence through spirituality in life

Time	Results
1 minute	behaviour purification
2 minutes	behaviour purification and control of the mind
5 minutes	beside the above, insight of the inner Self

This program is possible to implement in the time that we spend in a waiting room or in a traffic jam, in association with our rhythm or breath.

Several paths to attain God

Bhakti yoga, The Path of Devotion or Divine Love

This path particularly appeals to those of an emotional nature. Bhakti yoga is motivated chiefly by the power of love and sees God as the embodiment of love. Through prayer, worship and ritual he surrenders himself to God, channelling and transmitting his emotions into unconditional love or devotion. The sound incarnation of the Lord (the Supreme Soul) enters into the heart of a self-realised devotee. She hears in devotion the sixteen kinds of nature sounds. The most valuable of these sixteen is the Anāhata śabda, which comes from the inner source of the devotee. Chanting or singing the praises of the names of God is a substantial part of Bhakti yoga. The background and or the image of an incarnation determine the choice of the devotee. The preference and choice of the incarnation stipulate at the same time the density, charm, form, character and strength, which make these gods popular. The devotee identifies her or him with this Hero and becomes a hero. This method is similar to the choice of a partner. The aim in both cases is the interaction or approach.

All these forms of the Lord are certainly of the One without a form that is transcendental; they came about in the self from the modes of material energy with its elements. His devotees compiled by the wise man of God is, as a supplement to the Veda's, there for the ultimate good of all people, bringing success, happiness and perfection.

If a devotee sits on the floor or chair and recite names of the Lord in the morning and evening they will find relief from all miseries of life. A pure devotee of the Lord whose heart has once been cleansed by the process of devotional service never relinquishes the lotus feet of the Lord, for they fully satisfy him, as a traveller is satisfied at home after a troubled journey (BhT. 2.8.5, 6). The process of self-realisation is spirituality, knowledge, renunciation, spiritual power, sense control and freedom from false ego.

Karma yoga, the yoga of Action

Karma yoga is the path chosen by those with an outgoing nature. It purifies the heart by teaching you to act selflessly, without thought of gain or reward. By detaching yourself from the fruits of your actions and offering them to God, you learn to sublimate the ego. The goal is to divert the energy or impulse from its immediate goal to one of a more acceptable social, moral, or aesthetic nature or use to make the person nobler or purer. To achieve this, it is helpful to keep your mind focused by repeating a mantra while engaged in any activity. You have a right to perform your prescribed duty. Never consider yourself the cause of the results of your activities, and never be attached from not doing your duty. The Bhāgavad Gītā prescribes this goal of life in chapter 2, sloka 47.

There are three considerations here: prescribed or direct duties, capricious or variable work, and inaction. Prescribed duties are activities enjoined in terms of one's acquired modes of material nature. Capricious work means actions without the sanction of authority, and inaction means not performing one's prescribed duties. The Lord advised that Arjuna, disciple of Lord Kṛṣṇa in the Bhāgavad Gītā, not to be inactive, but that he perform his prescribed duty without being attached to the result. One who is attached to the result of his work is also the cause of the action. Thus he is the enjoyer or sufferer of the result of such actions. As far as prescribed duties are concerned, they can be split into three subdivisions, namely routine work, emergency work and desired activities. Routine work performed as an obligation in terms of the scriptural injunctions, without desire for results, is action in the mode of goodness. Work with results becomes the cause of bondage; therefore such work is not auspicious. Everyone has his right to pertain property or ownership in regard to prescribed duties, but should act without attachment to the result; such disinterested obligatory or necessary duties doubtlessly lead one to the path of liberation. One who has actually come to understand one's constitutional position as an eternal servitor of the Lord gives up all engagements save working in the society. This is also a sort of the Jñāna yoga or transcendental loving service to the Lord. Such devotional service is the right course of action for the living entity. Only misers desire to enjoy the fruit of their own work just to be further entangled in material bondage. Except for work for God, all activities are abominable because they continually bind the worker to the cycle of birth and death.

Rāja yoga, The Science of Physical and Mental Control

Rāja yoga is also called aṣṭāṅga yoga referring to the eight limbs leading to absolute mental control. It is often called the 'royal road' because it offers a comprehensive method for controlling the waves of thought by turning our mental and physical energy into spiritual energy. The chief practice of Rāja yoga is meditation. It also includes all other methods, which help one to control body, energy, senses and mind. The Haṭha yoga uses relaxation and other practices such as Yamas, Niyamas, Mudras, Bandhas etc. to gain control of the physical body and the subtle life force, called Prāṇa. When body and energy are under control, meditation comes naturally. More information you will find in chapter Yoga.

Pūjā

Pūjā can be described as a divine ritual performed at home and in a temple (Mandir) under the guidance of a professional, called Pujārī, or in the household without the guidance or presence of such a professional. The daily pūjā is called Nitya Pūjā and on special occasions Naimittike Pūjā and sporadically for instance to consecrate a house, it is called Kāmya pūjā. Pūjā was developed during the vedic era. As mentioned in the first verse of the Rig Veda, homa (fire offer) for the deities Homa and Agni (compare the Rig Veda verses Puruṣa śukta 6, 7, 8, 9, 10, 14, 15 and 16). They speak about the yajña (a manifestation of prayer ceremonies and lectures) but the deities are invoked and revered by means of a pūjā.

The pūjā being its religious part has been concluded as the basic theme of the yajña.

The ritual that has to be performed consists in the offering of a fixed sequence of services, accompanied by the recitation of mantras. The two standard forms are Pañcopācāra-pūjā or five services version and the Ṣoḍaśopacāra-pūjā or sixteen services version. I have to make an observation about the term standard. Hinduism does not possess a Pope who decrees from time to time, what should be done and what not. India is furthermore a large country with regional cultural idiosyncrasies. Last but not the least: time, assimilation and incorporation of foreign elements and ideas contributed towards shaping the rituals.

Like everything else in creation revealed religion is the determining factor, as moral guidance of humanity is subject to the universal law of development.

Wisdom therefore claims to be the final culminating phase in this preordained evolutional process. It is a fervent prayer, that keeping in advance to this Vedic code of heavenly guidance for moral, material, and in particular the essence of the spiritual conduct and fulfilment of mankind is a long felt event among our Hindu community. Thereby trying to earn higher virtues by adhering to the principles of our Vedic rituals and promote to keep alive our Vedic Spirit of Hinduism.

Jñāna yoga in Pūjā

Jñana yoga is the yoga of knowledge or wisdom. In order to practise this yoga wisdom of Hinduism is most important. Hinduism describes the Cosmos and the creatures within. This cosmic science gives techniques on how to come to self-realisation through the several paths of yoga and pūjā. Pūjā and yoga (wisdom and the Vedic code) affirms the doctrine that through the practice of certain disciplines one may achieve liberation from the limitations of flesh, the delusions of sense, and the pitfalls of thought and thus attain union with the object of knowledge. Such union, according to the doctrine, is the only true way of knowing. For most Yogis (those who practise yoga), the object of knowledge is the universal spirit or Brahm. A minority of atheistic Yogi seeks perfect self-knowledge instead of knowledge of God.

The visible cosmic manifestation is a demonstration of Puruṣa's own creative energy. Since the countless varieties of forms within this cosmic manifestation are simply a display of His external energy. This Virāṭrūpa (universal body) is not His real form. Above what we have described is incarnations and energy forms. For detailed information we refer to chapter Pūjā of this book. All the stars and planets are simply manifestations of His different energies, but originally He is one to who there is no second. Therefore there is nothing beyond Him.

This entire cosmic manifestation is therefore not false but is simply a temporary manifestation of His inconceivable energy. His name, form and bodily features are expanded in countless forms. No one can determine exactly how many forms exist, yet He Himself, in His incarnation as the learned scholar Kapila Deva, have analysed the cosmic manifestation as containing twenty four elements.

The objects of material enjoyment (sound, form, taste, touch and smell), the activities of the senses, the controllers of sensory activities (the demigods), the body, eternal time and egotism are all creations of His material energy. Those who's intelligence has become fixed by perfect execution of mystic yoga can see that all these elements result from the actions of His external energy. They can also see His transcendental form as Super Soul in the background of everything. He doesn't desire the creation, maintenance or annihilation of this material world, but He performs these activities for the conditioned souls by His creative energy. Exactly as a piece of iron moves under the influence of a Lodestone, inert matter moves when He glances over total material energy. Non-devotees simply count the different elements and remain ignorant of His actual form. Therefore all the ritualistic ceremonies of sacrifice are part of His transcendental body, and he is the only enjoyer of all sacrifices in the pūjā. Taking the philosophy of Vedānta the Jñāna Yogi uses his mind to inquire into its own nature. Hindu philosophy assumes that this entity as pure intelligence remains ever in its purity and only through a transcendent beginningless illusion appears to take part in or become associated with our experience. True knowledge or emancipation consists in the apprehension of the soul or self as pure intelligence and all else as extraneous to it. Before practising Jñāna yoga, the aspirant (micro cosmos) needs to have integrated the lessons of Hinduism or the (macro) cosmic science.

Wisdom guides the Ātmā or Soul

The body is material and hence can be analysed and described with ease since it is visible, touchable, defensible and measurable. But the soul is abstract and not visible. We have many terms to indicate it: spirit, ego, I, person, consciousness, the self, the superego, mentality etc. which makes it difficult for a full insight. Subramuniyaswami provides us with a few definitions in his book 'Dancing with Śiva. Jīva, he says means: living, existing; the principle of life and perception, the true human being. Jīva, he continues, was derived from the Sanskrit word 'Jiv' which means life. That is the individual ãtmã or the soul during its material state. The soul itself is the sound or the energy that lies hidden and enclosed by the three worlds Bhūh (physical), Bhūvah (astral) and Svah (transcendental). The ãtmã is part of the energy or Śakti from the essence of Param Śakti (Param Ātmā or God). One of the most fundamental teachings of Hinduism he says is that we are the Ãtmã and not the material body, emotions, external mind or personality. The soul has to acquire devas or bodies in the world to be able to make a positive contribution to it. Thus doing it strengthens its radiation and purifies it. The soul in a human being has already been purified to a certain extent since it finds itself in the highest creation on earth and its energy is in a position to steer its further purification.

The term Deva was derived from 'dih' that means to plaster, to mould, to form, to knead. The term is used in the Upaniṣads, in texts about yoga to denote the three bodies of the soul. Jīvana or life is a synthesis of soul and body.A Jīvanmukta is someone who has been purified during his lifetime. When a person dies the physical body (sthūla) perishes but the soul remains in the astral body (sūkṣma) and the causal body (kāraṇa). These are spheres, which cannot be seen with the eyes. The purpose of life is Viṣvagrasā or entrance of the soul in Śiva when its evolution has been completed. It is the reunion of the individual soul-body with the body of Śiva (Parameśvara in Śivaloka where it once originated). The individuality disappears when the soul Śiva, the creator, becomes protector: individual entity extends to universality. It becomes one with the Al: the Jīvā in Śiva.

Travelling path after death

Those persons that renounce the path of action take refuge in the path of wisdom, and adhere to the practice of austerity penance (the high level of density in the state of contemplation), after death travel through the path of devayāna the path of light. He is led through the different spheres by enlightened energies, such as Agni (the fire god) sitted on the Maṇipura cakra in the human being and on the Venus in the cosmos. This contact happens through the Third Eye. The process happens by the day, the bright half of the lunar months, Śuklapakṣa, the six months of the sun's passage to the northern solstice, the year, the devas, the Vāyu, the sun, the moon, the lightning, the region of Varuṇa, the region of Indra, and the region of Prajāpati.

He who goes by the devayāṇa, has not to come back again to this world, but remains in the Brahmā loka (Brahma-world) till the end of the cycle, where he attains complete absorption in Brahm with Brahmā. This process of emancipation is called karma-mukti or gradual or indirect salvation. This is a one way ticket to the Blue.

Those that renounce the path of wisdom, take refuge in the path of action and adhere to the performance of Vedīc austerity after death, travel through quite a different path. This is the medium level of density in the state of contemplation. This path is called the 'Pitṛyāṇa', (path of the manes or mind) or Dhūma Mārga, the path of darkness. He is led through the different spheres, such as those of smoke or darkness, night, the six months of the sun's passage to the southern solstice, year, the Pitṛloka, (i.e.) the world of the manes, to the moon, the ether, thence to the rain, and descends to thẹ plants, partaken by some one, enters in to the womb of mother and thus takes birth into this world of sufferings, in the form of human being.

Others, who are of ordinary knowledge and actions, do some charitable or good work in their lifetime but fail to realise God. When they depart they go, to Çandraloka by the third or Newatpatha. This is the low level of density in the state of contemplation. There they remain for the enjoyment of the fruits of their good Karma till its exhausted. Then the soul returns with some residue of their past Karma, to be reborn on this earth to undergo all the pains and pleasures of life of the lower animals, viz., as serpent, scorpion; centipede and so forth.

Cosmic and Bio Rhythm

In the cosmos, music and dance are conjointly in the action of The Comic Dancer to undertake a task for creating the cosmos. The great Musician and Dancer is Naṭarāja, the Hindu god Śiva performing the Cosmic Dance. In one hand he holds a drum symbolising creation and the rhythmic beat of time.

In the other, he holds the sacred fire, the symbol of destruction and metamorphosis. With his right foot he tramples the demon of ignorance; the left foot is raised to symbolise salvation. A third hand points to hope given by the raised foot, and a fourth hand is held in a gesture of blessing. An arch of flame surrounds the whole figure, representing Prakṛti (nature) brought to life by the animated figure of Śiva contained within. The dynamism of the dancing figure with its flying belt and flowing locks contrast with the tranquillity of its face and the hand raised in blessing. Śiva wears a male earring in one ear, a female one in the other, symbolising his dual nature (ardhanariśvara, half-man, half-woman). The Cosmic Dance takes place at Chidambaram, which symbolises the center of the Hindu universe; Chidambaram is also a symbol of the human heart.

The soul or ātmā is a sound or vibration. Sound is a physical phenomena that stimulates the sense of hearing. In humans, hearing takes place whenever vibrations of frequencies between about 15 and 20,000 hertz reach the inner ear. The hertz, or Hz, is a unit of frequency equalling one cycle per second. Such vibrations reach the inner ear when they are transmitted through air, and the term sound is something restricted to such airborne vibrational waves. Modern physicists, however, usually extend the term to include similar vibrations in liquid or solid media. Sounds of frequencies higher than about 20,000 Hz are called ultrasonic.

Music is a part of virtually every culture on earth, but it varies widely among cultures in style and structure. Definitions of music can change dramatically over a short time, as they have across the world during the 20th century. The music of India is a mosaic of different genres and levels of sophistication. At one extreme, classical music is performed in the urban concert halls for purely artistic reasons, and, at the other, many kinds of functional rural music accompanies life cycle and agricultural rites. In between are many other musical genres of different regions of the country, reflecting the diversity of its peoples, their life-styles, and their languages. The origins of classical music can be traced to the Nāṭya Śāstra (circa 2nd century AD), a Sanskrit treatise on drama, which encompasses music as well.

Can music exist without sound?

Some philosophers argue that music should be defined as a kind of "mental image" and that the physical aspects of sound are simply by-products of this image. If you think you can have a musical experience by imagining the sound of a piece of music, then you think music can exist without sound. But most musical experiences involve producing or listening to physical characteristics of sound such as pitch and timbre (quality comparable to texture or colour in sight).

The highest purpose of humans should be to purify their souls by cultivating intellectual virtues, refraining from sensual pleasures, and practising various religious rituals. For instance, children's Music is stylistically diverse music designed to appeal to children and music appreciation is learning about music to increase one's enjoyment of different musical styles, compositions, and instruments. The musical scale of ancient China, derived through arithmetic from a basic note, reflected the ancient Chinese conception of the organisation of the universe. Each degree of the scale was closely related to the cardinal points (north, south, east, west), the elements, the seasons, the planets, the months of the year, colours, materials, numbers, parts of the human body, animals, smells, and so forth. The Chinese found in nature eight different sources of musical sound: metal, stone, silk, bamboo, calabash, terra cotta, skin, and wood.

Many of the elaborate melody patterns of India, called ragas, are believed to have magical or curative powers. Ragas are traditionally played at specific hours or during specific seasons; it is believed that to depart from this timetable would be harmful to the performer and audience.

In some tribal societies, music appears to serve as a special form of communication with supernatural beings, and the prominent use of music in modern Christian and Jewish services may be a remnant of such a purpose. Music has always held an important role in religious rituals.

Music and dance

Art is an excellent aid when someone is trying to understand complex ideas from another culture. We can compare music and dance with our two hands. Dance, patterned and rhythmic bodily movements, usually performed to music that serves as a form of communication or expression. Human beings express themselves naturally through movement. Dance is the transformation of ordinary functional and expressive movement into extraordinary movement for extraordinary purposes; even a common movement such as walking is performed in dance in a patterned way, perhaps in circles or to a special rhythm, and it occurs in a special context. Dance may involve a fixed vocabulary of movements that have no meaning in them, as in much of ballet and European folk dance, or pantomime and symbolic gestures may be used, as in many Asian dance forms. Peoples of different cultures dance differently and for varying purposes; their varied forms of dance can reveal much about their way of life. Spirituality depends on happiness-attained by music and dance becomes a main part of the way of life.

Dance and human culture

Dance can be art, ritual, or recreation. It goes beyond the functional purposes of the movements used in work or athletics in order to express emotions, moods, or ideas; tell a story; serve religious, political, economic, or social needs; or simply be an experience that is pleasurable, exciting, or aesthetically valuable.

The body can perform such actions as rotating, bending, stretching, jumping, and turning. By varying these physical actions and using different dynamics, human beings can devise an infinite number of body movements. Out of the range of movements that the body is capable of performing, every culture emphasises certain features in its dance styles.

Besides giving physical pleasure, dancing can have psychological effects. Feelings and ideas can be expressed and communicated; sharing rhythms and movements can make a group feel unified. In some societies, dancing often leads to trance or other altered states of consciousness. Spirits can interpret these states as signalling possession, or they may be sought as a means to emotional release. A state of trance may enable people to perform remarkable feats of strength, endurance, or danger, such as dancing through hot coals. In some societies shamans dance in trance in order to heal others physically or emotionally. The modern field of dance therapy is developed as a means to help people express themselves and relate to others.

Sargam and Its Cosmic Meaning

Sargam is life rhythm in cosmic science. Life is a sum total of rhythms. Without rhythms, there is no music in life hence no life or music. Music is the cosmic or spiritual language which every creature produces. The seven musical notes are Ṣaḍja, ṛṣabha, Gandhara, Madhyama, Pañcama, Dhaivata and Niṣāda. The last note SA is the endless sound. Sound is everywhere, within and around us—a continuum of vital force and latent energy. Only a part of it can be heard: the world of manifest, audible sounds with their individual phonetic, morphological, and semantic distinctions occupy no more than a small fraction of the total field of sound; the greater part is within, unmanifested and beyond the grasp of conscious experience. The sounds that are uttered are subject to all the illusions of the phenomenal world; what these sounds mean, or suggest, is all-important. Consequently the source and the goal of sound are of greater intrinsic interest than the phenomenon itself.

Mātṛkā is the sum total of the fifty letters of the Sanskrit alphabet; for as from a mother comes birth, so from mātṛkā, or sound, the world proceeds. Śabda Brahmā, the "Sound or Nāda," "Logos," or "Word," is the Creator of the worlds of name and form. The Word is measured in four quarters. The wise who possess insight know these four divisions. Three quarters, concealed in secret, cause no movement. The fourth is the quarter that is spoken by Men (RV 1.164.45) Sound is not what one should desire to understand. One should know the hearer (Kauśitakī Upaniṣad 3.8). Bindu is of the nature of Nāda of Śiva, and Bīja of śakti, and Nāda has been said to be the relation of these two by those who are versed in all the Agamas (Sāradā-tilaka: ch. I). Nāda is comparable with the Golden Egg or Hiraṇyagarbha (the Ardha) as mentioned before.

The Trinity of 'Brahmā', 'Viṣṇu' and 'Maheśa' has been attributed the quality of being 'Nādātmak'. Music was synonimised with 'Brahmā' in the form of 'Nāda' and as such it was called "Nāda Brahmā". We worship "Nāda-Brahmā", that comparable bliss which is immanent in all the creatures as intelligence and is manifested in the phenomenon of this universe. Indeed through the worship of Nāda are worshipped gods (like) Brahmā, Viṣṇu, and Śiva, as essentially, they are one with it.

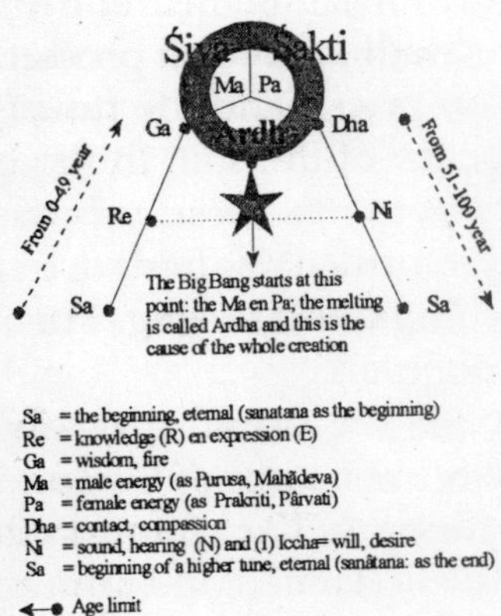

Figure 5: The seven musical notes in relation with the Big Bang

"Let us make our body sound" is a proverb. In each plan of action this expression is quoted: It sounds good. This is also the case when the ultrasounds in Brahmā or unmanifested God awoke with the idea to create. The Rig Veda explains this in the following hymn: 'O Fire-God, let my brilliance be all-pervading in the battle. While performing sacrifices, let us make our body sound. Let all directions bow to me. Let us overcome the enemies under your command (RV 10.128.1). These ultrasounds were primary in the rudimentary beginning and were called the Sabda Brahm. From this primary beginning the first practice scales of ultrasounds arose, these were the SA-RE-GA-MA-PA-DHA-NI-SA (DO-RE-MI-FA-SO-LA-TI-DO).

After these ultrasounds had converted the Big Bang arose. These notes divide the cosmos into several celestial planes and hierarchy. This is the conversion procedure, which has an Androgyne character. In this process of creation comes sound directly after space or ether and air. The sound ventilates further advancement in the development of the creation and creatures. In the figure this is expressed by means of three strengths which in the upward direction, the SA-RE-GA, and further these strengths come up for discussion again in the downward diagrid as DHA-NI-SA. These are the two legs of the human being of the two stairs in life. In the first range the SA is the Svāhā of devotion in sacrifice, as love and service of the people and the environment. The higher range in life is last SA. This is the Svadhā, which is produced as a last sound in the body. Later on priests and the future generations will produce rest and peace of the soul in the higher regions in the sky. Life exists between these two brackets SA's. The contents within these primary sounds are the karma of life. Life is standing up, shining and sinking. The Sanātana Dharma produces these three levels.

Sanātana Dharma is the primordial way of life. Dharma begins with the first SA as nature of God and ends in a God's nature with the higher SA. The upward diagrid (the first 3 tones) develops in the first half of life, which is drawn in yogic science for 49 years of the humans (7x7) life. This time of life is the time for growth, development and exploration of the world. The break-even point at the end, the downward diagrid, starts as a recurrence of exploration, development and growth in which development or knowledge increases in quality and proceeds in spirituality. Spirituality is higher consciousness for connection of this life with Heaven or God. Dharma of God is also Sanātana Dharma, which mean that the micro and macro cosmos are merging with Dharma. At a good biorhythm this lasts for a minimum of 49 years. The body and skin evaluate and evolve every seven years. This is renewing in people and must lead to renewal in the community.

In other words, people are born in pampers and come back in pampers. Rhythmic breathing brings music in life and the other way around. People can live healthy and longer lives due to the natural method of breathing: Prāṇāyāma. Studying the upward and downward diagrid, we see that in both circumstances development takes a central position. It is stipulated that development, knowledge and wisdom (Jñāna) are the core part of our life. This development takes place in each body, and hence also in the community as a large body. The two hands (upwards and downward) of people mean falling and standing up. These two streams make a family or parents. Without a father no mother exists and the other way around. The responsibility of each parent in the figure at the top and in society provokes feeding, education, accompaniment and control of a child. For an optimum increase it is necessary that the child gets the love of both parents. This ensures harmonious increase and development in the child and or the future. Pedagogical recipes are harmonics in the higher waves, which sounds in fixed intervals. Pūjā or sacrifice also consists of 16 celestial steps of worship, similar to the 16 harmonics as frequencies of the fundamental waves in nature. Therefore music stands for quality, in people as well as in a community. Love sounds like music in the ears of the people and or humanity. In this respect we refer to the primordial source of the cosmic science, as the Vedas. The Vedas mentioned that sound comes first in the body and takes a distinguished role in the body or cosmos.

Understanding the Spiritual World

Religious cultures provide their members with patterned ways of interacting with spiritual beings. Such communication is often the center of religious practices. Perhaps the most widely practised forms are prayers in the form of request, offerings and sacrifices, purification or penance, and worship. These rituals may be performed regularly, or in times of special need, when human beings find themselves dependent on forces of the universe beyond their control.We are all connected to one another through the divine presence that dwells within us. We have taken birth in a physical body to grow and evolve into our divine potential. We are inwardly already one with God. Our religion contains the knowledge of how to realise this oneness and not create unwanted experiences along the way. The peerless path is following the way of our spiritual forefathers, discovering the mystical meaning of the scriptures. The peerless path is commitment, study, discipline, practice and the maturing of yoga into wisdom. In the initial stages, we suffer until we learn. Learning leads us to service; and selfless service is the beginning of spiritual striving. Service leads us to understanding. Understanding leads us to meditate deeply and without distractions.

Finally, meditation leads us to surrender in God. This is the straight and certain path, the Sat Mārga, leading to Self

Realisation—the inner most purpose of life—and subsequently to mokṣa, freedom from rebirth. Religion can be a vital guide in helping the individual to explore his true nature. On the other hand, it can also be a negative influence contributing to narrow-mindedness and ego identification. The onus for inner growth lies with the individual. One does not need to be religious to be spiritual, and a religious person is not necessarily spiritual. Religion is an attempt at linking the soul with the divine. The individual soul is an image or reflection of the Supreme Soul. Just as the Sun is reflected in different pots of water, so also the Supreme Soul is reflected in different minds of different persons. Soul is spirit. It is immaterial. It is intelligence or consciousness. It is Caitanya. Individual soul is reflected Caitanya. It is this individual soul that departs from the body after its death and goes to heaven, with the senses, mind, Prāṇa, impressions, desires and tendencies. It is endowed with a subtle astral body when it proceeds to heaven. When the water in the lake is absorbed, the reflection of the Sun in the water merges in the Sun itself. Even so, "when the mind is annihilated through meditation, the individual soul merges itself in the Supreme Soul or Paramātmā. This is the goal of life."

Yoga: Āsana, Cakras and Kuṇḍalini

The Western reader may be surprised at the recurring reference to the Universal Spirit, to mythology and even to philosophical and moral principles. He must not forget that in ancient times all the higher achievements of man, in knowledge, art and power, were part of religion and were assumed to belong to God and to His priestly servants on earth. The Catholic Pope is the last such embodiment of divine knowledge and power in the West. But formerly, even in the Western world, music, painting, architecture, philosophy and medicine, as well as wars, were always in the service of God. It is very important as well as interesting that the reader should know the origin of āsanas and the knowledge of the cakras as well.

Patañjali defined āsana as Sthiram Sukhamāsanam (PYS 2.36), or freely translated: sitting in such a comfortable position that it allows for peaceful meditation. That is the concept of dehasamya. Dehasamya develops the awareness of our physical posture in different conditions. There are many people who sit for a long time on chairs and have lower back problems and shoulder problems.

The eight constituents of yoga are like eight steps of a ladder.[3] Yamas and Niyamas are related to every field of life, but Āsanas (physical postures) are related directly to the succeeding steps. Without attaining steadiness (Dṛiḍha Bhūmi) in Āsanas (physical postures), one cannot acquire success in yoga or super-consciousness (Samādhi). To attain success in Samādhi it is necessary first to attain proficiency in a few of these postures—Svastikā, Siddha and Padma Āsanas. It is said: "Health is the principal means of acquiring virtue, wealth, and liberation."

The famous yoga exponent B.K.S. Iyengar[4] has compared the eight components of yoga to the parts of a tree. Thus, he says: Yama is the root of the Tree of yoga. Niyama is the trunk. Āsanas are the branches. Prāṇāyāma corresponds to the leaves. Samādhi is the fruit. The virtues to be cultivated under Yama are:

1. Non-violence or abstention from harming others.
2. Truthfulness or abstention from falsehood.
3. Non-stealing or abstention from theft.
4. Sexual purity or abstention from sexual impurity.
5. Non-covetousness or abstention from greed.

The aim of the exercises with Haṭha yoga is to stimulate the cakras and to distribute the generated Kuṇḍalini energy throughout the whole body. Haṭha yoga is described in the yoga Upaniṣads as a means to attain physical and mental purification and balance. The Kuṇḍalini is the microcosmic form of universal energy, or more simply, the vast storehouse of static, potential psychic energy, which exists, in latent form in every being. It is the most powerful manifestation of creative force in the human body.

---

3. *First Steps to Higher Yoga:* Yogesvarananda Paramhamsa; Yoga Niketan Trust; India 1985.
4. *The Tree of Yoga;* B.K.S. Iyengar; Harper Collins Publishers; India 1988.

Pūjā

All religions teach that prayers and rituals are very important in devotion to God. The religions or lands may vary but this belief of importance of prayers is stressed in all faiths. Our ancestors have given us the gift of the rules of community worship in a Temple for the welfare of the people of the community as a whole and the prosperity of the world. They have given us the rules of prayers at home as essential for welfare of the individuals and their family. The basic and essential principle behind prayer is total surrender to God who fills the universe by His glory and is present everywhere and that without His command even an atom will not move. Pūjā, being its religious part so to speak. Only when this part has been concluded the basic theme of yajña is treated. In almost every Indian home a lamp is lit daily before the altar of the Lord. In some houses it is lit at dawn, in some, twice a day at dawn and dusk—and in a few it is maintained continuously (akhanda dīpa). All auspicious functions and moments like daily worship, rituals and festivals and even many social occasions like inaugurations commence with the lighting of the lamp, which is often maintained right through the occasion.

Light symbolises knowledge, and darkness symbolises ignorance. The Lord is the "Knowledge Principle" (Caitanya) who is the source, the enlivener and the illuminator of all knowledge. Hence light is worshipped as the Lord Himself. Knowledge removes ignorance just as light removes darkness. Also knowledge is a lasting inner wealth by which all outer achievements can be accomplished. Hence we light the lamp to bow down to knowledge as the greatest of all forms of wealth. Knowledge backs all our actions whether good or bad. We therefore keep a lamp lit during all auspicious occasions as a witness to our thoughts and actions.

Hinduism

Hinduism is the term given to those who practise a way of life. It has evolved from the word 'Sindhu', which means sea, and also refers to the Indus river. The word travelled through

Persia as 'Hind', and into Greek and Latin as 'India', the geographical designation for this subcontinent.

Hinduism is the largest religion in the world due to Buddhism, which is a branch of this religion. It boasts of a respectful era. Some scholars maintain that it is as old as humanity. Others declare that it originated some 6000 years ago in India. We don't have to get into a discussion whether Aryans or Hindus are a part of the original civilisation. Recent archaeological findings cast doubt on this theory. Ed. Viswanathan,[5] points out that according to recent excavations there already existed a highly developed culture of cities in India with paved roads and underground sewers before the invasion of the Aryan nomads from which he concludes that Hinduism already existed before the Aryan conquest and settlement and that the invaders merely absorbed and blended the cultural achievements of the conquered peoples with that of their own.

Since ancient times, Hindu thought has transcended geographical boundaries and influenced religious and philosophical ideas throughout the world. Persian, ancient Greek, and ancient Roman thought may well have been influenced by Hinduism. Three other religions that originated in India branched off from Hinduism: Buddhism, Jainism, and Sikhism. In the 19th century German philosopher Arthur Schopenhauer read both Hindu and Buddhist scriptures and based much of his thinking on them. In the United States, 19th century writers such as Ralph Waldo Emerson and Henry David Thoreau drew on Hinduism and its scriptures in developing their philosophy of transcendentalism.

More recently, civil-rights leader Martin Luther King, Jr., studied the teachings of Hindu leader Mohandas Gandhi on non-violent protest. In the sphere of popular culture, rock musician George Harrison embraced Hinduism during the 1960s, and some members of the United States counterculture explored Hinduism and Buddhism, as did the Beat poets (Beat Generation).

---

[5] *Am I a Hindu; The Hinduism Primer*, Viswanathan; Ed (Edakkandiyil); Rimer Gopsons Paper Ltd. Noida; India, 1993: p.22.

Millions of Westerners today practise meditation or yoga to achieve relief from stress or physical fitness, indicating Western receptiveness to Hindu practices. This is not to say that there are no beliefs and practices that may be identified as Hindu, but rather that Hindu tradition has concerned itself largely with the human situation rather than the Hindu situation. Instead of basing its identity on separating Hindu from non-Hindu or believer from non-believer, Hinduism has sought to recognise principles and practices that would lead any individual to become a better human being and understand and live in harmony with dharma. Dharma is an all-important concept for Hindus. In addition to tradition and moral order, it also signifies the path of knowledge and correct action. Because of Hinduism's emphasis on living in accordance with dharma, anyone who is striving for spiritual knowledge and seeking the right course of ethical action is, in the broadest sense, a follower of Sanātana dharma.

In the manner of science, Hinduism is constantly experimenting with and assimilating new ideas. Like science, it is far less concerned with the origin or history of ideas than with their truth as demonstrated through direct experience. Hinduism's openness to new ideas, teachers, and practices, and its desire for universality rather than exclusivity, set it apart from religions that distinguish their followers by their belief in particular historical events, people, or revelations.

Saintly figures such as Gandhi have periodically renewed Hinduism throughout its history and kept it abreast of the times. Because Hinduism has no central orthodoxy, and no belief in the need for one, renewal of its tradition has invariably come from sages in every age who base their knowledge on experience of the divine. Universal Consciousness pre-existed everything and it pervades or passes through all that exists including every individual like a thread, which passes through each pearl in a pearl necklace (BhG. 7: 7).

Chapter 1
Hinduism

The Origin

The history of Hindus is the history of a civilisation, which has developed in its natural state, without interruption, since antiquity. Its age is dated to be more than five thousand years. Hence Hindu history is a prototype of how human civilisation would have looked, if civilisation all across the globe had been allowed to develop democratically in its natural state. This is why we need to study civilisation, history and culture.

The evolution of this Civilisation can be considered to be natural and continuing as there is no last messiah in the Hindu worldview. In fact this is what distinguishes Hindu Civilisation from the rest. And this is why Hinduism is called a Living Idea, guided by the sum total of human wisdom that is not considered to be embodied in one person, or one book, or one period of human history. Recent archaeological findings cast doubt on this theory. Many authors of Hinduism point out that according to recent excavations there already existed a highly developed culture of cities in India with paved roads and underground sewers before the invasion of the Aryan nomads from which he concludes that Hinduism existed before the Aryan conquest and settlement and that the invaders merely absorbed and blended the cultural achievements of the conquered peoples with that of their own.

The term "Living Idea" means a continuity of freedom of thought from which emerge multifarious Hindu Principles. Two instances of Hindu Principles that symbolise the outcome of freedom of thought are the pronouncements made not today, but five thousand years back by unnamed Ṛṣis (Hindu ascetics) that, "This world is one family" (*Vasudhaiva Kuṭumbakam*) and that "The Universal Reality is the same, but different people can call it by different names" (*Ekam Sat Viprāḥ Bahudhā Vadanti*). In these two proclamations made in ancient Hindu India, we see the seeds of globalism and freedom of thought, five thousand years before the world was to become the global village of today. Thus in its true essence, Hinduism is a stridently assertive rational-humanist line of reasoning. At the level of practice, the outlook of Hinduism boils down to upholding righteousness (Sat-guṇa) and fighting ignoble attitudes (Dur-guṇa). Taking poetic license, we can describe the practitioners of this outlook as (*Hīnam Nāṣāyati Iti Hinduhu*) "Those who uphold righteousness and fight ignobleness are Hindus." Thus, far from being a narrow nationalistic doctrine, Hinduism is in its true essence, "a timeless and universal compilation of human wisdom." Hence it is also called *Sanātana* which means, something that is 'forever continuing'.

Hindu Traditions

Hindu tradition encourages Hindus to seek spiritual and moral truth wherever it might be found, while acknowledging that no creed can contain such truth in its fullness and that each individual must realise this truth through his or her own systematic effort. Our experience, our reason, and our dialogue with others especially with enlightened individuals provide various means of testing our understanding of spiritual and moral truth. And Hindu scripture, based on the insights of Hindu sages and seers, serves primarily as a guidebook. But ultimately truth comes to us through direct consciousness of the divine or the ultimate reality. In other religions this ultimate reality is known as God. Hindus refer to it by many names, but the most common name is Brahmā.

We can divide Hindu philosophical thinking in three eras (two in fact). But for analytical purposes it seems better to distinguish three.

1. The era of the Vedas (from 1200 to 700 BC)
2. The era of the Upaniṣads (700 BC to 200 BC)
3. The era of the Sūtras (700 BC to 200 BC)

The first era is often termed Vedism or Brahmism. The second era is the real Hinduism of present day. The first era gradually passed over into the second era whereby elements of the first era were absorbed and integrated. Dr. Israel Selvanayagam [cf. Israel Selvanayagam, Vedic Sacrifice, Challenge and Response, Passim, Manohar 1996] in his mentioned dissertation delves deeply into evolution which for instance Yajña underwent as a result of transition. According to this scholar, in the Vedic era sometimes animals were sacrificed, but under the influence of the Ahiṁsa idea (non-violence) of the Puranic period, the character of the sacrifice changed. The idea of non-violence is also denoted in the Rig Veda (RV 1.94.2; 1.101.4). The emphasis came to rest on the bringing of immaterial offers. In the case of yoga we can observe the same evolution, according to the author. Yoga, a Vedic creation, changed from a material sacrificial act into an immaterial one under the influence of Patañjali's system, where concentration, meditation and contemplation play a major role.

The very first mantra of the Rig Veda is about the Homa. This was part of the Yajña. The idea was to cajole nature and to influence it ecologically. It was also meant to open the Ajña or third eye. Here we see a direct connection between Yajña and Ajña.

In the era of the Upaniṣads a radical re-interpretation of the sacrifice takes place, without rejection of the Yajña. The idea becomes, to strive for self-realisation through Ātmā-Yajña (internal offer). The Havankuṇḍa or sacrificial pit is figuratively speaking moved from the yard to the inside of the body. There various cakras are present as energy centres, which generate power for mokṣa or redemption. The doctrine of Karma-saṁsāra (Karma-world) as spiritual heritage motivates to total salvation or liberation instead of temporal sojourn in Svarga (Paradise). God Brahmā is the quantitative total of reality. Cosmic consciousness and self-realisation can be achieved by actualising those internal powers. For this the path of Yoga is developed. But to remain on the safe side next to Ātmā-Yajña (yoga) Vedic rituals (Pūjā) are also practised, thereby creating a fusion between rituals and ethics. The external and internal worlds are thus correlated with the micro and macro cosmos. There is interest for Buddhism, Jainism and Sikhism. Kāmā or sex is considered inimical on the spiritual path. Ahiṁsā or non-violence becomes one of the virtues under the reign of king Ashoka.

The era of the Sūtras goes hand in hand with the era of the Upaniṣads. The codification of the Vedas takes place in the Dharmśastras accentuating their authority. The inherent potency of the Yajña-ritual is stressed. Habits of Dāna (gifts), Tapas (to chant inwardly) and Tīrtha (pilgrimage) become prominent. A phase of socio-religion commences and a synthesis between bhāgavata and Brahmin forms the basis for Vaiṣṇavism. The Bhagavad Gītā includes karma (Pūjā, Dānā, Tapas) and yoga. The Gītā is the quintessence of the Mahābhārata that is in turn part of the Bhāgavatam. The Gītā declares that Jñāna yajña stands higher than Dravya-yajña, in other words yoga (inner wisdom: knowledge of the Vedas) should be considered more valuable than material performances. The priests with knowledge of the Vedas are now the Gurus and the Yajamāna (sacrifice holders). The chief householder now seeks his salvation by means of Pūjā or Yoga. The devotee offers flowers and love. Associations such as the Ārya Samāj and the Bharata Samāj come into being preaching the return to the beginnings of the vedic tradition. There are movements to devise shorter versions of rituals. Some go so far that hardly anything remains of the old religion. They have a wide appeal. Modern man leads a hectic existence and chooses for less money and time consuming rituals.

Sanskrit as Religious Language

All major religions have a sacred language for their rituals. The Jews have Hebrew, the Catholics Latin, the Muslims

Arabic, and the Hindus have Sanskrit. All the languages mentioned are extinct, not being spoken anymore in day to day speech. Sans means holy and krit: practice or radiation. It is alleged that all modern languages were derived from Sanskrit. The pronunciation must be melodious and must give the impression of singing. That's why it is also known as Mṛdubhāṣaṇa, which can be translated as: agreeable or joyous language. Its sacredness is brought forth while humming when the inner mind manifests itself in the physical body; a perception of the astral body, more or less like the voice on a tape-recorder that can be heard without the speaker's presence. Sacred volumes claim that melodious chanting of hymns may positively influence one's karma. Legend has it that Sanskrit was the result of sounds produced by God Śiva on a drum called Damarū (Śiva's drum) and were picked up by Ṛṣis in meditation. Another opinion is that God gave it as a gift (Dhanvantri) to man.

The alphabet denoted as Devanāgari has 48 characters and 9 numerals. Devanāgari means city or village of gods. That is a spiritual abode of sounds, gutturals, numbers etc. in short a place of harbour for language. Synonymous with this is the term 'gauwn'. Gauwn means village. Gauwn also means a dressing gown that covers and harbours the body. Behind each letter stands a deva or a devi. By joining letters, words, mantras or hymns are created: which are of a higher order than the individual letters. The whole universe is embedded in the syllable AUM. This word is also equal to the numeral 3. OM establishes unity between letters and numerals in the nagari (village). While the milk-ocean was being churned by the devas and demons with the assistance of the gods, written language arose out of nowhere and was presented by Dhanavantri to mankind for preservation of knowledge and wisdom. There is an old saying: "scripta manet." What is written is lasting, what is said, evaporates. Thanks to the alphabet great works like the Mahābhārata and Rāmāyaṇa could have been preserved for posterity. An echo of this system we find in the academic world where meritorious persons are rewarded with a honorary degree.

Monotheism

The Hindu way is not only in history within the contexts of psychology and spirituality of symbol, but also directly demonstrates how it participates in the revelation of the ultimate human destiny. Every kind or size of energy in the cosmos is an identity and simultaneously an entity. The nature doesn't copy. The pious creates his own spiritual identity with a blueprint of a cosmic entity. The universal democracy produces 'androgynies' (human and deity) to guide each soul to the final destination, the Ultimate Reality or God. This is comparable with a child and a personal teacher based on personal patterns of thoughts and images of God. We refer to the Atharva Veda where the ascetics denote the cosmic truth: "I place in the hands of spiritually advanced persons, in diverse ways, these good-natured well-behaved, venerable, serviceable subjects. May God, the Averter of sin, grant me the blessing which as I anoint you, my heart desireth" (AV 2968).That's why Hinduism has a considerable number of Gods, Goddesses, and demigods. All are energies of One. We illustrate the diversity of this uniformity.

A goldsmith decides to establish a jewellery store. He is, his own manager. He makes the jewels, sells them, repairs them and demolishes them to make new ones when they are out of fashion. He is in short, manager, bookkeeper, salesman, jeweller, repairman, demolisher and handyman. Should he appear for every other duty behind another counter the visitor to the store might conclude having to do with more than one person. And yet it's the same man. A sixteen-shaped diamond stone oriented with its diagonals, verticals and horizontals, produces divers images of the same stone. Lord Viṣṇu for instance is depicted as a dwarf, as a fish, as a warrior etc. But it's the same God. To sum up, it may be said: one bucket of water is a large number of small and big drops from different shapes and contents.

In Hinduism the situation is more or less similar. It is the same God who appears in different shapes on earth that dependent upon the mission He has undertaken to fulfil. As the Bhagavad Gītā puts it: "whenever there is a decay of Dharma (righteousness) and outbreak of Adharma (non-righteousness), I descend Myself to protect good, to annihilate the wicked and to re-establish Dharma. I am born from age to age." When God comes in life form on earth we say that He is an avatār. He also appears during dreams or meditations of saints, ṛiṣis wise men or chosen men in many forms and under many names. This is rather confusing. Let me clarify this idea with an example for the benefit of those who still fail to grasp the notion.

Hinduism proceeds from the idea that God is without form. In many scriptures He is seen as pure energy. The Upaniṣads describe Him as Neti-Neti, "not this and not this." In the Bhagavad Gītā (7.8) where Lord Kṛṣṇa serves as charioteer for his disciple Arjuna He says after a request to be seen in his true form: "I can not be seen with the eyes you have got. But I will equip you with a godly eye, to behold my mystic self." Whereupon He revealed himself to Arjuna who saw an image of incredible magnificence with uncountable mouths and eyes adorned with beautiful clothes and beautiful ornaments etc. (See verses 9-15).

No human being would ever be able to reproduce this vision. Idols are created depicting ordinary people (sometimes weird-looking) as an aid in the religious process; to focus devotion on God, since ordinary people are incapable of conceiving anything without a form. In the foregoing paragraph I have already explained how the different images were conceived. It is therefore a fallacy to conclude that it is the idol or rather the material from which it is made that is being worshipped, which by the way would place Hinduism in the category of animism (a primitive religion) that attributes a soul to all objects. By means of the Prāṇa-Pratiṣṭhā-ritual the God that is being symbolised by the idol is asked to take possession of it.

Hindu Thought in Ancient Times

Since ancient times, Hindu thought has transcended geographical boundaries and influenced religious and philosophical ideas throughout the world. Persian, ancient Greek and ancient Roman thought may well have been influenced by Hinduism. Three other religions that originated in India branched off from Hinduism: Buddhism, Jainism, and Sikhism. In the 19th century German philosopher Arthur Schopenhauer read both Hindu and Buddhist scriptures and based much of his thinking on them. In the United States, 19th century writers such as Ralph Waldo Emerson and Henry David Thoreau drew on Hinduism and its scriptures in developing their philosophy of transcendentalism.

More recently, civil-rights leader Martin Luther King, Jr., studied the teachings of Hindu leader Mohandas Gandhi on non-violent protest. In the sphere of popular culture, rock musician George Harrison embraced Hinduism during the 1960s, and some members of the United States counterculture explored Hinduism and Buddhism, as did the Beat poets (Beat Generation). Millions of Westerners today practice meditation or Yoga to achieve relief from stress or physical fitness, indicating Western receptiveness to Hindu practices. This is not to say that there are no beliefs and practices that may be identified as Hindu, but rather that Hindu tradition has concerned itself largely with the human situation rather than the Hindu situation. Instead of basing its identity on separating Hindu from non-Hindu or believer from non-believer, Hinduism has sought to recognise principles and practices that would lead any individual to become a better human being and understand and live in harmony with dharma. Dharma is an all-important concept for Hindus. In addition to tradition and moral order, it also signifies the path of knowledge and correct action. Because of Hinduism's emphasis on living in accordance with dharma, anyone who is striving for spiritual knowledge and seeking the right course of ethical action is, in the broadest sense, a follower of Sanātana dharma.

Hinduism entered the English language in the early 19th century to describe the beliefs and practices of those residents of India who had not converted to Islam or Christianity and did not practise Judaism or Zoroastrianism. In the case of most religions, beliefs and practices come first, and those who subscribe to them are acknowledged as followers. In the case of Hindu tradition, however, the acknowledgement of Hindus came first, and their beliefs and practices constitute the contents of the religion. Hindus have highly individual regional and religious identities. Hindus themselves prefer to use the Sanskrit term Sanātana dharma for their religious tradition. Sanātana dharma is often translated into English as 'original or eternal tradition' but the translation of dharma as 'tradition' or 'religion' gives an extremely limited, even mistaken, sense of the word. Dharma has many meanings in Sanskrit, the sacred language of Hindu scripture, including 'moral order,' 'duty,' and 'right action.'

Dharma

Dharma is one of the four boons within the four stages of life. The Atharva Veda formulates the following hymn: "1 bestow on thee four boons, through four diverse sources, filled with the power of supplying food, vigour and nourishment. May all these forces enhancing pleasure reach thee in domestic life. May thou acquire completely these qualities strengthening the soul in diverse ways" (AV 859).

The four boons are Dharma (virtue), Artha (wealth), Kāmā (desire) and Mokṣa (salvation). The four sources are called, viz. Brahmcārya (celibacy) Gṛihastha (married life), Vānaprastha (the life of a recluse), Sanyāsa (the life of complete, renunciation) or the four Vedas. Dharma concerns the bases of the forthcoming actions in all four stages of life. Celibacy is the state of being unmarried, with abstinence from sexual activity. According to the Veda there should be plenty of butter, honey, milk, curd and water in the house of a married person. This is required in the stage of Gṛihastha. This kind of food is defined as spiritual food, mental vigour, and intellectual nourishment. In the third stage the married person leaves domestic life behind and seals the life of the senses. In the last stage of life one should renounce worldly desires and all their attachments. This stage is known as Sanyasi, means 'death' (San) of 'desires' (Yasi). Only one thought is in mind that *I am the spirit that always denies and I renounce all the deceits of the world, the flesh, and darkness.*

Major Groups of Dharma

How does one know in what measure his acts and deeds will influence his karma? The answer is given by the concept of dharma. Some scholars describe it as: stability, maintenance, harmony, equilibrium, and adherence to tradition and customs. Dharma is valid for both human beings and nature. Dharma makes the sun rise every morning. The sun behaves according to its dharma. It is dharma that makes people give alms. The term is derived from the Sanskrit dhri, which means: to maintain, to bear, to keep, to rule, to determine. Dharma rules the cosmos and maintains it. It determines the behaviour that is most conducive to spiritual progress. Dharma determines the just and righteous path. The scholars that have occupied themselves with this concept have categorized the concept in four major groups. Ṛta dharma, varṇa dharma, aṣrama dharma and svadharma. Each group has its subclasses.

1. Ṛta: Universal law. The inherent order of the cosmos. The laws that comprise and rule creation, functions, processes, thoughts and observations.
2. Varṇa Dharma: Law of the own kind. Social duty. Varṇa can mean race, tribe, appearance, character, colour, social class etc. This dharma describes one's duties and responsibilities within a country, society, community, class, profession or family. They are embodied in religious and moral laws.

Sub-groups of Dharma

A further sub-classification of dharma is in ṣīaḍa dharma, strī dharma and Puruṣa dharma.

1. Ṣīaḍa dharma (principles of good behaviour) holds for everyone irrespective of creed, age, class or gender. In the Manu śāstra it is described as: dhairya (Patience); kṣamā (forgiveness); dama (self restraint); asteya (not stealing); śauca (cleanliness); indriyanigraha (control of the senses); dhī (intelligence), vidyā (love for learning); satya (truthfulness); akrodha (absence of anger).

2. Strī dharma (specific duties of the wife). Traditional behaviour, modesty, silent power, religiosity, dignity, willingness to care for the family; heeding of vocation; to provide for social stability, education of the offspring to become good citizens of tomorrow.
3. Puruṣa dharma (specific duties of the husband). Correct behaviour, wisdom, leadership, integrity, maintenance of the family. The married man has to look after the well-being of his family.
4. Āśrama dharma (duties during the life-stages). There are four stages in life: 1. Brahmcāṛī (student); 2. Gṛhastha (head of the family); 3. Vānaprastha (older counsellor) and 4. Saṅyāsa (monk, hermit). They walk more or less parallel with the four major human objectives: dharma (righteousness); artha (riches, wealth) kāmā (joy, pleasure) and mokṣa (liberation). Every stage has its dharmas: gṛihastha dharma, saṅyāsa dharma etc.
5. Āpatti dharma (behaviour in cases of emergency). This dharma says that behaviour in calamitous situations should be governed by wisdom. Emergency situations can demand that one deviates from the normal rules of behaviour provided that the deviation is not made for ones own benefit but for the benefit of others.

Svadharma

A special kind of dharma is Svadharma, which is determined by the sum total of karmas, accrued from the past and the cumulative effect of the other three dharmas. It is the individualised dharma, ruled by someone's talents and abilities, desires and inclinations, religion, family and guru, mental and emotional state. The Bhagavad Gītā says (18.47): "It is better to fulfil your own svadharma poorly, than to fulfil the dharma of another perfectly. By fulfilling the duty which one's nature prescribes (svabhāva) one does not sin (kilbiṣa)." Everyone and everything is born in a culture and dies too in the same culture.

Hinduism accepts all four Puruṣārthas, as mentioned above in the Āṣrama dharma—the four major human objectives—as valid goals of human endeavour. It does not look down upon Kāmā or Artha, as indicated by the Kāmasūtra, a work on sexuality from about the 4th century A.D., and by the Arthaśāstra. The latter text by Kautilya, a minister to a king of the 4th century B.C., discusses how a king should wield political and economic power. Khajuraho is the place where the Kāmasūtra has been pictured.

They depict hundreds of figures in a variety of poses. Some poses are sexual in nature, while others are believed to be symbolic and have yet to be deciphered by archaeologists. Several sculpture-adorned temples devoted to Hinduism and Jainism are found in Khajuraho, which is located in north-central India.

The Nature of Hinduism

Hinduism, as it comes across in this book, is a robust, joyful religion, amazingly in step with the most advanced thinking of modern times, in love with life, deeply human as well as humane, delightfully aware of your personal life's needs—or so it seems, for the teaching in this book is no abstraction: It is down-to-earth and pressingly immediate. Due to its antiquity, the absence of a higher authority, like a Pope, who from time to time decrees what should be considered true faith or heresy, the fact that India in the course of time was ruled by many other nations, and its capacity to absorb other ideas, (new philosophies and rituals simply being added to old ones), the body of beliefs has grown to huge proportions. The main characteristic of Hinduism is its tolerance towards other faiths or, as the Bhāgavad Gītā teaches us (4.11): "Whatever and whichever way men approach Me, even so do I accept them; whatever paths they may choose finally lead to Me." And further: "In whatever form a devotee seeks to worship Me with faith, I make his faith steadfast." The famous Swami Vivekānanda who lived around the beginning of this century and travelled widely through the Western world to deliver lectures, put it thus: "We believe not only in universal toleration, but we accept all religions as true. As different streams having different sources, all mingle their waters in the sea, so different paths which men take through different tendencies, various though they appear, crooked or straight, all lead to God." Thanks to this principle, in the course of its existence many wise men, sages, wizards, etc. have felt free to add to Hinduism, creating side streams called darśans (philosophical movements), which some people might consider new religions, but which in fact only slightly deviate from the main stream and some even creating new mainstreams.

To mention a few of the first:

1. Śaivism. Worship of God Śiva.
2. Vaiṣṇavism. Worship of God Viṣṇu.
3. Śaktism. Worship of mother Goddesses.
4. Tantrism. More or less the same as above. It makes use of geometrical figures called maṇḍalas and yantras.

And to mention a few of the latter:

1. Buddhism. This religion rooted in Hinduism was spread by Gautama Buddha (560-480 VC) in the rest of Asia after serving for a time as the state religion of India during the reign of King Ashoka. It rejects the caste system, one of the cornerstones of Hinduism. The branch Buddhism with its emphasis on universal love and non-violence, has had a sobering influence on a significant part of the human species.
2. Ārya Samāj comparable to Protestantism in Christianity. Dayananda Sarasvati (1824-1883) claims to represent ten percent of all Hindus founded this religion in 1875. It preaches return to the original Vedas and rejects idol worship. In his book Satyārthaprakaśa the founder says: "Nowhere in the Vedas is mention made of idols."
3. Guru Nānak who lived from 1469 to 1538 founded Sikhism. It combines Hinduism with Islam. Sikhism was born in the Punjab area, which now falls into the present-day states of India and Pakistan.
4. Jainism. This was founded by Mahavira Vardhamana around 500 B.C. It rejects the authority of the Vedas altogether.

The often conflicting viewpoints which are being entertained and the enormous quantity of literature on the matter makes the grasping of Hinduism for the outsider not only quite a job but rather hazardous as well.

Hindu Civilisation

Men and women commonly divide work duties in their own culture and society. In chiefdoms and civilisations, households have to produce enough to support themselves and their leaders. In civilisations, many people specialise in offering a variety of services and producing a variety of goods. Each occupation is commonly associated with a different level of status, usually referred to as an economic class. Duty must also be self-sufficient. Most people also depend on technologies. "May spacious Agni, Lord of Duty, gladly, vast Agni, Duty's Lord, accept the butter." The Yajur Veda specifies productions as 'spacious', support as 'duty' and self-sufficient as 'butter'. "All-hail! Hallowed by Svāhā, with the beams of Sūrya, strive for his central place among the kinsmen" (YV 10.29: 425). In some tribes, however, people known as big men might earn a degree of higher status and respect than others by demonstrating bravery or bravado. These big men of chiefs must prove that they are closest in descent to the founding ancestors of the highest ranked clans within chiefdoms. They live as full-time rulers who may not have to work at productive duties. Chiefs have the power to collect some of the goods people produce, such as food, and redistribute them in times of need or use them in ceremony.

Ideology

In every society, culturally unique ways of thinking about the world unite people in their behaviour. Anthropologists often refer to the body of ideas that people share as ideology. This act is entrusted according to the Yajur Veda to the great Guru, Bṛhaspati. Particular beliefs often tie in closely with the daily concerns of domestic life, such as making a living, health and sickness, happiness and sadness, interpersonal relationships, and death. People's values tell them the differences between right and wrong or good and bad. Ideals serve as models for what people hope to achieve in life. The Yajur Veda indicates the improvement of domestic life as "grow in strength and swell to greatness." The butter's rapid flow delights his spirit! Bṛihaspati extend this act of worship. May he restore the sacrifice uninjured. Here let all Gods rejoice. OM! Step you forward. This is the stick for kindling you, O Agni. By means of this grow strong and swell to greatness. May we too grow in strength and swell to greatness. O Agni, you who win food, I cleanse you, you who have hastened to the food, Food-winner (spoil, wealth, the prize) (YV 2.13-14). Ideology can be broken down into at least three specific categories: beliefs, values, and ideals. These three elements make part of worship. People's beliefs give them an understanding of how the world works and how they should respond to the actions of others and their environments.

Comprehensive and Universal Tradition

Hindu tradition aims at comprehensiveness so far as religious beliefs and practices are concerned. First, it wishes to make the riches of Hinduism available to the Hindu and to any genuine seeker of truth and knowledge. But it does not limit Hindus to their tradition. Instead, it encourages them to explore all avenues that would lead to a realisation of the divine, and it provides a system with many paths for such realisation. A latest historical date means that people are still brilliant of mind to keep knowledge and to transfer this orally. Drawing the knowledge on paper means become unable to remember. We don't have to prove the age of the Hinduism. Recently Nasa discovered the Adamsbridge that goes back to the period of King Rama (see figure 6: Adamsbridge). This is over 1,700,000 years ago. Rama is a Hindu God incarnation in the Treta Yuga (the third era) as the king.

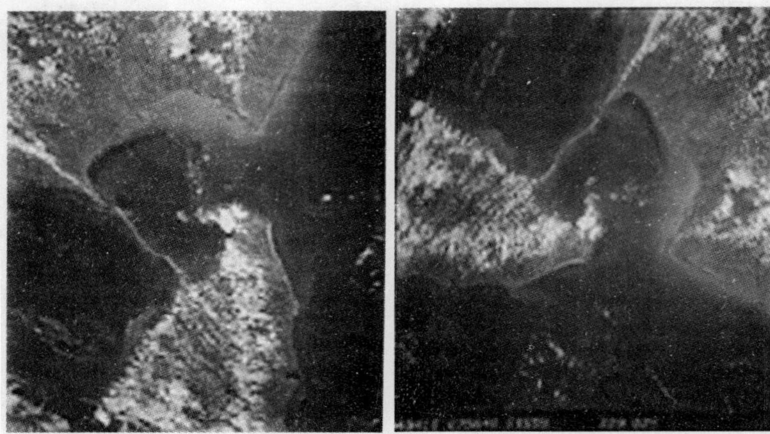

Figue 6: Adamsbridge

Science and Hinduism

Hinduism is constantly experimenting with and assimilating new ideas. Also like science, it is far less concerned with the origin or history of ideas than with their truth as demonstrated through direct experience. Hinduism's openness to new ideas, teachers, and practices, and its desire for universality rather than exclusivity, set it apart from religions that distinguish their followers by their belief in particular historical events, people, or revelations.

Hindu Teachings

Within Hinduism there are various schools of thought, which Hindu scholars have systematized in different ways. These are six systems, viz. Nyāya, on rigorous logic, Vaiśeṣic, on atoms and the structure of matter, Sāṁkhya on numbers and categories, Yoga on meditation techniques, Mīmāmsā on the analysis of sacred texts, and Vedãnta on the nature and experience of spirituality. Vedãnta is Theism and Sãmkhya is Materialism. While the Vedãnta School was theistic, believing in the existence of God, Yoga is a system of transforming and absorbing higher power from the gods and achieves liberation by increase of the density of our soul or micro god. The discipline uses both physical and mental faculties to arrive to its spiritual aims. All of these schools have enriched Hinduism with their individual emphases. Their teachings are usually summarised in texts called Sūtras or aphorisms. These sūtras can be memorised easily and recited as a means of gaining spiritual focus. In many scriptures we find a lot of histories which are based on mythology. Indian mythology is a potpourri of energies. This energy becomes gods, demons, abstract concepts, and other supernatural entities depending on their task in the cosmos. The primary entities change as time passes, with new 'sediments' of entities being added on while the lower layers dwindle in importance. The difference is the density. The commonality among all these sediments is the general character of the Hindu gods and goddesses. Gods and goddesses are beings who far outstrip mankind in intellect, power, longevity, and, most importantly, spiritual insight. Divinities are beings that exist with perfect spiritual understanding. It is the achievement of this spiritual understanding, or ecstasy, that the 'good-hearted' man is attempting to achieve through correct thought, action, and sacrifices.

Yoga Science

The last hundred years of scientific and philosophical thought have caused dramatic upheavals in how we view our universe, our spiritual beliefs, and ourselves: the total of the spiritual universe. Yoga is a process of the merging between the individual soul with the All Soul. This process contains four steps, viz. entering the sphere of God, look like Him, be close and adopt His desire and become a unity with Him. Practically this means to come to a Country, integration in the Country, contribute in the development and become a citizen or getting the nationality of the Country. With the advent of Darwinism, relativity, nihilism, and existentialism, traditional religious dogmas have been challenged as never before. Increasingly, people are wondering if enduring spiritual and moral truths even exist. Hinduism is a delightful way of life for Hindus and non-Hindus, and for people who are interested in spirituality, moral truths and the deeper meanings of the Vedic values, it demonstrates genuine compatibility of scientific and religious values, and how science and our most cherished moral values actually enrich and reinforce one another.

The term 'yoga' also means "making a compromise with the beauty of nature." Beauty is sweet like honey for every creature in nature. Beauty or Śriṁgāra is related with the ceremonial rites and rituals in the life of a devout Hindu. In fact, there are no vital actions birth, initiation, marriage, death etc. which can be allowed to be performed without its appropriate rite or Saṁskāra. The Solah Śrīṁgāras symbolises the culmination of the basic feminine urge for "beautification." Śrīṁgāra, the painting and decorating the body to enhance it has been an elaborate art of Hindu society. It was not a mere cosmetic process but had an under-current of deeper significance—a philosophy. The true fruit of the technique of yoga is not a material achievement or performance. The practitioners are interested in keeping the head and the heart clean through the harmony of breath. The fruit of your action will tell you whether you are on the right path or not.

Darśnā or Philosophy

Philosophies, as mentioned earlier interacted closely with religions and Hinduism, Buddhism, Jainism all show traces of ideas borrowed from the different philosophical schools which strictly speaking were parts of no religion.

While these philosophical schools played an all-important role in influencing the development of Indian religions, these philosophical schools themselves did not evolve into separate religions. They could not so evolve, as they were intellectual traditions without any mass following. The lack of mass following had a positive effect as it kept the spirit of quest alive and disallowed the emergence of rigid commitment to certain ideas, which prevented them from taking on the form of religion. Philosophical schools whether theistic or materialist remained distinct from religions proper. We shall explain in brief the nature of these different philosophical traditions. All the religions and philosophies we have so far discussed originated in ancient times in India. All the religions have a concept of Liberation as final distiny.

The Bhāgavatam (10.14.58) gives an impression of the unity and the way to liberate human beings from bondage. "For one who has accepted the boat of the lotus feet of the Lord, who is the shelter of the cosmic manifestation and is famous as Mukunda, or the giver of mukti, the ocean of the material world is like the water contained in a calf's footprint (Param-padam), or the place where there are no material miseries, or Vaikuṇṭha, is his goal, not the place where there is danger in every step of life."

Learned transcendentalists who know the Absolute Truth call this non-dual substance Brahm, Paramātmā or Bhagavān (Bh.T. 1.2.11). These three terms are mainly used in daily rituals and performances, or Pūjā.

The performance of pūjā is the core of worshipping God and an aspect of Karma Yoga. Its purpose, in essence, is to propitiate the eternal and boundless God in any of its manifestations. The act is performed by giving a general royal reception through various oblations and offerings (clothes, decorations, feast etc.), accompanied by chanting of hymns or mantras. The sacrifice which is extended on every side by the threads (of created things) spread out by the worship of the gods for a hundred and one (years).

Very popular in modern society is the philosophy of the Ásanas. The positions are performed for health and a good physical condition as the practice of sport is one of the means to stay healthy and to function with vigour and alertness, so we need the capacity to manage effectively in the surrounding world and the ability to control one's own life. One's health and character are reflected in its breathing pattern. In the performance of Āsanas, two avenues or paths are involved. One is the evolutory, expressive or exhibitive path, taking the self towards the body, towards the pores of the skin, towards the periphery. The other is the involutory, intuitive or inhibitive path, where the vehicles of the body are made to move towards the self.

By performing the āsanas the centres of the body will be activated and stimulated for our physical and mental progress.

Vedānta

Vedānta is the only philosophical tradition that remains alive today. The reason is that unlike any other philosophical school, Vedānta has been fully integrated into Hindu religion. Vedānta literally means "end of the Vedas" but it is interpreted as "culmination of the Vedas." The founder of Vedānta tradition is said to be the Vedic Seer Vyāsa, but its most well known exponent was Ādi Śankarācārya. There were others too like Sāyanācārya, Madhavācārya and many others. The Vedānta system virtually represents Śankarācārya's interpretation of the Sūtras. The Sūtras are a collection of rituals and practices that have been sanctioned in Vedic literature. The essence of Vedānta philosophy is that all human beings have souls (Ātman). And although physically all beings have a separate existence, their souls are actually not separate. They are merged into one supreme soul (Param-Ātmah) or the absolute soul (Brahmā). This unity of different souls is called Advaita or non-dualism (also called Monism). The doctrine of Advaita is central to Vedānta philosophy. The visible and palpable universe around us is considered to be unreal (Mithyā which is but an illusion i.e. Māyā), while that which is the supreme reality the absolute soul (Brahm) cannot be perceived by our normal senses of sight, smell, hearing or touch. Vedānta philosophy continues to be very popular among Hindu philosophers and is a subject at many discourses at temples. There are many contemporary names associated with this philosophy.

Sāṁkhya

The Sāṁkhya school is relatively materialistic as compared to Vedānta. The founder of the Sāṁkhya School is considered to be a philosopher, named Kapila. The term Sāṁkhya could be derived from Sāṁkhya meaning 'numbers'. This could be so as Sāṁkhya philosophy divides the universe into 25 principles (tattvas). The first 8 tattvas comprise of the material universe and are termed as Prakṛti. One tattva (principle) is the motive power of the universe, which is looked upon as the soul or spirit and is termed Puruṣa. The remaining 16 tattvas are the result of Puruṣa acting upon Prakṛti and they constitute the material universe with all its movements of rotation, revolution, gravitation. Thus everything begins with matter (Prakṛti) but this matter in itself is inert or dead, it is activated by the stimulus provided to it by the motive power (Puruṣa) and the result of this is the active universe with its twinkling stars and rotating planets of which we are a part. The Sāṁkhya system of ideas is thus not entirely theistic as it assumes the existence of both matter and motive power to begin with. The universe is not looked upon as the creation of a supreme creator. But the Sāṁkhya doctrine is neither entirely materialistic. According to Sāṁkhya, matter (Prakṛti) which exists without any creator having created it, but is inert until it is activated by the motive power (Puruṣa).

Evidently the Sāṁkhya doctrine tried to explain the existence (or creation) of the universe by extending the idea of sexual procreation to the entire universe. Incidentally, Puruṣa literally means 'man' or male and Prakṛti is one of the names of the Mother-Goddess.

Incarnation or Avatāra

Brahmā that is, Brahmā with attributes generally takes the form of one of three main Hindu deities: Brahmā, Viṣṇu, or Śiva. These personified forms of Brahmā correspond to three stages in the cycle of the universe. Brahmā corresponds to the creative spirit from which the universe arises. Viṣṇu corresponds to the force of order that sustains the universe. Śiva corresponds to the force that brings a cycle to end destruction acting as a prelude to transformation, leaving pure consciousness from which the universe is reborn after destruction. Other forms of Īśvara widely worshipped by Hindus are Śakti, the female aspect of divinity, and Gaṇeṣa, the elephant-headed deity associated with the removal of obstacles.

Brahmā also may choose to take birth in a knowable form, or avatāra (incarnation), to uphold dharma and restore balance to the world. Kṛṣṇa, a well-known avatāra of Viṣṇu, appears at times to save the world. Rāma, another well-known avatār of Viṣṇu, is the subject of the Hindu epic Rāmāyana (Way of Rāma). Whether Nirguṇa (no form) or Saguṇa (with form), Brahmā represents the ultimate reality (sat), ultimate consciousness (cit), and ultimate bliss (ānanda).

Majority of Hindus choose a personal deity, a Saguṇa form of Brahmā with whom they can feel a direct personal connection. Devotion to this deity can take a number of forms, including prayer, ceremonial worship, chanting of the deity's name, and pilgrimage to sites sacred to the deity.

The Hindu god Viṣṇu appears on earth in ten incarnations called avatāra, to destroy injustice and save humankind. Sacred Hindu writings called the Puranas describe these incarnations. These incarnations and their Hindu names are: fish (Matsya), tortoise (Kūrma), boar (Vārāha), man lion (Narasiṁha), dwarf (Vāmana), axe-wielding human (Paraśurāma), ideal person (Rāma of the Rāmāyaṇa), all-attractive perfect person (Kṛṣṇa), the enlightened (Buddha), and a future incarnation (Kalki).

In context with the mainfestations of Lord Viṣṇu all of creation arises from Brahmā, according to Hindu teaching. Puruṣa as Brahmā means man or mankind and also a cosmogenic figure, the creative source, the primeval male (B.G. 15:14), who envelops the whole universe and who represents totality (S.Br. 11.1.6, 1-2; Ait. Up. 1.1-4; RV 7.104.15). Brahmā is both the efficient cause of the universe (creator) as well as the material cause (substance of which the universe is created). For this reason, all of creation is divine and deserving of our respect.

Soul or Ātmā

We as individuals too are a part of this changing universe. Our bodies are constantly undergoing change, while our minds, formed of thoughts and feelings, are also in a state of flux. According to Vedānta, however, our self consists of more than mind and body. At its core lies the unchanging ātmā, our innermost, transcendental self, as opposed to the material self (our body, thoughts, and feelings) that is part of the universe. The ātmā is our true self. But we lose sight of it because of our passionate involvement with our material self and its search for happiness in this universe. The universe can never provide perfect and permanent happiness, however, because it, like our material self, is in a state of constant flux. We attain true happiness only through an awareness of our ātmān and the discovery of its true relationship with Brahmā.

Mantra or Formula

A mantra is a word or a combination of words which, if correctly recited, leads over the ocean of rebirth. In simple terminology: a mantra is a formula which is recited with the objective to ask for the solution of problems, removal of sorrows; the fulfilment of spiritual or worldly desires such as prosperity, the punishment of an enemy etc. By means of the mantra the powers of gods, devas etc. are invoked and propitiated.

Mantra-vidyā teaches that the universe was created from an idea of God, by the projection of his word Aum. It is nāda or sound. That's why mantra, nāda and Veda are intertwined. Brahmā is the highest reality and nothing else but the cosmic word AUM. The blowing on the conch shell and the ringing of the temple bell represent cosmic sound and vibration. The first universe came forth from AUM and was the Causal Universe. From 'That' came the Astral Universe, and from that the Material Universe. This threefold must be kept in mind because it plays an important role in Hinduism. Creation was caused by the word AUM (three letters). God is a triumvirate of God Brahmā (the Creator), God Viṣṇu (the preserver) and God Viṣṇu (the destroyer). God Brahmā has created everything. He himself was born from the navel string of lord Viṣṇu.

The Upanishads explain AUM as standing for the whole universe and its parts, for its past, present and future. From this original vibration originated all manifestations.

"Aum is Brahmā. Aum is Brahmā's word. Aum is the Brahmā-sound. (Śabda-Brahmā). Aum is the sound that constructed the universe. During cosmic destruction the universe passed over into Aum. Aum has no beginning. Aum has no end. Aum was there before time was created. Aum stands above space, time and causality. Aum surpasses past, present and future. Aum stands above the underworld, the earth and the ethereal regions. Aum stands above sattva (glitter), rajas (passion) and tamas (darkness). Aum surpasses Brahmā, the creator, Viṣṇu, the preserver and üiva, the destroyer. Aum is the greatest (Parātparaḥ)."

The Vedas abound with mantras of great power originating from nāda or sound. That's the reason why every mantra has a particular nāda or sound intonation. In case the intonation is unknown the mantra may not produce the desired result. That's the reason too why the Rig Veda mantras must be differently recited from those of the Sāma Veda. Not only must the sound be known but also the words. A faulty pronunciation will not produce good results; worse still might deliver an outcome quite opposite to that asked for.

In order to propitiate a God, mantra-kriyā (inward and outward worship) and bhakti (devotion) are essential. If a person recites a mantra without bhakti or commitment, this is done mechanically the God will not look favourably upon this. That's why the modern practice of some persons to use cassettes must be dissuaded for this will not create cosmic energy. If someone recites a mantra or meditates on it with dedication but without knowledge of its esoteric significance and without showing outward signs of worship or signs of inward worship, such as relinquishment of the ego and desires, the outcome will not be perfect. But if mantra-kriyā and bhakti are blended the outcome will be beneficial.

Mind Force

Mind power in meditation is compared with horsepower. That's why we have to find 'horses' (SV 1212) to go forth in our activities, continuously, and in great quantity. The order to find horses means "become warriors" and "fort-destroyers." The mind can be attacked by a lot of enemies (RV 8.1.7) and these cause a lot of pain and unhappiness. One of the pains is sexual lust that poisons a man's happiness. A Roman philosopher and poet, Lucretius calls this lust bitterness in his poem De Rerum Natura "In the midst of the fountain of bliss there arises something bitter, which stings him even amid the very flowers." Life can become bitter, hard and cruel. Fighting with these influences is a battle to conquer everyday. Mind control is the same like winning a battle on the field (SV 1215), and conquering the wealth of the enemies (RV 9.63.7). The enemy of daily life is stress that can contribute to some respiratory disorders. For example, stress can trigger an attack of asthma. Wheezing, panting, and a feeling of being suffocated characterise asthma attacks. In addition, emotional stress can cause or aggravate many skin disorders, from those that produce itching, tickling, and pain to those that cause rashes and acne. Winston Churchill (1874 - 1965) once said about the mental disorder in the human mind. "This is not the end. It is not even the beginning of the end. But it is, perhaps, the end of the beginning." If we don't do anything about this, the individual will suffer for a long time. For a daily practice I would say: Early to bed and early to rise, makes a man healthy, wealthy, and wise.

Prosperity is only an instrument to be used, not a deity to be worshipped. The wealth of the enemy 'anger' is peace to give (SV 1215), of 'hate' is brotherhood and friendship (RV 10.10.1), of 'illusion' is knowledge and wisdom (AV 4239), of 'egoism' is worship and high praise (RV 1.94.1). A German theologian, Martin Luther (1483-1546) said "Wealth has in it neither material, formal, efficient, nor final cause, not anything else that is good; therefore our Lord God commonly gives riches to those from whom he withholds spiritual good."

Mahatma Gandhi adds in this thinking "Increase of material comforts, it may be generally laid down, does not in any way whatsoever conduce to moral growth."

Even the philosophy of pacifism has been propounded throughout history on grounds of morality, divine will, or economic and social utility. And the term 'brotherhood' is a subject of peace. Equality is an ethical aspiration that cannot be realised without recourse either to despotism or to an act of fraternity.

This wealth is the result of the serious efforts (AV 4548) which gives prosperity and happiness. We frame this high wealth—the chariot which travels to the Gods—with our mind (SV 1.2.66). The mind travels by air (SV 1214), that's why we have to train ourselves to control the air forces or breath, also called yoking the horses.

Air is also one of the economic goods and must be in scarce supply. Air does not normally have economic value because it is freely available. Air that is artificially conditioned is economically valuable, however, because it is relatively scarce. Think about the modern technique of gaining electricity from the air, viz. windmills. Wind is created when air that has been warmed over sun-heated land rises, leaving a vacuum in the space it once occupied. Cooler surrounding air then rushes in to fill the vacuum. This movement of rushing air is what we know as wind. The windmill is a machine that converts wind into useful energy. This energy is derived from the force of wind acting on oblique blades or sails that radiate from a shaft. Another example is a wind turbine generator that converts shaft power into electrical power.

In the Rig Veda mantra, Indra is called the result of serious efforts, the electrical power. Another part is that people can make indirect use of solar energy (Indra) that has been naturally collected. Earth's atmosphere, oceans, and plant life, for example, collect solar energy that people later extract to power technology. The mantra stimulates the scientist and technicians to investigate the truth. The oceans also collect and store solar energy, favoured by Indra (SV 1211). A significant fraction of the Sun's radiation reflects or scatters from the water's surface. The remaining fraction enters the water and rapidly diminishes with depth as the energy is absorbed and converted to heat or chemical energy. This absorption creates differences in temperature between layers of water in the ocean called temperature gradients.

The mind should not be affected mentally or morally by the above-mentioned 'enemy', that's the reason why yoga teaches us to withdraw on the right time. This is called a return of a chariot from the west to the east (SV 1217). From west to east means that the radiant energy from the Sun is transformed to potential energy of water in streams and rivers. People can tap the power stored in the water cycle by directing these flowing waters through modern turbines. Power produced in this way is called hydroelectric power.

If you don't return you will be afflicted or attacked with a deadly or disastrous effect. The mind is very impulsive because thoughts can come very suddenly and strongly, just like a demon that withholds the rain (SV 1211). A demon refers to beings whose special powers placed them between people and the gods. These beings had the ability either to improve people's lives or carry out the punishment of the gods. Demons usually are known as familiar creatures as vampires, which suck the blood of living victims. Another variety of demon, the Japanese Oni, is said to bring on storms. Kill the vampire and control the storms in the mind, which is the teaching of yoga.

Let the mind become just like Indu, the grant heroic fame. Indu is the great Indra, the god of the atmosphere, storms, rain, and battle, and the most powerful foe of various demonic powers preventing the rain and the dew from fructifying the earth. Because of those impulses, the mind becomes just like a horse that's unable to leave a forest (SV 1220) because of imprisonment. Indra killed the demon Vṛtra, who imprisons the waters. The Sāma Veda calls these imprisonments dark black clouds and the black path (SV 1218). Impulses should be brought under conditions for effective use, to gain control over for a particular end: liberation. A scientist tries to harness waterpower and the energy of the sun (as mentioned above), in the same way a yogi tries to control the 'horse' just like a pious and liberal prince.

The Law of Karma

The concept of karma is fundamental in Hinduism and without a thorough understanding of it one will not be able to understand Hinduism. Some scholars have compared it with 'sin' in Christianity. But it is more than sin. Sin means something bad. Karma means both bad and good. The term is derived from the Sanskrit Kri, which means 'to do'. Karma is the algebraic sum (the total of negative and positive) of the deeds and thoughts of a human being during his lifetime. Good deeds and thoughts produce a positive karma. Bad deeds and thoughts are a negative karma. The concept of karma teaches that every individual within the cycle of birth and rebirth accumulates a quantity of karma. A negative karma leads to rebirth on a lower plane. A good karma leads to rebirth on a higher level. Ed. Viswanathan puts it like this: 'If a person lived as a rotten individual in his last life, then his soul will take birth in a home where people will be leading rotten lives. If he lived a pious life, then he will be reborn in an ideal home where both parents will be pious and happy (loc. cit.p.140). Karma can be described as a neutral law belonging to the inner cosmos in the same manner that the law of gravitation belongs to the outer cosmos.

Reincarnation and Karma

There is much inequality and suffering in the world next to much happiness and opulence. How do we account for that? What to think for instance of the never ending tribal warfare, hunger, killings and starvation, malnutrition and diseases in Africa? They were first tormented by slavery, then by colonialism and now by tribal wars and sicknesses like aids. In the past the biblical story of Ham was taken as corroborative evidence that the Lord cursed the Africans. For those who are unfamiliar with the story: Noah the man who had escaped the flood with his ark had gotten drunk from drinking wine and had fallen nakedly asleep. His son Ham had laughed at the sight when he saw his father in that state, the other two sons had covered their father with a coverlet. Noah had cursed Ham saying that his sons and offsprings would be the servants of the offspring of his brother Shem (the Semites) and Japhet (the whites): "a servant of servants shall he be unto his brethren" says the Bible. The people who used that argument neglected to study the Bible farther. Because a few chapters later the Bible continues with saying that the descendants of Ham created Babylon and it were there of all places that the Jews were led into slavery. That's why the argument is seldom heard nowadays.

Hinduism does not believe that God curses people. The Bhagavad Gītā (5.15) tells us that He is not responsible for our actions and deeds. We are the ones that determine how we live our lives. Our karma simply adapts itself to our deeds, actions and thoughts. On the basis of that, we will return in a place on earth befitting us. Every creature reincarnates. The accumulated karma determines on what level. Place of birth, degree of happiness, prosperity, or station in life can provide an indication about the load of karma that a creature carries with him from his previous life. Or graphically said: the light that someone radiates is a function of the voltage of the battery that he carries within him.

It is fashionable to blame colonialism for the state of affairs. People who use that argument shut their eyes for the fact that Ethiopia only for a very short time (less than ten years) has been a colony and happens to be one of the most backward and wretched of African nations. The concept of karma can serve to explain the inequalities around the situation of the African people and us.

Action and Its Consequences

Karma is a crucial Hindu concept. According to the doctrine of karma, our present condition in life is the consequence of the actions of our previous lives. All the karma and sacrificial rituals eulogised and prescribed in the Vedas are only aids in this spiritual path (or frail rafts) and are of secondary importance (RV 10.82.7). The choices we have made in the past directly affect our condition in this life, and the choices we make today and thereafter will have consequences for our future lives in saṁsāra. An understanding of this interconnection, according to Hindu teachings, can lead an individual toward right choices, deeds, thoughts, and desires, without the need for an external set of commandments.

The principle of karma provides the basic framework for Hindu ethics. The word karma is sometimes translated into English as 'destiny,' but karma does not imply the absence of free will or freedom of action that destiny does. Under the doctrine of karma, the ability to make choices remains with the individual.

We are subject to the 'law' of karma just as our physical movements on earth are subject to the law of gravitation. But just as the law of gravitation does not take away our freedom to move about, the doctrine of karma does not leave us unfree to act. It merely describes the moral law under which we function, just as the law of gravitation is a physical law governing our being.

When we cause pain or injury, we add to the karmic debt we carry into our future lives. When we give to others in a genuine way, we lighten our karmic load. In the Gītā, an important Hindu text, Kṛṣṇa states that the best way to be free of debt is by selfless action or by dedicating every action as an offering to Kṛṣṇa himself. In addition, human beings can purify themselves of karmic debt through different yogas (disciplines), kriyās (purification processes), and bhakti (devotions). Large among these forces is ṛta, the concept of cosmic order.

Reincarnation Revisited

The concept of soul is connected with the notion of reincarnation. The acceptance of the existence of reincarnation is both ancient and modern. The old Egyptians believed in it. All the great Greek philosophers like Pythagoras, Plato, Aristotle and Plotine believed in it. The Tibetans believe in it. The theosophical societies believe in it. The Catholic faith in the past also believed in it until it was declared as heresy at the second council of Constantinople which was celebrated in 553 A.D. According to a recent survey quoted by Ed. Viswanathan (p. 145) a quarter of the Westerners also believe in it. Without the aid of the doctrine many phenomena cannot be explained. How can we explain the eating technique of newly born children or animals? The minute the child feels the nipples of the mother's breast against its lips it starts sucking. Where did it learn that? Only Hinduism is in a position to explain that. It states that we unknowingly and without being aware of it, carry with us the heritage of good and bad deeds and thoughts from our past life. The Garuṛapurāṇa (a book describing life after death) teaches us that somewhere in the cosmos there resides a cosmic judge, called Dharmarāja. He makes decisions about our destiny which he does on the basis of the data accumulated by his assistants, called Guptacāras, who register all our thoughts and deeds. If the sum total is positive we return to earth on a higher level. If the sum total is negative we will go for a worse life form. This leads us to an inquiry into the concept of karma, one of the pillars of Hinduism, which I shall undertake in the following paragraph.

The Chain of Lives or Saṁsāra

We normally think of ourselves as coming into being when we are born of our parents and as perishing when we die. According to Hinduism, however, this current life is merely one link in a chain of lives that extends far into the past and projects far into the future. The point of origin of this chain cannot be determined. The process of our involvement in the universe the chain of births and deaths is called Saṁsāra.

Saṁsāra is caused by a lack of knowledge of our true self and our resultant desire for fulfilment outside us. We continue to embody ourselves, or be reborn, in this infinite and eternal universe as a result of these unfulfilled desires. The chain of births lets us resume the pursuit. The law that governs Saṁsāra is called karma. Each birth and death we undergo is determined by the balance sheet of our karma that is, in accordance with the actions performed and the dispositions acquired in the past.

Heaven

Hinduism knows both heaven and hell. Hell is called Naraka. This is not a permanent state. Naraka means literally: belonging to mankind (nara). This is an abode of darkness, a territory of Antarloka or inner world, a fearful place where demoniacal creatures sojourn until they are freed from the negative karmas created by them; a place where they are punished for the crimes committed in their former lives. Subramuniyaswami describes it as a state of the mind expressed in feelings of hatred, repentance, rancour, fear, envy and self-denial. Catholicism considers suicide a mortal sin and therefore commits perpetrators directly to hell. Hinduism condemns suicide (Prāṇatyāga, i.e. sva-deha-ghata). Not as a mortal sin, but because it creates negative karmas. It permits euthanasia (prayopaveśa) in case death is imminent and legislation allows it. Heaven is denoted as Mokṣa. Purpose of life on earth is to go to heaven to reach Samādhi or reunion with God. This is only achieved after purification on earth. Earth therefore resembles purgatory of Catholicism. Purification is not that easy. At dead the body dies but the soul never dies. It returns to the earth but in another body. Or, as the Bhāgavad Gītā tells us (2.22): 'In the same manner someone discards his old clothes to put on new ones, the soul discards the old body to enter into another one.' The soul goes on entering an endless number of bodies (a human being, an animal, a fish, an amoeba, and even a tree), until it has exhausted all negative karmas attached to it. This process is known as reincarnation. It can go on for eight million four hundred thousand times as the sacred volumes teach us.

Recompense or Depths

Every human being is born in a culture and has a storehouse of acts, gathered in previous lives, which is known as a granted chariot (body) or a wheeled pleasure carriage. The mind is the driver of this chariot and needs intellectual or spiritual light. A human being with an enlightened mind means a religious man who has been trained to believe in the truth, which conscientiously fulfils his moral and religious duties, and at the same time has been successful in his philosophical studies. The soul distributes from this chariot the threefold 'being' in life, viz. Will, Joy and Desire. The Will is related with the mind resulting in strength and brightness to struggle (RV 8.93.9). All human behaviour is motivated by the will to power. In its positive sense, the will to power is not simply power over others, but the power over oneself that is necessary for creativity. Such power is manifested in independence, creativity, and originality. Joy is related with the fame (worship) resulting in reward and praise which offers a real, specific goal that a person can work toward. Desire is related with gifts (SV 1223) resulting in the pleasure in settled and ancient places of heaven. A gift here is meant to be something given for worthy behaviour and act; and not the madness of bodily desire and the transport of sensuous enjoyment or sensual pleasure. With this kind of desire we end in the dissolution of all our parts and the antiquated smell of corpses. Yama, the God of Death declares that there is the path of joy, and the path of pleasure. Both attract the soul. Who follows the first comes to good; who follows pleasure reaches not the End. The two paths lie in front of man. Pondering on them, the wise man chooses the path of joy; the fool takes the path of pleasure (Kaṭḥ Up. 2.1-2). Civilized people cannot fully satisfy their sexual instinct without love and duty. Duty cannot be contrasted with pleasure, nor work with play. When duty is pleasure and work is play, and the person doing his duty and being virtuous, then the human being is operating at the same time seeking his pleasure and being happy. An English poet, Thomas Traherne (637 - 1674) writes in Centuries of Meditations "You never enjoy the world aright, till the sea itself floweth in your veins, till you are clothed with the heavens, and crowned with the stars: and perceive yourself to be the sole heir of the whole world, and more than so, because men are in it who are every one sole heirs as well as you. Till you can sing and rejoice and delight in God, as misers do in gold, and kings in sceptres, you never enjoy the world." The Greek philosopher, Epicurus (341-270 BC) formulates freedom by saying that "when we say that pleasure is the goal, we do not mean the pleasures of the dissipated and those which consist in the process of enjoyment, but freedom from pain in the body and from disturbance in the mind."

Every act of a human being has to be recompensed (RV 4.55.2)—called slaying the demon Vṛta (RV 4.42.7) and driving off the godless (SV 1213)—because they are obstructions or enemies in this life. The prevailing clarity and fine proportions of its performances, achievement in building up, developing a natural way of life without obstacles, and the ability to discharge a difficult task, is called driving away from the godless. Success is to be measured not so much by the position that one has reached in life as by the obstacles which he has had to overcome while trying to succeed. George Mason (1725-1792), former U.S. statesman, indicated that all men are by nature equally free and independent, and have certain inherent rights, of which, when they enter into a state of society, they cannot by any compact deprive or dispossess their posterity; namely, the enjoyment of life and liberty, with the means of acquiring and possessing property, and pursuing and obtaining happiness and safety.

After eliminating the obstructions there will be no darkness, but only light and the flowing Soma (nectar) will be there. Soma covers will, joy and desire, and becomes devotion. No need to chase other kind of material enjoyments in life, because the mind will be vigorous (RV 8.93.7) and free of bondage or mightier (SV 1222). The Indian national leader, Mahatma Gandhi (1869-1948), describes the freedom of bondage as follows: "My service to my people is part of the discipline to which I subject myself to in order to free my soul from the bonds of the flesh (...) For me the path of salvation leads through the unceasing tribulation in the service of my fellow countrymen and humanity."

There will be no darkness and every pleasing aspect of life will shine brighter. Every thought of the mind will be recognised (clean) as water. This life-water is called the gracious song and Soma (RV 9.61.25) which means the chariot is a flute (song) and a flow of nectar. Francis Bacon (1561-1626), English philosopher, writes in his essay *Of Goodness and Goodness of Nature* "If a man be gracious and courteous to strangers, it shows he is a citizen of the world." The place of this flowing water has been called the settled place of the deities (RV 6.51.2): liberation. In this society liberation is associated with democracy. The former U.S. President, John Fitzgerald Kennedy (1917-1963), formulated in a speech in the Republic of Ireland, Dublin Castle the term 'democracy' as follows: "Democracy is a difficult kind of government. It requires the highest qualities of self-discipline, restraint, a willingness to make commitments and sacrifices for general interest, and it also requires knowledge."

Life Sources

The ancient Hindu scriptures, the Upaniṣads, contain a line, which has been made the motto of the Indian Republic: 'Satyameva Jayate', Only truth wins. The same thought is expressed in the Biblical line: 'Magna est veritas, et praevalet', Great is Truth, and it prevails. A quotation from the poet W.H. Auden, about the cultivation of the virtue of truthfulness: "Only the free have disposition to be truthful, Only the truthful have the interest to be just, Only the just possess the willpower to be free."

Satyagraha

Mahatma Gandhi was inspired with the verses in the Bhagavad Gītā (2.62, 63) and made a deep impression on his mind, and they still ring in the ears of many followers. "If one ponders on objects of the sense, there springs attraction; from attraction grows desire, desire flames to fierce passion, passion breeds recklessness; then the memory all betrayed lets noble purpose go, and saps the mind, till purpose, mind, and man are all undone." In the present world, full of hatred, bitterness, cruelty, racial discrimination, communal tensions, inequities, human degradation and erosion of values, Gandhi is more relevant today than at any other time. In the context of the present situation, there is an imperative need to recapture the spirit and human touch of Gandhi. Students at all grade levels and in every domain of science should have the opportunity to use scientific and spiritual inquiry. And to develop the ability to think and act in ways associated with inquiry.

Gandhi coined the word 'Satyagraha' to define his philosophy. Satyagraha means "holding on to truth." Satyagraha has been described as a threefold force of truth, love and soul force." Since God is Love, Truth and Love are also identical. In daily life we hear by radio people are singing the song: "Prema Ke Pūjāri Ham Hai Rasa Ke Bhikhari, Ham Hai Prema Ke Pūjāri, Ho Ho Prema Ke Pūjāri, Kahan Re Himalayā Aisā Kahan Aisā Pāni, Yehi Vo Zameen Jispe Duniya Divāni.

Thus cultivating the virtue of truthfulness really means that we have to hold on to Truth, Goodness, Love and Beauty and reject outright all that is untrue or false and all that which generates hatred or ugliness. God being Truth, holding on to Truth brings us nearer to God and invests us with some divinity.

Water is Life

Water is the major constituent of living matter. From 50 to 90 percent of the weight of living organisms is water. This aspect is called Apāva, which means "who sports in the waters." Water is necessary for life on earth. All organisms contain it; some live in it; some drink it.

A name of the same importance as Nārāyaṇa, and having a similar though not an identical application. According to the Brahm Purāṇa and the Harivanśa, Apāva performed the creator Brahmā, and divided himself into two parts, male and female, the former begetting offspring upon the latter. The result was the production of Viṣṇu, who created Virāj, who brought the first man into the world.

According to the Śrīmad Bhāgavatam (12.13.1) the whole creation started with Brahmā, then Varuṇa (water). Sūta Gosvami said: "Unto that personality whom Brahmā, Varuṇa, Indra, Rudra and the Marutas praise by chanting transcendental hymns and reciting the Vedas with all their corollaries, pada-kramas and Upaniṣads, to whom the chanters of the Sāma Veda always sing, whom the perfected yogis see within their minds after fixing themselves in trance and absorbing themselves within Him, and whose limit can never be found by any demigod or demon-unto that Supreme Lord I offer my humble obeisances.

God creates with the Big—Bang or OM as seed and the dissolution goes back to the seed or Nara-Nārāyaṇa. Nārāyaṇa is also the source of the Nara or human. Human is a prototype of God. A new creation starts with the same process viz. a wheel or circles in which every point is a life in the cycle of birth and death. We can expose this with the primal seven sounds in the nature, viz. SA-RE-GA-MA-PA-DHA-NI. Everything starts with SA and goes back into SA. The cycle of creation and creatures continues as the primal scale of music in karma or Ṛta sequences. For human is a life of hundred years for the karma and for Brahmā life is one Kalpa (4,320,000,000 years) for his karma. The tunes SA-RE- etc. are icons of our karma in life. The progress is cumulative, so it sounds different. But the end is as the beginning—SA, a lower, and as a higher scale. The Bhāgavad Gītā (8.13) denotes that "After being situated in this yoga practice and vibrating the sacred syllable Om, the supreme combination of letters, if one thinks of the Supreme Lord and quits his body, he will certainly reach the spiritual planets." The seed of All is the All in the Seed a A or One Character. This is the Primal Sound.

The Tree of Life

Cosmic science describes the process of seed to tree (banyan tree). The Lord said in the Gītā (15.1): "It is said that there is an imperishable banyan tree that has its roots upward and its branches down and whose leaves are Vedic hymns. One who knows this tree is the knower of the Vedas."

The entanglement of this material world is compared here to a banyan tree. For one who is engaged in fruitive activities, there is no end to the banyan tree. He wanders from one branch to another. The tree of this material world has no end, and for one, who is attached to this tree, there is no possibility of liberation. The Vedic hymns, meant for elevating oneself, are called the leaves of this tree. This tree's roots grow upward because they begin from where Brahmā is located, the topmost planet of this universe. If one can understand this indestructible tree of illusion, then one can get out of it. This process of extrication should be understood.

Turning Point

Now, the basic principle of devotional service is detachment from material activities and attachment to the transcendental service of the Lord. The root of this material existence grows upward. This means that it begins from total material substance, from the topmost planet of the universe. From there, the whole universe is expanded, with so many branches, representing the various planetary systems. The fruits represent the results of the living entities activities, namely, religion, economic development, sense gratification and liberation. Now, there is no ready experience in this world of a tree situated with its branches down and its roots upward, but there is such a thing. That tree can be found beside a reservoir of water. We can see that the trees on the bank reflect upon the water with their branches down and roots up. In other words, the tree of this material world is only a reflection of the real tree of the spiritual world. This reflection of the spiritual world is situated on desire, just as a tree's reflection is situated on water. Desire is the cause of things being situated in this reflected material light. One who wants to get out of this material existence must know this tree thoroughly through analytical study. Then he can cut off his relationship with it. This tree, being the reflection of the real tree, is an exact replica. Everything is there in the spiritual world. The Vedānta take Brahmā to be the root of this material tree, and from the root, according to Sāṁkhya philosophy, come Prakṛti, Puruṣa, then the three Guṇas, then the five gross elements (Pañca-mahābhūta) then the senses (Daśendriya), mind, etc. (AV 2250, 2251). In this way they divide the whole material world into twenty-four elements.

If a person knows the Vedas, it is assumed that he knows how to cut off attachment to this material world. If one knows that process, he actually knows the Vedas. One who is attracted by the ritualistic formulas of the Vedas is attracted by the beautiful green leaves of the tree. He does not exactly know the purpose of the Vedas. The purpose of the Vedas, as disclosed by the Lord Himself, is to cut down this reflected tree and attain the real tree of the spiritual world.

God and Man

Life is similar to the waves in the ocean; the rhythm in the scale of music. It is a matter of ups and downs between quality and inequality. Devas need a physical body to liberate themselves from the astral and carnal body. Mokṣa or salvation is the cornerstone in heaven too as it is on earth. Expertise shows that when human is trying to build a temple of love, high powers (demons) supply stones. The architecture of Love uses the mirror image of heaven on earth. For the procedure we take a look at the mirror image of God from the universe to the earth, the spiritual universe.

We find a draft in the Atharva Veda how to create a cosmopolitan look alike (AV 2493-2518).

"Protection of the world, and Omnipotence, the two forces of God, are the two horns of the cow of the universe; the Sun is the head, Fire the forehead, Air the joint of the neck (2493). Soma, the king of herbs, is the brain, Sky is the upper jaw, and Earth is the lower jaw. Lightning is the tongue, the Winds are the teeth, Revati is the neck, the Kṛttikās are the shoulders, the Summer is the shoulder-bar. The whole universe is life-breath. The throat is the heavenly region. The earth is the seating place. The revolving Sun is the breast. Atmosphere is the belly. Jupiter is the hump. Vast quarters are the breastbone and cartilages of the ribs. The rearịng forces of fire and air are the backbones; the subtle elements of fire and air are the ribs. Prāṇa and Apāna breaths are the shoulders, the cloud and the Sun are the back-legs, and desire for victory and praise efficacy is the forelegs. Lightning is the buttock parts, Air the tail, the purifying substances like fire and air the hair. Priestly rank and princely power are the hips, and military strength is the thighs. Retention and prosperity are the two knee-bones, males the legs, females are bits of the feet, Earth is the hoof. Thought is the heart, intelligence is the liver, and law the pericardium. Hunger is the belly, corn is the rectum, and clouds are the inward parts. Wrath is the kidneys, enthusiasm the testicles, offspring the generative organ. River is the womb, clouds, the lords of rain are the breasts, and thunder is the udder. The all-embracing sky is the hide, the herbs are her hair, and the stars her variegated spots on the body. Godly persons are her entrails, ordinary men are her bowels, and learned guests her abdomen. Devils are the blood; low, wicked, stupid persons are the undigested contents of the stomach. The rain-cloud is her fat, her resting-place her marrow. Sitting He is fire, when He hath stood up He is day and night. Standing eastwards God is full of glory, standing southwards He is full of justice. Standing westwards, He is the Supporter; standing northwards he is the Creator. Pervading in all objects of the universe, He is the Creator and Ruler of all. God is Friend when He looks upon mankind with an eye of mercy. He is full of joy when he pervades all objects. In meditation He is the Friend of the learned. In concentration (Samādhī) He is the Protector of mankind, Free from all bonds He is Omnipotent. God fashions the whole universe. He gives shape to animate and inanimate creation. He bestows joy on all. He, who knows this Omnipresent God, is worshipped by men of grades, ranks, speaking and non-speaking souls (2518)".

The Ayur Veda is a branch of the Atharva Veda that explains how to live a youthful and healthy life. The recipes are the homeopathy of this science, also included is a life with yoga.

Spirituality and Reality

The real picture of life is "get up, stand up and come up for spirituality or reality." Lots of people don't know the real purpose of life and are out of the circle of life, the reality. Vedānta opens in the third book with the Sūtra (3.4.1): "The end of man (is attained) by this (the independent knowledge of the Self ordained in the Vedānta): such being the word of the Veda. This refers to men in general and not specially to one who knows Brahmā (3.4.13), and that even if it be conceded by virtue of the context that it refers to such a person it implies only a permission and not an injunction to perform works, for the purpose of praising knowledge, as is shown by the words "Na Karma Lipyate Nare", "work does not taint the man" (Īśopaniṣad, mantra 2).

Philosophers quote this type of people with the song: 'Zindagi Ka Safar, Hai Ye Kaisa Safar, Koi Samjha Nahi, Koi Jana Nahi. If there is now Sāṁskāra or sacrament in life, 'we throw away the baby with the bathwater'; the sacrament is consecrating the inner life values or inner sheats (Kosha Kalānuvartana).

Dissolution (Mokṣa)

Every beginning has an end. "What was the station? What was the material? How was (it done)? So that the beholder of all, Viśkarman (was) generated and disclosed heaven by his might" (RV 10.81.2). The entire cosmic rhythm changes in this stage from a speed train into a stop train. Step by step the dissolution is taking over the arena of the universe. In the Yajur Veda we find the footprint of the Viśvakarman, in moderation with the rhythm of the kettledrum of Śiva, the Choirmaster. He is the One who 'stopped,' or "has sat down in Agni" for dissolution. The 'wealth' desired by Viśvakarman is heaven, "by the wish to become many," or, "by the desire to create again and again." (YV 17.17). In the next creation the same process starts over and over again. Read below how the process continues after the creation. The next process is the churning of the ocean, giving birth to all the creatures:

"When the Supreme appeared as Lord Kūrma, a tortoise, His back was scratched by the sharp-edged stones lying on massive, whirling Mount Mandara, and this scratching made the Lord sleepy. May you all be protected by the winds caused by the Lord's breathing in this sleepy condition. Ever since that time, even up to the present day, the ocean tides have imitated the Lord's inhalation and exhalation by piously coming in and going out."

New Birth

Above it is said that after Pralaya (dissolution), the creator made all things again. "Having eyes everywhere, and having a face everywhere, having arms everywhere, and having feet everywhere, he traverses (heaven) with his arms, (earth) with his swift-moving (feet), and exists a god without companion generating heaven and earth" (RV 10.81.3). It is now asked—where was the scene of action, what were the materials, and how was the work performed? In this world, a potter must have his shop, his clay, and his wheel; so what site, matter, and implements have Iśvara?

"The Ṛṣi, the Hota, our father who is offering all these worlds has taken his seat; desiring wealth by pious benedictions, the first inventor has entered inferior (beings)" (RV 10.81.1). "By sacrifice the gods worshipped (him who is also) the sacrifice; those were the first duties. Those great ones became partakers of heaven where ancient deities the Sādhyas abide" (RV 10.90.16).

"The Ral's face is hidden by a vessel formed of golden light, The Spirit yonder in the Sun, the Spirit dwelling there am I. OM! Heaven! Brahmā!" (YV 1975)

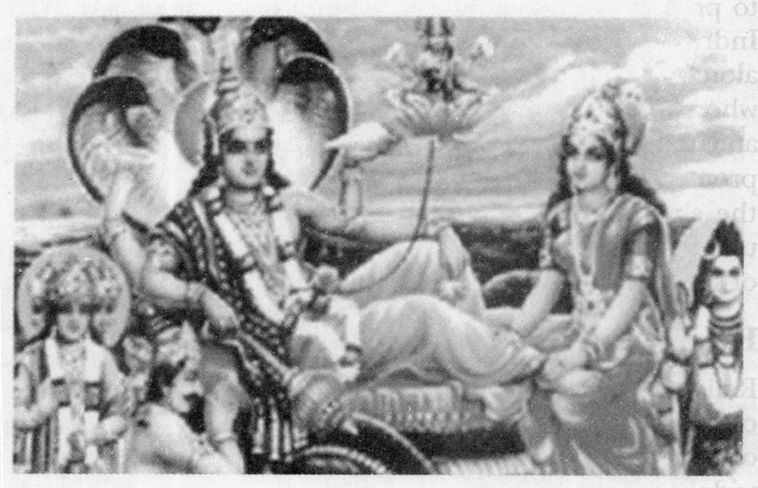

Figure 7:Śerasāgara
(THE HAPPY END OR BEGINNING)

Chapter 2

Understanding the Spiritual World

Religion is a worldwide phenomenon that has played a part in all human cultures. Since the beginning of time, human beings have been intrigued by the spiritual world. These unseen forces have manifested themselves as gods, spirits, ancestors, or other sacred forms that we sort to interact with in a sacred manner. The Rig Veda enumerates some fruits of religious acts in order to protect the human being against destruction: "We enjoy, Indra, through your guiding protection, desirable affluence along with descendants and reputation: grant us, sovereign, who rule over (earthly and heavenly) riches, vast, desirable, and infinite treasures. We invoke on this occasion for his present protection, that Indra who is attended by the Maruts; who is the showerer (of benefits); augmenting (in prowess); the unreviled of foes, radiant, ruling, all-subduing, fierce, the giver of strength" (RV 5.19.10-11).

Heaven

Religious cultures provide their members with patterned ways of interacting with spiritual beings. Such communication is often the center of religious practices.[1] Perhaps the most widely practised forms are prayer in the form of request, offerings and sacrifices, purification or penance, and worship. The Sāma Veda calls it nourishment: "For him in the ancient sacrifice thrice seven milch kine milk forth the right mixture; he makes four other beautiful waters for purification when he is nourished with the sacrifices (SV 560, 1423). Thrice seven

[1] History of Civilizations of Central Asia volume I to III; Dani, A.H., Masson, V.M.; Motilal Banarsidass Publishers Pvt. Ltd.; Delhi; 1999.

milch kine may signify the 12 months, the 5 seasons, the 3 worlds and the sun. The four waters are the Vasatavart waters and the three Ekadhana waters."

These kind of rituals may be performed regularly, or in times of special need, when human beings find themselves dependent on forces of the universe beyond their control.[2] Gods are believed to make their will known to humans in a variety of ways, including prophecy, states of trance, dreams, visions, divination, healings, special signs and miracles, intuition, mystical experiences, or the embodiment of special individuals. An example in the Rig Veda is given: "I bow, Rudra, to you, approaching (our rite), as a boy to his father when pronouncing a blessing upon him: I glorify you, the giver of much (wealth), the protector of the virtuous; do you, thus glorified, bestow healing herbs upon me. Maruts, I solicit of you those medicaments which are pure; those, showerers (of benefits), which give great pleasure; those which confer felicity; those which (our) sire, Manu, selected; and those (medicaments) of Rudra which are the alleviation (of disease), and defence (against danger)" (RV 2.33. 12-13). In primitive cultures, it was believed that heaven is a place where gods or other spiritual beings dwell.[3] It is also the state of perfect supernatural happiness in the afterlife where divine justice and judgments are passed. Life after death was considered a shadowy continuation of life on earth.[4]

Jewish mystics believed the heavens were contained in the seven spheres of the firmament. They found in the Persian doctrine of resurrection a hope of release from Sheol to a new life on earth or in the heavens.

Aristotle declared that all (polytheistic) religions united in placing the abode of the gods in the most elevated place in the universe. Such regions were, in classical times, considered closed to ordinary mortals.

---

[2] Introduction to Religious Philosophy; Masih, Y.; Motilal Banarsidass Publishers Pvt. Ltd.; Delhi; 2002.

[3] Ancient Indian Rituals and their Social Contents; N. N. Bhattacharyya; Manohar Publishers & Distributors; New Delhi; 1996

[4] Beginnings of Life, Culture and History (vol I); Kulkarni, S.D., Vedavyasa, Shri Bhagavan; Itihasa Samshodhana Mandira (BHISMA); Bombay; 1988.

The belief of Christians is that, since the resurrection of Christ, the souls of the just who are free from sin are admitted immediately after death into heaven, where their chief joy consists in an unclouded vision of God known as the beatific vision.[5]

In the Koran, Muslims adopt the concept of the seven heavens of the firmament, differing in degrees of glory from the abode of the Most High down to the first, or most earthly, paradise.[6]

Nirvana, the heaven of Buddhism, is a state of extinction of all desire and of union with Brahma, the creator god, achieved by perfecting the soul in the course of its successive transmigrations.[7] The Rig Veda summarises all thoughts: "Beholding the up-springing light above the darkness, we approach the divine Sun among the gods, the excellent light" (RV 1.50.10). Here we have an allusion to a spiritual sun. The darkness, it is said, implies sin, and the approach to the sun intimates reunion with supreme spirit. We go to the best light, which means that we become identified with spiritual light (sayujyam gacchamah; and again, the worshipper becomes identical with that which he worships (tam yatha yathopasate tad eva bhavati).

Hindus believe that the universe is a great, enclosed sphere, a cosmic egg that contains concentric heavens, hells, oceans and continents. The word bhu stands for earth and gola stands for sphere. The syllable aṇḍa Brahmāṇḍa oval was known. The credit for discovering the Arabic numerals that are customarily in use is attributed to Indians.[8] The concept of zero is beyond doubt an early Indian contribution. There are several such examples which are cited in support of the intellectual dynamism that existed in the past in the scientific

---

[5] The World's Great Religions; Hutchinson, Paul; Golden Press, Inc.; New York; 1958.

[6] Classical Indian Ethical Thought; Tiwari, Kedar Nath; Motilal Banarsidass Publishers Pvt. Ltd.; Delhi; 1998.

[7] Comparative Ethics in Hindu and Buddhist Traditions; Hindery, Roderick; Motilal Banarsidass Publishers Pvt. Ltd.; Delhi; 1978.

[8] An integrated theory of the earth; Murthy, S.R.N.; Kalpatharu Research Academy; Bangalore; 1987.

disciplines.[9] We shall now comment briefly about the sixth and the last Vedāṅga which is called kalpa. After a spiritual aspirant acquires knowledge in the disciplines, mentioned below, he is considered to be ready for action. Accordingly, this limb of the Vedas spells out in detail the practical know-how of the various rituals.[10] As this is something which takes meaning only when directly instructed by a teacher, we shall not dwell on this subject further. We have so far mentioned the four Vedas, viz. Rig, Yajur, Sāma, Atharva, and their Vedāṅgas, parts of the Vedas. The remaining four sub-disciplines are called upagas, which mean subsidiary limbs. These are Mimāṁsā, Nyāya, Purāṇa and Dharma śāstra.[11]

Human life is also cyclic. After death, the soul leaves the body and is reborn in another body. This condition of endless rebirth is called 'samsara'. The precise quality of the new birth is determined by the accumulated merit and demerit that result from all the actions, or karma, that the soul has committed in its past life or lives. The Rig Veda mentions the results of karma as follows: "Performer of good deeds, flow quickly round the terrestrial region, giving (riches) to the worshipper and the shaker (of the libation); do not deprive us of the wealth that enriches our dwellings; may we be invested with abundant wealth of divers kinds. O Indu, bring us quickly (wealth) with a hundred gifts, with horses, with a thousand gifts, with cattle and with gold; measure unto us abundant riches and food; come, purified one, to (hear) our praise" (RV 9.72.8-9). Karma accrues in this way. They also believe karma can be counteracted by expiations and rituals, ultimately attaining release (mokṣa) through the renunciation of all worldly desires. The slogan in the Yajur Veda gives an image of renunciation: "Enveloped by the Lord must be This

---

[9] Cyclic Universe, Creation, Evolution, Involution and Dissolution of the Universe, vol. 1 The Unsolved Riddle; Panda, N.C.; D.K. Printworld (P) Ltd.; Delhi; 2002.

[10] Hindu Spirituality. Vedas through Vedanta; Sivaraman, Krishna (ed.); Motilal Banarsidass Publishers Pvt. Ltd.; Delhi; 1989.

[11] Hindu World (volume 1&2); Walker, Benjamin; An encyclopaedic survey of Hinduism; Harper Collins Publishers India; Delhi; 1995.

All—each thing that moves on earth. With that renounced enjoy yourself. Covet no wealth of any man' (YV 1959).

The New Age Movement is a amalgam of diverse spiritual, social, and political elements. It aims at transforming individuals and society through spiritual awareness. The New Age offers a utopian vision, an era of harmony and progress.[12] The movement took root in the 1980's, bringing feminist, ecological and spiritual concerns into the mainstream. A large market for natural goods, crystals, meditation and healing aids, books, magazines, audio and video tapes, workshops and retreats emerged in the United States and other countries holistic thinking has continued to influence medicine, psychology, relationships, right livelihood, animal welfare, the environment and the promise of world peace.[13] The Vedas add in this context: "May Indra and Agni be (with us) with their protections for our happiness: may Indra and Varuna, to whom oblations are offered, (be with us) for our happiness: may Indra and Soma be (with us) for our happiness, our prosperity, our good: May Indra and Pūṣaṇa be (with us) in battle for our triumph" (RV 7.35.1; YV 36.11).

Authority of the Sacred Books

Every religion has its sacred books with explanations about creation and the Creator, with rules of conduct and about how rituals should be performed. Christianity has the Bible, Islam the Koran, Hinduism the Vedas. The wordings are not always quite clear since they are mostly the revelations of God to a chosen one who had to remember them, pass them on or commit them to paper. And besides that they were delivered in times of antiquity with other languages and usages etc. which have long since become extinct.[14] Those books came to us in

---

[12] Victor Raj, A.R.; The Hindu Connection, Roots of the New Age; Concordia Publishing House; St. Louis; 1995.

[13] The Holistic Way to Health, Happiness and Harmony; V.K. Subramanian; Shakti Malik Abhinav Publications; New Delhi; 1996.

[14] The Holistic Way to Health, Happiness and Harmony; V.K. Subramanian; Shakti Malik Abhinav Publications; New Delhi; 1996.[14] Ritual and Mantras: Rules Without Meaning; Staal, Frits; Motilal Banarsidass Publishers Pvt. Ltd.; Delhi; 1996.

translated form and everyone knows how hazardous translations can be. That's the reason why sacred books, as is the case with the rules of law even in present times, cannot be studied or understood without the aid of commentaries, interpretations and explanations. For this reason Catholics were forbidden in the past to read the Bible, a prohibition that was only repealed in recent times. Hinduism is in this regard even more complicated than the other religions. It is older, hence has had more time to evolve. Religions have produced thousands of wise men and women who have occupied themselves with religious matters and who have added-and still add-the product of their inspiration, meditation and thoughts to the already vast body of knowledge.

A Concept of Life

We are all connected to one another through the divine presence that dwells within us. We have taken birth in a physical body to grow and evolve into our divine potential. We are inwardly already one with God. Our religion contains the knowledge of how to realise this oneness and not create unwanted experiences along the way. The peerless path is following the way of our spiritual forefathers, discovering the mystical meaning of the scriptures. The peerless path is commitment, study, discipline, practice and the maturing of yoga into wisdom.[15] In the beginning stages, we suffer until we learn. Learning leads us to service; and selfless service is the beginning of spiritual striving. Service leads us to understanding. Understanding leads us to meditate deeply and without distractions. Finally, meditation leads us to surrender in God. This is the straight and certain path, the San Mārga, leading to Self Realisation-the inmost purpose of life-and subsequently to mokśa, freedom from rebirth. "Only by knowing God, one can attain salvation" (YV. 31.18).

Religion can be a vital guide in helping the individual to explore his true nature. On the other hand, it can also be a

---

[15] The Concept of Man, A study in comparative philosophy; Radhakrishnan, S., Raju, P.T.; Harper Collins Publishers; Delhi; 1997.

negative influence contributing to narrow-mindedness and ego identification. The onus for inner growth lies with the individual. One does not need to be religious to be spiritual, and a religious person is not necessarily spiritual. Religion is an attempt at linking the soul with the divine. The individual soul is an image or reflection of the Supreme Soul. Just as the Sun is reflected in different pots of water, so also the Supreme Soul is reflected in different minds of different persons. Soul is spirit. It is immaterial. It is intelligence or consciousness. It is Caitanya. Individual soul is reflected Caitanya. It is this individual soul that departs from the body after its death and goes to heaven, with the senses, mind, Prāṇa, impressions, desires and tendencies. It is endowed with a subtle astral body when it proceeds to heaven. When the water in the lake is absorbed, the reflection of the Sun in the water merges in the Sun itself. "The supporting Brahm holds the heaven and earth both. He holds this wide atmosphere also (AV. 10.7.35). Even so, 'when the mind is annihilated through meditation, the individual soul merges itself in the Supreme Soul or Paramātmā. This is the goal of life.

Unfortunately, it is now common for religious adherents to conform to the observance of certain rites and rituals, the performance of deeds of merit, the wearing of particular apparel, or the recitation of specific mantras (hymn) and verses with little or no knowledge of the underlying spiritual principles.[16]

The Human Body, a Microcosm of the Universe

In the process of fertilisation, two cells combine to initiate the cycle of life. The cosmos contains linear and solar energy. All creatures are dependent on these two forms of energy for survival and growth. After fertilisation, the cell divides, resulting in eight to sixteen cells, at which point the substance for the body begins to develop.

According to ancient Ayurvedic physiology, the Rig Veda(10.90.15), Yajur Veda (31.65), the human body consists of a number of material substances called *dhātu*, which were

[16] Science and Mysticism, The Essence of Vedic Philosophy; Kesavan H.K. New Age International Publishers; Delhi; 1997.

formed as a result of the natural processing of digested food. These elements manifest themselves and function as follows:

- Rasa, the alimentary juice or chyle; originates from digested food, finds its place in the heart, flows from the heart through twenty-four ducts, and thus feeds the whole body. At the end of five days rasa is transmuted into rakta or blood, and in thirty days into sperm or egg cell.
- Rakta, or blood, is generated from rasa. An imbalance of the humours (doṣa) can spoil blood and make it frothy, black, blue, green, slow, fast or noxious. Rakta was once regarded as a fourth humour but this classification was soon abandoned.
- Māṁsa, or flesh, is blood processed by the natural fires and condensed by the bodily winds. It is specialised in the form of muscles, about five hundred in number.
- Meda, or fat, is flesh further processed by the natural fires and deposited in a single layer under the skin and in a triple layer under the belly.
- Asthi, or bone, is fat processed by the natural fires and dried and hardened by the bodily winds. The number of bones listed varies between 300 and 360, with most authorities favouring the latter and finding a relationship between the bones and the number of days in the year.
- Majjā, or marrow, is the oily 'perspiration' of the bones, concealed to moisten the dryness of the osseous framework.
- Śukra, or semen, originates from the marrow. It is present all over the body, but concentrated in the testicles. It is regarded as a form of psychic heat and plays an important part in occultism.
- Ojas is the essence of all seven substances. It is the divine light or aura of our physical body.

Fundamentally, human beings embody the mysteries of the cosmos. Man is a microcosm containing all the multifarious elements of the universe, including a spark of divinity.[17] This

---

[17] The Hindu quest for the perfection of man; Organ, Troy Wilson; Munshiram Manoharlal Publishers Pvt. Ltd.; Delhi; 1994.

mortal framework consists of three parts: the gross, subtle and causal bodies; Bhūr, Bhuvah and Svāh. These three bodies house the soul enclosed in one or more kāla's, also known as 'sheaths' that enfold the selves as follows:

- *Sthūla-śarīra*,the 'gross-body', an organic vehicle of flesh and blood, made up of five gross elements called *bhūta* (earth, water, fire, air, ether), which resolve into their initial state at death.
- *Liṅga-śarīra* 'sign-body', which is also called *sūkṣma-śarira*, "subtle- or non-physical body" houses the jīvātmā or soul.
- *Kāraṇa-śarīra* or "causal body" reflects that the human being functions in two distinct forms of experience, as male and female, and these two genders constitute the dual principles of our androgynous nature.

Hence the characteristic organs, the liṅga (penis) and yonī (vagina) are regarded as the most significant of the personal components, since they are the agents of fusion and the means of reconciling the polarities in a single harmonious unity.[18] The first fusion is between the moon and the sun energy (cold and warm) and the second between the two parts of the body (female and male). We can see the functions of these two parts of our body. In cases of paralysis, for example, he is paralysed on the right side. The two 'parties' balance each other out.[19]

The koṣas[20] are tubes in the body that can be described as follows:

- *Annamaya koṣa*: the power of the tree to extract food from the soil.
- *Prāṇamaya* koṣa: the power to be able to move. The fly which can find food and fly about.
- *Manomaya* koṣa: the power to react to danger alongside the power to seek food and movement. This is the intuitive power, which birds also possess.
- *Vijñānamaya* koṣa: the intellect that is somewhat inactive, as with apes and cows.

---

[18] Wisdom, The Absolute is Adorable; Nataraja Guru; D.K. Printworld (P) Ltd.; Delhi; 1995.

[19] Hinduism and Scientific Quest; Iyengar, T.R.R.; D.K. Printworld (P) Ltd.; Delhi; 1997.

[20] All About Hinduism; Sri Swami Sivananda; The Divine Life Society; Himalayas; India; 1993.

- *Ānandamaya* koṣa: the power to express happiness and peace through laughter and bliss as distinct from the other four powers, and the power to be able to meditate and contemplate, as in the case of human beings. This is compared with Siddhi or secret power; prāpti, the fulfilment of all desires.

Dr. Premācārya Śāstrī explains that the following three koṣas are only possessed by persons who are advanced on the spiritual level (the enlightened ones):

- *Ājñājani* koṣa: the very learned possess the power of wisdom, creativity etc. in the society. See also section siddhi (prāpti).
- *Vipinmani* koṣa: being born with wisdom and being able, as a child, to perform wonders.
- *Sankṛmina* koṣa: the godly power in the human being.

Sacraments

Religious cultures ascribe spiritual significance to every stage in life through ritualistic rites of passage. For example, children are blessed at birth or given a special religious name. Rites of entry into adulthood also connect the individual to the sacred traditions of their culture.[21] In Thailand, young men become sons of Buddha through a ceremony in which they re-enact key parts of His search for enlightenment.[22] In Jewish bar mitzvahs and bat mitzvahs, adolescents read from the Torah, the primary scripture of Judaism. Christian youths participate in First Communion, partaking of the Eucharist for the first time. Weddings and funerals are two other ceremonies of passage laden with sacred meaning. Every aspect of life-eating, working, marrying, bearing children, suffering and dying-can be accorded religious significance.[23]

---

[21] Hindu Samskāras, Socio-Religious Study of the Hindu Sacraments; Pandey, Rajbali; Motilal Banarsidass Publishers Pvt. Ltd.; Delhi; 1993.

[22] Introduction to Buddhism; Kelsang Gyatso, Geshe; Motilal Banarsidass Publishers Pvt. Ltd.; Delhi; 1992.

[23] The Religions Hidden Cults of India; Macmann, Sir george; Neeraj Publishing House; Delhi; 1982.

As human beings, we have a duty to the world at large (apart from loving one's neighbour, helping one another, showing forgiveness etc.), and to our own inner world (rest, peace, harmony, vital breathing and inner balance). The Atharva Veda calls it "the awakening of fire": "The Fire has given me this glory, brilliance, fame, force, vigour, longevity and strength (AV 19.37.1). Honouring the deep spiritual significance of the sacraments keeps us young and healthy, and helps improve the quality of life.[24] Given below is a partial list of the sacraments that Hindus observe:

- *Sīmānta,* the parting of the hair of the expectant mother between the fourth and eighth months, which symbolises the preparation for the event of birth.
- *Nāmakarna,* the ceremony of giving the child a name–usually performed between the birth and the 12th day after birth.
- *Niṣkramāna,* the "first outing", when the child is taken outdoors for the first time, usually during the fourth month. A square portion of the courtyard is plastered over with cow-dung and clay before the child is carried out to the sound of conch-shells and the chanting of hymns. He is placed facing the sun and the rite is therefore sometimes called the *sūryadarśana* or sun showing.
- *Annaprāśana,* "food eating", is when the child is fed with solid food for the first time. It is generally performed in the sixth month.
- *Karnavedha,* 'ear piercing', is performed on children of both sexes to permit the wearing of rings in the ear lobes. This takes place between the tenth day and the 12th month after birth, but is best done during the ninth month.
- *Cūrākaraṇa,*or tonsure, when the hair on a boy's head is first shaved. The ceremony takes place between the ages of one and seven. Several samskārs are associated with education.

---

[24] Aspects of Hindu Morality; Jhingran, Saral; Motilal Banarsidass Publishers Pvt. Ltd.; Delhi; 1999.

- *Vidyārambha,* when the boy is taught the alphabet, usually at the age of five.
- *Upanayana,* when the child is invested with the sacred thread at the age of eight. This also commences his formal education.
- *Vedārambha,* when the child starts his study of the Vedas, the cosmic science, at the age of ten.
- *Samavartana,* any time after the age of fifteen, when the youth returns home after the completion of his studies.
- *Vivāha,* the sacrament of marriage, which ends with the rite of fifteen *samarpana* or consummation.
- *Antyeṣṭi* or 'final' ceremonies performed after death, are the last rites of the Hindu and include the obsequies and the *śrāddha* (devotion) rites for the soul on its journey to heaven in the subtle- or non-physical body, which houses the *jīvātmā* or soul.

Developing Inner Qualities

At the age of eight, the child has received the most important purifying sacrament and leaves his home for study. This may be universally known, although it is not practised by all cultures. The bodily growth phase has stabilised and hence education and training is projected to take place independently. Through institutional training, the child is educated and trained in specific fields that provide knowledge and wisdom with deep rooted principles.[25] This can be compared to the military and police academy in the west. In the east we find institutes, which also train people in non-violence. Spirituality has gradually become a way of life, a melting together of diverse cultures, religions or movements. The crucial elements being non-violence, tolerance, Ahiṁsā, or non-violence is the highest virtue for the layperson. The futility of violence has been repeatedly demonstrated by the great wars of history, which have invariably resulted in thousands of dead bodies, widows and broken bones and

---

[25] Hinduism: The Anthropology of a Civilization; Biardeau, Madeleine; Calcutta, Chennai, Mumbai; Oxford University Press; 1997.

homes. Yet we do not learn. The Veda also proclaims peace by saying: "Don't kill the cow, because she is holy and venerable" (YV 13.43).

The great Buddha proclaimed that non-violence or non-injury to others is our supreme duty.

Mahatma Gandhi has, in our own lifetime, demonstrated the power of non-violence. He believed in the doctrine of non-violence not as a weapon of the weak but as a weapon of the strongest. He used it successfully as a weapon against the British in India, but the spirit of non-violence is to be found in all religions. It is clearly present in the teachings of Buddhism, Christianity, Hinduism and Islām. Martin Luther King Jr. in his Nobel Prize acceptance speech declared: "The choice today is not between violence and non-violence. It is either non-violence or non-existence."

Violence is as malefic in individual lives as in the case of nations. It has to be eschewed in thought, speech and action. Everyone knows that violence only breeds enmity, danger and death. Yet, it is a pity that most of the movies shown on television and in theatres glorify violence as the means to fight evil. The hero with the gun is the model for emulation by our children. The voice of the gun became sound of money. Discerning social researchers and psychologists are unanimous in their view that violence in the visual media encourages violence in society.

The Language and Dharma

The elements of a language are normally categorised into seven main groups of five elements each, making the total of 35 (Tattvas). The 36th element is the most powerful part of the female energy called Lalita. The seven main groups being: material, impression, action, sense, the empirical individual, limitation of Māyā and verities. The five materials within each of these seven groups are as follows:

- The five main materials: *earth, water, fire, air and space.*
- The five impressions: *scent, taste, sight, touch and hearing.*

- The five end products of action: *excretion, sex, grasping, moving and speaking.*
- The five instruments of sensing: *smelling, tasting, seeing, feeling and hearing.*
- The empirical individual: *nature of the individual, false egoism, knowledge, mind, and manhood.*
- Limitations of Māyā: *action, knowing, desire, time and fate.*
- The five verities (deeper insights): *consistent, wisdom, will, strength and the destroyer.*

The existence of languages therefore is basic and vital to the perpetuation of human civilisations.

Siddhis

The imprints left on the subconscious mind (from this or previous lives) color all of our experiences: our nature, responses, states of mind, etc. In addition, sacraments create deep and positive impressions on the individual. The Atharva Veda sums up the functions of the mind: Manas (Sensation and Motivation), Cetas (Consciousness and Thinking), Dhi (Attention), Akuti (Feeling and Emotion), Citti (Recollection), Mati (Intelligence), Śruta (Learning), Cakṣas (Perception) (AV 6.41.1).

Science mentions that the brain is the control centre for movement, sleep, hunger, thirst, and virtually every other vital activity necessary for survival. All human emotions-including love, hate, fear, anger, elation, and sadness-are controlled by the brain. It also receives and interprets the countless signals that are sent to it from other parts of the body and from the external environment. The brain makes us conscious, emotional, and intelligent.[26] The human brain has three major structural components: the large dome-shaped cerebrum (*top*), the smaller somewhat spherical cerebellum (*lower right*), and the brainstem (*centre*). Prominent in the brainstem are the medulla oblongata (the egg-shaped enlargement at centre) and the thalamus (between the medulla and the

[26] Breath, Mind and Consciousness; Johari, Harish; Rochester, Vermont; Distiny Books; U.S.A.; 1989.

cerebrum). The cerebrum is responsible for intelligence and reasoning. The cerebellum helps to maintain balance and posture. The medulla is involved in maintaining involuntary functions such as respiration, and the thalamus acts as a relay centre for electrical impulses traveling to and from the cerebral cortex. Most high-level brain functions take place in the cerebrum. The cerebrum receives information from all the sense organs and sends motor commands (signals that result in activity in the muscles or glands) to other parts of the brain and the rest of the body. Motor commands are transmitted by the motor cortex, a strip of cerebral cortex extending from side to side across the top of the cerebrum

Modern analysis of consciousness of the German Psychologist Wilhelm Max Wundt with the task of psychology was the study of the structure of consciousness, which extended well beyond sensations and included feelings, images, memory, attention, duration, and movement. This introspective approach was fully developed by the American Psychologist Edward Bradford Titchener at Cornell University. Setting his task as that of describing the structure of the mind, Titchener attempted to detail, from introspective self-reports, the dimensions of the elements of consciousness. For example, taste was 'dimensionalized' into four basic categories: sweet, sour, salt, and bitter. This approach was known as structuralism. Consciousness theory today mention-the concept of a direct, simple linkage-between environment and behaviour became unsatisfactory in recent decades, the interest in altered states of consciousness[27] may be taken as a visible sign of renewed interest in the topic of consciousness. That persons are active and intervening participants in their behaviour has become increasingly clear.

The Sanskrit word siddhi means power, accomplishment, and perfection: extraordinary powers of the soul, developed through consistent meditation and deliberation. Through the process of Self Realisation, those powers unfold naturally

---

[27] The Spectrum of Consciousness; Wilber, Ken; Motilal Banarsidass Publishers Pvt. Ltd.; Delhi; 2002.

according to the needs of the individual. There are eight classical powers:

1. *aṇimā*: Aṇimā (atomisation) enables the devotee to become infinitely small in order to understand the inner nature of atoms and molecules that form the building blocks of this universe. The human body is a micro-concept of the macro cosmos. Both are composed with 27 elements. This power can be gained by deep meditation on the heart centre. In this state the devotee can attain invisibility and can enter the most difficult of substances (similar to the property of neutrinos, an energy radiated by the Sun which permeates through all substances. At any instance, over a hundred billion neutrinos pass through any individual's body).
2. *mahimā*: Mahimā is the opposite of the first, and allows the devotee to become vast so as to be able to see the cosmic structure of stars and galaxies, and penetrate beyond space and time to experience the ultimate Reality'. In this state the devotee can make himself/herself infinitely large. This power can be gained by meditating on the essence of the intellect (mahat), the first transformation of the primeval state of nature (prakriti).
3. *laghimā*: In this state the devotee can achieve super-lightness or levitation; leave the body at will and do astral projection. Control over the element earth gives the ability to make the body as light as air for astral travel and to shine with a golden aura. Deep meditation on, and identification with the element air is the origin of this siddhi.
4. *prāpti*: In this state the devotee can bring anything within reach to fulfill all his desires. Prāpti is gained by meditation on the creative power of the universe. The devotee concentrates on the medulla oblongata, the egg-shaped enlargement in the centre of our brain. The vital reflex centres are located here, which

continue functioning even when the cerebrum is severed from it. Concentration of the medulla oblongata, with the achieved mahimā, gives the devotee complete satisfaction. A similar feeling at a lower state can be experienced by the use of hard drugs. The drug user becomes an artist (Vibhavān). The drugs artificially keep the poise of the body yearning for repeatedly pleasant sensation. In the *prāpti* the dancer becomes the dance and the Vibhavān keeps on dancing in search of the rhythm.

5. *prakāmya*: Prakāmya is to develop an irresistible will that can compel others to obey one's wishes. Meditation on the space element (throat) leads to this siddhi, and the ability to hypnotise is a form of this power. The devotee engages the attention of a subject and assigns certain tasks to him or her while uttering monotonously, with muscle relaxation, eye fixation, arm levitation, concentration on one's own breathing. In this state the devotee can be anywhere at will, he can either be in the skies or under the earth.
6. *iśitva*: Iśitva is the power to control nature. One may look upon the marvels of modern science and technology as mild examples of this siddhi. In this state the devotee can attain supremacy to a level just below that of the gods. He can manipulate the sub-potencies of māyā, the world of illusions.
7. *vaśitva*: Vaśitva is the ability to control or animate nature and to influence the behavior of men and animals. Iśitva and Vaśitva are gained by meditation on the creative power of the universe. In this state the devotee is unimpeded by the three modes of nature.
8. *kāma-avasajitva*: Kāma-avasajitva allows the devotee to take any form at will and to fulfill all desires. This power is attained by meditating on the principle of primeval ego (ahaṁkāra) and is quite common. One frequently hears of saints and religious leaders who can feed thousands of devotees on just a pot of rice.

The devotee can obtain anything from anywhere, to the highest possible limit.

The eight magical powers are by-products of yogic discipline. When the various stages of yoga are perfected and one goes deeper into meditation, the eight occult powers come naturally.[28] Though they are called 'magical' and 'occult', they are in fact only highly developed and perfected aspects of the energies of the human mind: the energy of wisdom (jñāna Śakti), of will (icchā Śakti) and of consistent action (kriyā Śakti).

These mystic perfections are considered to be naturally existing and unexcelled within this world. As the devotee attains power over one siddhi after another he will find that, along with psychic experiences, he also acquires magical powers. Many gurus who exhibit magical abilities are usually stuck at the Lālanā centre, between the throat and the Ājñā centre (centre of knowledge), the third eye, between the eyebrows. Lālanā is the secret cakra for female energy or the tongue, situated at the base of the palate (tālu) region just behind the uvula. The rising mystic perfections should be made to pass through the Lālanā centre on its way to the knowledge centre. Cakras are vortexes of energies that we have in our bodies. They are present in the ethereal body and in related locations of the physical body.[29] The Sanskrit word for this vortex is moving wheel. The cakra brings into the body the universal energies that we need in order to remain living. The seven main cakras function as pathways for energy to be taken in, metabolised and sent to the major nerve centre nearest each one. They have the following impact fields: material, impression, action, sense, the empirical individual, limitation of Māyā and verities (see section: The Language and Dharma).

We describe the process of how mystic perfection can be achieved, and what the nature is of such perfection, controls

---

[28] Concentration and Meditation; Sri Swami Sivananda; Tehri-Garhwal; The Divine Life Society; U.P.; 1994.

[29] Chakra's Energy, Centers of transformation; Johari, Harish; Rochester, Vermont; Destiny Books; U.S.A.; 1987.

of the mind by intensely concentrated meditation, the illusory identification with material objects, knowledge and activities as follow:

One who worships the Lord in His atomic form pervading all subtle elements, fixing his mind on that alone, obtains the mystic perfection called animā. Other powers can also be achieved.[30] For example, we can learn to see the past, present and future; to tolerate heat and cold; to know the minds of others; to control the influence of fire, sun, water, poison, etc. Siddhis enable us to develop magical or mystical powers. The practice of achieving these kinds of powers is called *siddha yoga.*

Ten other secondary mystic perfections arising from the modes of nature have been cited by the enlightened ones. These are the powers of freeing oneself from hunger, thirst and other bodily disturbances, hearing and seeing things far away, moving the body at the speed of the mind, assuming any form one desires, entering the bodies of others, and dying at will.

The Art of Living

The art of living teaches us that we are all residents of two worlds: the external world of relationships, work, family and community, and the internal world of our deepest spiritual reality. Living skillfully demands that we balance these two worlds, the greatest and most challenging achievement.

Man and God

Human beings are spiritual creatures endowed with the same qualities and capacities of the Creator. In principle, we are gods, but many of our divine qualities are dormant. We must activate and be activated and integrate our potentials into the fabric of our lives. The potentials are compared with those of craftsmen (gods). "Śilpa (crafts) is concerned with all gods" (YV 24.5; 29.58). The Rig Veda proclaims to be craftsmen: "O Fire-God, you, being worshipped, make us famous craftsmen, so that we may obtain prosperity. We may make our project

---

[30] Spiritual Experiences; Shri Swami Sivananda; A Divine Life Society Publication; Delhi; 1995.

flourishing and prosperous with the new industry. Heaven and Earth, along with the other Gods, protect us from all calamities" (RV 1.31.8).

The Five Dimensions of Power

We can only experience God when we transcend the mind and our senses on the wings of love and devotion. The union of our souls with God is true religion. Once we understand His will and live in accordance with it, we understand the purpose of practising our faith. Spirituality will then unfold through five distinct stages of consciousness known as kāla's:

1. *Nivṛttikāla:* "sphere of perdition, destruction; returning," the level within aśuddha māyā of physical and near-physical existence, conscious, unconscious and sub-subconscious mind. Reference can be made to Sigmund Freud and his description of the Id, Ego and Super Ego.

2. *Pratiṣṭhakāla:* "sphere of resting, tranquility," the level within ashuddha māyā (odic energy) of intellect and instinct. In this stage, the head is hard at work searching for places of rest.

3. *Vidyākāla:* "sphere of knowing," the level within Śuddhaśuddha māyā (actinodic energy) of sub-super conscious awareness of forms in their totality in progressive states of manifestation, and of the interrelated forces of the actinodic energies. The mind further impedes the entrance into the spiritual. This stage is still physical. The eyes begin to weep, not from grief but from joy.

4. *Śhāntikāla:* "sphere of peace," the level within śuddha māyā where forms are made of inner sounds and colors, where reside great devas and rishis who are beyond the reincarnation cycles. This is the stage where we reach the zero point, which is in the third eye and is the resting place. It is following intensive prayer that one experiences rest, peace, and harmony. In this stage, tears begin to roll down the face and the nose becomes moist and may also begin to flow.

5. *Śāntyātītakāla:* "sphere beyond peace," is an extremely rarified level of śuddha māyā (actinic energy) in which super-consciousness expands into an infinite inner space, above the medulla oblongata,

the realm of the Gods. At this point one experiences an extraordinary flow of cosmic energy. A smile appears upon the lips and the enjoyment of cosmic energy is eternal.

Perfection

The number nine represents perfection. There are nine planets in our solar system, and nine female forces in the cosmos. In Hinduism, these forces are called Durgās.

The square root of 9 is 3. With this perfection, the spiritual value of this number doubles, 3x3=9. The immaterial essential value is 9, while the material essential value is 3x3x3=27 (3^3). This number is the logarithm of the external nature which must support and nurture the inner nature. Just as the earth is comprised of 3 layers, so is every kind of body composed of three layers. Each contains nine types of elements. This format is identical with all creatures. With respect to this, human beings are also gods, because our body is made up of 27 elements. At the time of death, of the 27 elements the following 10 elements are disfunctional, namely, earth, water, fire, air, and ether and the other five most important types of air for vāyas which keep everything alive in the body are: prāṇa-apāna- samāna, udāna and vyāna. These 10 elements constitute the elements physical body. After death, the soul along with the rest of the 17 elements which together form the astral and the causal body, go to heaven.

The number nine engulfs actions or the active forms of numbers enclosed in it. This number must demonstrate perfection because one plus eight is once again nine and between one and nine one finds combinations that total up to nine. Any arbitrary large number multiplied by nine produces a number whose digits add up to nine. This number is an exponential function with three parameters characterized by three properties:

1. It is the largest number in the series.
2. It accommodates and controls all internal combinations.
3. It holds all variables constant when multiplying with other numbers. It is a passive as well as an active parameter. The core message remains present in the same way the vibrations

of sound (soul) are present in each body even though this body is in the form of a human being, animal or plant. All figures below 9 are subordinate to 9. The number 9 is thus the mother who bears vibrations in her. With a bang, the parts become knots which can cause another bang. In fact in Psychology it is asserted that: *the total is more than the sum of the constituent parts.'*

Moving around the model in a clockwise or counterclockwise, all figures end with 9. This implies that as we circulate through life, we will always arrive at 9. If you multiply the number 9 by any number, the sum of its digits will always be 9:

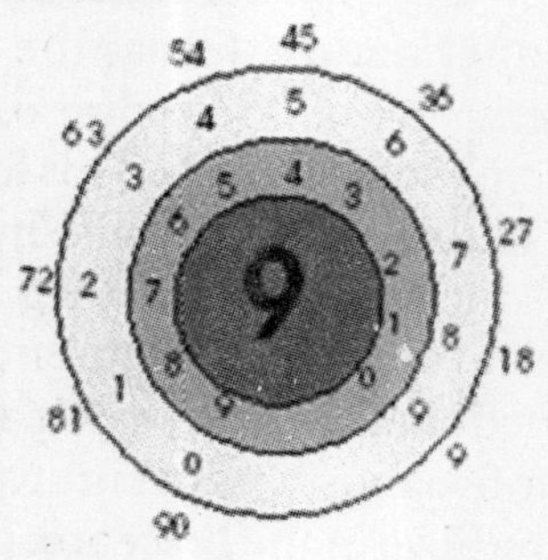

1 x 9 = 9
2 x 9 = 18 (1 + 8 = 9)
3 x 9 = 27 (2 + 7 = 9)
4 x 9 = 36 (3 + 6 = 9)
5 x 9 = 45 (4 + 5 = 9)
6 x 9 = 54 (5 + 4 = 9)
7 x 9 = 63 (6 + 3 = 9)
8 x 9 = 72 (7 + 2 = 9)
9 x 9 = 81 (8 + 1 = 9)
10 x 9 = 90 (9 + 0 = 9)

9 x 478542135 = 4306879215
4 + 3 + 0 + 6 + 8 + 7 + 9 + 2 + 1 + 5 = 45
4 + 5 = 9

The number 9 represents cosmic energy, while the number 8 is associated with physical energy:

1 x 8 = 08 (8)
2 x 8 = 16 (7)
3 x 8 = 24 (6)
4 x 8 = 32 (5)
5 x 8 = 40 (4)
6 x 8 = 48 (3/12)
7 x 8 = 56 (2/11)
8 x 8 = 64 (1/10)
9 x 8 = 72 (9)
10 x 8 = 80 (8)

If we talk about the number 8, then we're mentioning physical energy. Number 9 is cosmic energy. Watch the last numbers:

When we start with 8, and go from 8 to 2. The calculation is being compared to a period of 10 years. As the diagram describes, spiritual life starts at the age of 40. The end could be 80 years. In accordance of the yoga teachings, humans can live for 49 up years and 49 (7^2) down years. The right side of the diagram gives the development of life and the left side the time. In the senile period, people can think that they reached the perfect number and that feeling goes down very fast. Death is near.

Chapter 3

Yoga

The Meaning of Yoga

The word Yoga comes from the Sanskrit word "Yuj" and literally means union, the union implied being the union of the individual soul with the Supreme Spirit, God (RV 1.34.9; 3.27.11; 4.24.4). The Supreme Soul is Infinite, Omniscient and Omnipotent. It is an embodiment of knowledge and bliss. The individual soul is under bondage through ignorance and limiting adjuncts such as mind, body and senses. It is mere appearance. It is illusory (Māyā). When it attains knowledge of the Imperishable, it is freed from limiting adjuncts and bondage. Just as the bubble becomes one with the ocean, so also the Jīva becomes one with the Supreme Soul when ignorance is destroyed.[1] A dead body cannot speak, cannot walk, and cannot see. It remains like a log of wood after the soul has departed from the body. It is the soul that enlivens, stimulates, moves and directs the body, mind and the senses. Yoga is, in this matter for the prevention of disease, protection of health and beauty and prolongation of life. The Supreme Soul is self-consciousness, self-awareness, self-delight, self-knowledge and self-existence. It knows itself and knows others. It is self-luminous and illumines everything. Hence it is caitanya. Matter does not know itself. It does not know others. Hence it is Jara or insentient. The Supreme Soul is formless, attributeless, all-pervading indivisible, decayless, timeless and

[1] *Introduction to Tantra Sūtra*; Sir John Woodroffe; Ganesh & Company; Madras; 1997 (page 127):

spaceless. There is neither time nor day nor night in the Sun itself, although it creates day and night. So is the Supreme Soul. Soul is Infinite, Eternal, and Immortal. The Supreme alone exists. This world of names and forms is illusory. It is superimposed upon the Supreme Soul, just as snake is superimposed on the rope. Bring a light; the snake in the rope vanishes at once.[2] Yoga is a creative technique to Self-Integration. This is a practical guide who can help to master suffering and harness latent powers.

The word Yoga derived from the root Yuj "to join" in Sanskrit, is in grammar Samdhi. In logic (avayavaśakti) it is the power of the parts taken together. In its most widely known and present sense, can Yoga be translated as the 'union of a human soul (Jīva) with a divine soul or Supreme Spirit (Śiva)' (RV 10.30.11; 10.114.9).

Although many people associate the word Yoga with a physical discipline, in its original Hindu meaning Yoga refers to any technique that unites the seeker with the ultimate reality. The result of the technique is to achieve mastery over the mind and body, leading to self-realisation.

While physical fitness buffs may seek such a union by practicing Haṭha yoga, people with different personality traits have other choices. For the action-oriented person there is Karma yoga, the Yoga of action, which calls for a life of selfless deeds and actions appropriate to the person's station in life. In the Nārada Purāna it has been said that without Kriyā Yoga, it is not possible to attain or practice Jñāna Yoga (Nrd. P. Vol. I.5.31). Read more about Kriyā Yoga in the paragraph Patañjali Yoga. All types of yoga do not represent tightly sealed compartments, they are merely convenient classifications. They are sometimes called Mārgas (paths), suggesting that the same destination can be approached via different routes.

Yoga in the classical method is a Darśana, or doctrine, that is theistic and emphasises purification through meditation. At this stage of extreme purification or 'Self-Realization', the

[2] What becomes of the soul after Death; Swami Sivananda; A Divine Life Society Publication; Tehri-Garhwal; U.P.; 1997 (page 14 - 24).

soul or Jīva or Ātmā and the spirit are found to have merged together (Mund. Up. 3.1.3; Kaṭha Up. 4:15). A yogi, or practitioner of yoga, meditates in order to achieve true bliss, which involves a complete withdrawal from the world. Yogis assume the bodily posture that affords them the most stability and the least effort. Effective meditation relies on careful control of respiration and intense focus on a single object. The yogi strives to transcend body and matter through consistent meditation.

Yoga, One of the Six Systems

The six systems of Hindu philosophy are Nyāya, on rigorous logic, Vaiśeṣic, on atoms and the structure of matter, Sāṁkhya on numbers and categories, Yoga on meditation techniques, Mimāṁsā on the analysis of sacred texts, and Vedānta on the nature and experience of spirituality. The discipline uses both physical and mental faculties to arrive to its spiritual aims. Yoga is a system of transforming and absorbing power from the gods and to achieve liberation by raising the densities of our soul. The soul is a constantly vibrating sound, a bit of a piece of the Big Bang. When this density is raised, we are able to use, besides the physical body the invisible or astral body to travel in the cosmos. Those are processes which are used to discover man's inner essence, which is a part of the Supreme. There is an ignorance of the identity between the Soul and the Supreme Soul due to Avidyā. Jñāna or knowledge attains the realisation of such identity. The energy is Avidyā (nescience or illusion) because She binds, and Vidyā (knowledge) because She liberates and destroys the Saṁsāra (phenomenal existence). By the saying cited from the Patañjali-sūtra three modifications of Avidyā are indicated-viz., ignorance, egoism, and happiness. God Himself in the Atharva Veda mentions the importance of Jñāna yoga: "I equip with Knowledge and luster, the divine, virtuous, enterprising, powerful unborn soul. With the help of death, learned soul, keeping in a view the Exalted Joyous God, may we, advancing spirituality seek for salvation, the abode of purity" (AV 4.14.6: 698). He proceeds in hymn (AV 4.14.9: 70), O man, robe well, with thy mature, vast force, the Soul, that assumes different forms in different births, feels with all its organs, and is equipped with mature knowledge. Advance from here to the Most Exalted God, and with thy four feet (Dharma, Artha, Kāma and Mokṣa) stand firmly in the world.

Man's aim of life on earth is to ultimately become one with his Creator. It takes some people a very long time to reach this state and some attain it only after as many as 8,400,000 reincarnations. Only then the Ātmā (soul) becomes a Muktātmā (liberated soul) or Puruṣa (elevated soul).The individual has achieved his Mukti (salvation) and ceases to exist in the visible world. His ātmā is not more in a body but in the universe, it has gone up from the temporal into the eternal.

There are four means, or if so preferred, 'ways' to shorten time: knowledge of the Holy Scriptures, accumulation of positive karmās, regular prayer and regular practice of yoga. Patañjali, who lived in India around 500 A.D., is generally considered the founder of this method. In his book Yoga-Sūtras he stated that the aim of yoga should be to make the soul return to its essential nature, separate from all matter. Besides yoga there is another method for purification, and that is 'pūjā'. Pūjā is divine sacrifice of materialistic or non-materialistic way of services with devotion. Both yoga and pūjā have been built from several aspects. A number of the aspects in both forms of performance promote inner growth.
Buddha teaches his noble truths, in four ways:

1. Existence is suffering.
2. The desire of existence is the origin of suffering.
3. The destruction of this desire of existence is the destruction of suffering.
4. The noble eightfold path to the destruction of suffering is: right faith, right resolve, right speech, right action, right living, right effort, right thought and right meditation.

Meditation

Meditation is usually understood as a devout reflection on Creation or the Creator. The withdrawing into oneself and losing oneself in meditation and systematic reflections of a positive nature can therefore improve the quality of the practitioner and can have a positive radiation towards society. If the tiny caterpillar can realise its aim of life intuitively, then how much higher, can man reach with his superior mind? In other words, man can become a super human being by making use of this technique. This, in its turn, can be of importance to attain liberation faster or even to travel in the mind throughout the entire universe.

It is common to adapt the following posture in meditation: sitting on the ground; the right foot on the left thigh and the left foot on the right thigh; the heels pressed against the abdomen; the body, neck and head kept upright. This is called the lotus position (Padmāsana). The lotus is important in Hinduism. Every God or Goddess is portrayed on a lotus flower. What does this mysterious flower signify?

Edakkandiyil Viswanathan states in his book *Am I a Hindu* that the Lotus is the symbol of purity, its blossoms are actually the blossoms of consciousness. That is the reason why our spiritual centres or cakras (energy centre, wheel or vortex) are compared with lotuses. God, in the Sahasrā cakra, is Light. The lotus blossoms, thanks to sunlight, our cakras blossom because of the Divine Light. This learned writer states further that the lotus has an esoteric meaning: in the manner that the lotus remains pure, floating on water, although its stem is in the mud under the water, so also the yogī's mind, living in the mud of this world, amidst the waters of karma, should remain pure and untouched, floating on the water, turning to the sun of knowledge in order to bloom in the cosmic consciousness or super sensory experiences. "The devotees install in the very recesses of their hearts through showering meditation, the adorable and perfect God, who is existent even before the creation of the universe. The learned person, the yogis with special spiritual powers and the self controllers get united with Him in deep meditation (RV 10.90.7; YV 3109; AV 4549)". The lotus position gives balance and disengagement when we meditate, sitting in that lotus position.

The entire creation is already in an embryonic state present in the lotus which emerges from the navel of God Viṣṇu and from which God Brahmā may start the creation. The lotus seed serves as a model for the planets. The devotee when meditating because his liberation, at that moment embryonic in process, is in keeping with the creative process of God Brahmā keeps this embryonic state in mind. The upright back and the head together become the magical lotus flower in which the creation as well as the creatures are stored, a replica of the entity; small wonder that the various cakras portray their qualities in lotus petals.

The eight-petalled Maṇipūra lotus, under the heart-cakra or the Anāhata-cakra, is the seat of the new soul or baby as a Haṁsa (Hansa) or swan and God lives in the Soul. One should therefore meditate on the Cosmic Puruṣa in the depth of the heart, in the heart centre, and in correlation with the Soul. The eight petals stand for the eight guarding deities (Dikpālakas): Indra (Lord of the Heaven), guardian of the east, Agni, the fire god of the south-east, Yama of the south, Nirṭi of the south-west, Varuṇa of the west, Vāyu of the north-west, Kubera of the north and Śiva of the north-east. In the midst is the finite centre of consciousness, the Jīva or the Individual Soul. Cosmic consciousness is spread from within and without the heart to the thousand-petalled lotus at the top of the brain.

The Individual Soul, surrounded by Māyā (deceit), karma (acts from the past) and Ahaṁkāra (ego) remains in misery as a result of the identification with the body, mind and the intellect, which is the development of Prakṛti or the kinetic nature. Therefore meditation on the Supreme Reality reveals the Light of Truth, which drives away the darkness of ignorance (avidyā) and breaks the ties of desire, which has arisen from such ignorance.

Meditation on Godhead

That which is luminous, That which is smaller than the atoms, That in which are set the worlds and their peoples, That is this; It is Brahmā immutable; life is That; It is speech and mind. That is this, the true and real; it is That which is immortal; it is into That, that thou must pierce, fair son, into That, penetrate (Mund. Up. 11.1.2). The object of meditation here is the eternal Godhead Itself. It is the luminous Light. It is smaller than the smallest (Aṇoraṇiyān) and greater than the greatest (Mahatomahiyān). He is the Ākshāram Brahm, i.e. the Indestructible Word. So when we are asked to meditate on the eternal Puruṣa with His Cosmic Form, we are asked to meditate on the eternal Word that is God, which is "Aum". It is impossible for a weak body and a weak mind to practise such meditation. Of course, a lesser type of meditation makes one strong for higher types. Therefore, to attempt the highest type discussed in the Upaniṣad is only for the very strong in all respects. For when the Light descends and nectar flows, the body and the mind should have the power to receive it; if the body and the mind are not strong enough, then various disorders take place. One who meditates is really a strong warrior in life's battle to win a victory over the mind, which is tenacious, and the senses, which are turbulent. If he wins, his is the Kingdom of Heaven.

The true fruit of yoga is not a material achievement or performance. Yogis never measure the intake of oxygen. That is not what they are interested in. The yogi's interest is to keep the head and the heart clean through the harmony of breath, and this is achieved through the practice of prāñāyāma. The fruit of your action will tell you whether you are on the right path or not.

Nectar of Life

There is a very fine story in the Purāṇas which, speaks of amṛa-manthana, or nectar churning, where the nectar of life was drawn out by the churning of the ocean. The demons and the angels were fighting each other for the establishment of dharma, or virtue. The angels followed the policy of virtue, and the demons favoured vice. As the demons were stronger than the angels (RV 1.168.7: 1815), vice was increasing in the universe, so the angels approached Brahmā and Śiva who advised them to ask Lord Viṣṇu, the protector, for guidance to establish virtue. Lord Viṣṇu's advice was that they should churn the ocean to bring out from it the elixir of life. As distribution was his concern, they could then leave the rest to him.

Mount Meru was thrown into the ocean to serve as a churning rod, and the king cobra, Ādiśeṣa, was used as a rope to move the mountain. The demons, being stronger, took hold of Ādiśeṣa's head, and the angels held the tail. While they were churning, the mountain sank down into the ocean, so they could not churn at all. So Lord Viṣṇu took the form of Kūrma, the turtle, and went down to the bottom of the ocean to lift the mountain so that they could churn again.

This churning of the mountain is nothing but inhalation and exhalation is inhalation of the Sea. Like the mountain churning the ocean, the spine acts as a churning rod for breathe in our body. When inhalation and exhalation take place, the spine sends energy flashing forwards, backwards, upwards and downwards to produce the elixir of life, or jīvātma, in our system. Lord Viṣṇu in this story is the same as Puruṣa, the soul, in human beings. Viṣṇu in the form of our innermost self, or ātmā, causes us to breathe and thereby draws on the external energies, which at their gross level, contain the nuclear energies of the elixir of life. Thus we grow in health and harmony and increase our span of life by drawing the hidden energy from the ocean of the universal atmosphere.

Philosophically speaking, inhalation is the movement of the self to come into contact with the periphery: the core of being moves with the breath and touches the inner layer of the skin-the extreme frontier of the body. This is the outward or evolutionary process of the soul. Exhalation is the return journey: it is the involuntary process, where the body, the cells and the intelligence move inwards to reach their source, the ātmā, or the core of the being. This evolutionary and involuntary process within each individual is prāṇāyāma.

Thus, in each cycle of breath, we have two paths towards understanding the existence of God. They are known as pravṛtti-mārga, the path of creation, and nivṛtti-mārga, the path of renunciation. Pravṛtti-mārga, the outward path of creation, is in inhalation, and nivṛtti-mārga, the inward path of renunciation, is in exhalation. On the basis of this philosophy, the yogis were trained to reach a balance between these two states. Thus abhyāsa, practice, and vairāgya, renunciation, are brought together in cohesion in the practice of kumbhaka, which is usually translated as retention.

Kumbhaka is retention of breath, intelligence and self, where the lifted Lord-the core of the being-in the inhalation is held by the practitioner as long as he or she can maintain it. This is ātmā-dhyāna-meditation on the soul. One does not simply hold the breath by physical retention, but holds on to the very self, which was raised up and elated through the inhalation. The moment one lets the self sink, the retention of breath becomes merely physical and mechanical, and is not true kumbhaka at all. In inhalation, as mentioned before, the self comes to the surface, like Lord Viṣṇu who, after descending to the bottom of the ocean, lifted the mountain to churn the ocean again. To maintain the stability of the lifted self is true kumbhaka. It is a purely divine state of practice in which inhalation (Pūraka), retention (kumbhaka) and exhalation (recāka), are all involved. In kumbhaka, the self becomes one with the body and the body becomes one with the self. It is the divine union of body and mind in inhalation, exhalation and retention.

If you look at breath in the form of the respiratory system, it is physical. But when the action of the breath on the mind is studied and understood, it becomes spiritual. Prāṇāyāma is the bridge between the physical and the spiritual. Hence prāṇāyāma is the hub of yoga.

Ojas, the Spiritual Energy

In order to be able to practice yoga one should have 'Ojas'. The already on many occasions quoted book: Am I a Hindu says the following about this: Ojas "is the spiritual energy which is stored in the brains". Through elevated thoughts, meditation, japa, worship and Prāṇāyāma, sexual energy can be converted into Ojas-Śakti and be stored in the brains. This energy can be used for reflections and spiritual ends. Anger and the energy of the muscles can also be turned into Ojas.

Someone who has a large amount of Ojas in his brain can do considerable spiritual work. He is intelligent, has a magnetic aura around his countenance and radiant eyes. He can influence people, his addresses are impressive, his speeches poignant. He has an awesome personality. Śrī Śankara, an Akhanda-Brahmācārya (celibate) performed miracles through the power of his Ojas. He performed Dig-vijaya and held disputes and high-minded debates with competent scholars in various parts of India. A yogi always fixes his attention on the accumulation of this sacred energy by continuous chastity.

A yogi must avoid the two extremes of affluence and renunciation. He must not fast or torment his body. He who does this can, according to the Bhagavad Gitā, never become a yogi. But one who does not work cannot become a yogī either.

The yogi says that by practising āsanas, you can bring awareness to an extension equal to that of consciousness. This is total awareness.[3] This is meditation. Consciousness is always present in our finger, but most of the time we are not aware of it, so the consciousness of the finger is dormant. You should know the difference between consciousness and awareness. Consciousness exists everywhere in the body. When you are walking, if a thorn touches your foot, what happens? It pricks, and you immediately feel the pain, so you cannot say that consciousness was not there. But until the thorn pricked you, you were not aware of your foot. The consciousness in your foot was dormant, but the moment the foot was pricked, it was brought to the surface. To awaken that dormant consciousness is awareness. Your consciousness is six feet long, or five and a half feet long in your body-it is as long as your body is tall. But awareness is small. Awareness may extend two feet, one foot, one inch or half an inch. When awareness fades, concentration fades, intelligence fades, and consciousness also fades. But the moment you are attentive, your intelligence is concentrated. This concentration is dhārana, and when that intelligence and awareness do not fluctuate but remain constant, that is meditation.

[3] The Tree of Yoga; B.K.S. Iyengar; Harper Collins Publishers India Pvt Ltd.; New Delhi; 2000.

Patañjali Yoga System

Yoga is one of the six classic systems of Hindu philosophy, distinguished from the others by the marvels of bodily control and the magical powers ascribed to its advanced devotees. The difference between the individual soul and the Supreme soul is that the individual soul has become impure through cravings, desires, egoism, pride, greed, lust and likes and dislikes. Yoga also means 'yoke' as mentioned in "*Seer of the Fifth Veda*' by Bruce M. Sullivan (p. 35), as a word which is etymologically related and conveys well the idea of exertion. Because yoga means an effort, any effort, the term is used very widely, often without intending any reference to ever, and particularly in the passages about Vyāsa, the word yoga does seem to refer to a spiritual discipline based on the Sāmkhya philosophy and similar to Patañjali's yoga system. Hence it is finite (Paricchinna), it is endowed with limited knowledge (Alpajña) and limited power (Alpa-Śaktimāna).

Yoga is a spirit-or lighting mechanism. Yoga awakes the inner part of the human being, feeds it mentally and makes it healthy. Because of this the soul is able to live a balanced and long life. The inner rhythm of the body is coordinated with that of the cosmos. The soul is the action in the body in which vibration is a constant. It is supervised by the Puruṣa and Yama, the death, as long as there is a difference in the vibration between it and death, the human body is mortal. Yoga is a method which raises the ultrasound in the soul and is able to free the soul even from death. As soon as the spirit is intensified by yoga, the fire ignited in people is the same as the fire of a sacrifice ignited. Also the yogi performs ritual ceremonies and both: the yogi and the pūjā are systems to clean the inner body and the cosmos. Instead of pūjā the Purohita or priest frequently functions as a celestial agent between people and cosmos (god).

The ancient seers of India have bequeathed to mankind invaluable secrets of the inner world of man and the outer universe and the inter-links between the two. The veracity of this is being slowly but surely validated by the faltering advances of modern science. One of the most valuable works in this regard is the Yoga Sūtras of sage Patañjali.

The Yoga system of Patañjali constitutes one of the six systems of Indian philosophy. It is the most concise among all the six (Patañjali's work comprises only 164 verses) but is the most important, since it gives practical steps for self-realisation. The Yoga system of Maharishi Patañjali has eight components:

- The Yama: has the following components: do not cause sorrow, or kill, not even in the mind. Be truthful, do not covet, be chaste, do not accept anything from anyone. This purifies the mind, the Citta. Do not cause harm to any creature by thought, word or deed. There is no greater virtue than non-violence (Ahiṁsā). For man there is no greater happiness than the acquisition of a non-violent attitude towards all creatures. A yogi must not cause harm to anyone by thought, word or deed. Mercy will then not be bestowed upon him alone, but will reach further, embracing the entire world.
- Niyamas: virtuous behaviour, contentment, and purity from within as well as from without. Fixed rules for sleeping and awakening. Fixed habits as study.
- Āsana : the right postures to reinforce the muscles and the joints and to make the spine and all other bones more resilient. Not only does a good posture benefit a person's build but it benefits his internal organs, his glands and his nerves as well. Because the āsanas release physical and mental tensions, they also make unprecedented sources of energy accessible.
- Prāṇāyāma is proper breathing. The word Prāṇāyāma consists of two parts, Prāṇa and yama. Prāṇa is the life force (vitality) in the body. Yama means 'not killing' or 'keeping alive'. Prāṇāyāma is the systematic control of the Prāṇa or breathing systematically in order to come to rest and to avail oneself of more oxygen from the breathed air. With proper respiration technique the body is supplied with new vitality and the mind is brought under control. Because of this, one feels calm and refreshed. And hence the ability to concentrate is being developed.
- Pratyāhara is bringing the Indriyās or senses under control of the will. The organs of the senses work outwards and get in touch with external objects.

- Dhāraṇa: Meditation, being lost in thought or musing. Concentration, with open or closed eyes, on the lotus of the heart or on the centre of the head. When meditating, a special group of waves arises; negative waves roll back and disappear in the end. Finally a few waves remain at the back of the mind. If the mind can be concentrated on the centre of the head during 12 seconds, this is a dhāraṇa.
- Dhyāna: a dhyāna consists of twelve dhāranas. If the mind can be concentrated on that spot during 144 seconds, this is called a dhyāna.
- Samādhī: contemplation, enjoying being in a state of bliss. If the mind can be concentrated on the centre of the head during 1728 seconds (28,8 minutes), this is a samādhī. A samādhī consists 12 dhyānas.

The proportion between dhāraṇa, dhyāna and samādhī is one of 1:12:144. The word samādhī consists of two parts: samā and dhī. Samā means: 'merge into' and dhī comes from buddhi or wisdom. Samādhī therefore means 'merge into wisdom'. When there is no need of a basis anymore, when the entire mind is only one (1) single wave, it is called samādhī. Deprived of all means such as particular spots and centres, only the essence of the thought remains. The successful yogī is in control of the small wave of the Prāṇa which represents our own energy, mentally and physically. Only when we have succeeded in controlling this small wave, we may be able to control the entire Prāṇa. The *yogī* who has mastered this, has reached perfection. He is no longer under any power. He has become almost omnipotent, almost omniscient.

The great sage Patañjali has described Kriyā Yoga (purificatory Yoga) in the second chapter of his Yoga-Darśana (Philosophy of Yoga) to introduce general aspirants to the practice of Yoga. Purificatory action, study and making God the motive of action, IS the Yoga, of action (PYS 2:1).[4]

---

[4] Yoga Sūtras, with the commentary of Vyasa and the gloss of Vachaspati Misra, translated by Rama Prasada; Munshiram Manoharlal Publishers Pvt. Ltd.; New Delhi; 1998.

The word 'tapas' has been translated as purificatory action, because 'tapas' means that which burns up impurities.

The word Īśvarapraṇidhāna has been translated as the devotion to God being the motive of action. The same word in the first chapter (I. 23) has been translated as feeling the omnipresence of the Lord. The root meaning of the word 'praṇidhāna ' is the placing of anything under another to the fullest extent (pra = fullness, ṇi = under and dhāna = placing). In the chapter on trance the word can only mean the contemplation of Him as the substratum of all phenomena. Hence 'Īśvarapraṇidhāna' as a means of achieving trance can only mean the habituating of the mind to feel the omnipresence of the divine principle. Table 2 shows every aspect of Kriyā Yoga in relation with the three *paths of yoga.* As a branch of the Yoga of action ' praṇidhāna' must have special reference to action which would be out of place in contemplation. It has, therefore, been translated here as above. The root meaning, it is easy to see, runs through both these meanings. Purificatory action has been taken up (as a factor of the Yoga of action). This is considered an action worthy of performance, as it purifies the mind when not impeded. Study is the repeated utterance of purifying words, like the AUM and others; or, the reading of the teachings about absolute spiritual freedom (Mokṣa). Devotion to God and making Him the motive of all actions means dedication of all actions to the Highest Teacher, or the renunciation of its fruit.

Table 2: The evolutionary stages (Avasthā) in Sādhana, according to the three main texts on Yoga

Gītā	Yoga	Yogānga	Śakti	Elements of Prakrti involved
Karma	*Tapas*	*1. Yama*	*Prakṛti sakti*	1.Behaviour *(ācāra)* *Character(svabhāva)*
		2. Niyama *3. Āsana* *4. Prāṇāyāma*	*Pritvi (earth)* *āpa (water)*	2. Organs of *action* Senses *of perception* 3. Mind *(manas)* 4. Breath *(prāna)*
		5. Pratyāhāra	*āpa(water)* *Teja (fire)*	5.Mind *directly controls the senses* of perception
Jñāna	*Svādhyāya*	*6. Dhāraṇā*	*Vāyu (air)*	6.Intelligence *(buddhi)* Ego *(ahamkāra)* Consciousness *(citta)*
		7. Dhyāna	*ākāsa (ether)*	7. Conscience *(Dharmendriya Antahkarana)*
Bhakti	Isvara Prani-dhana	*8. Samādhi*	**Purusa sakti** *Ojas sakti (the light of the soul)*	*8. Soul (ātmā prasādana)*

Source: Yogacārya B.K.S. Iyengar, Astadala Yogamala, Allied Publishers Limited, New Delhi, 2000.

The Art of Yoga

Art is based on repose, reflection, science and philosophy. Art and beauty are free from bonds imposed by place, time, age, sex and religion. Art is developed with the help of science and the background of philosophy. In a sense an artist is a scientist as well as a philosopher. Yoga is no exception to this rule. Indians consider all forms of art as yoga.

The body is the abode of the soul and the instrument for the expression of spiritual life. So, instead of renouncing the material basis, the yogi accepts it as part of the spiritual problem. Elaborating on the topic of āsana the yogi realises that our body has a dignity of its own as much as the mind. It is the temple of the yogi as well as the artist.

Yoga encompasses everything from the skin of the body to the soul and takes the yogi and the artist from the plane of the body towards the plane of the spirit. The yogi or the artist develops the integration of thoughts with will-power (Manobala) and maintains harmony within and outside him. He draws inspiration from the touch of the Divine, and with spiritual strength uses his technique and skill to produce a synthesis of divine expression and divine beauty (Divya Saundarya). Yoga is an art of opening the unconscious parts of our being, which will enable us to feel the direct touch of cosmic consciousness, sometimes inspire ourselves with the touch. We cannot look upon man as a physical machine to which spiritual life is attached from the outside.

The first chapter of the Patañjali Yoga Śāstra, in fifty-one aphorisms, gives what may be called the theory or the science of Yoga. An ardent and intelligent person can learn enough from this chapter alone to become a practical Yogin. But for men of ordinary intellect, more detailed teaching is necessary; the second chapter enters into such teaching. It may be called the art of Yoga, the technique of it. The art of Yoga consists in bringing under control and purifying the three lower vehicles of man, namely the body, the mind and the spiritual Self, the astro-physical, mental, and the causal bodies. The astro-physical body is to be purified and brought under control by what are called ascetic practices; early rising, bathing, fasting, bearing hardships, etc., in short, all that go under the name of Tapas or austerities. The mental body must be purified and strengthened by study, by acquiring knowledge. An ignorant person cannot be a Yogi. The causal or spiritual body is to be developed by entire devotion to God. Thus an atheist cannot be a true Yogi

The aim of yoga is to attain perfection of the intellect, both of the head and the heart, so that the artist becomes devoted, true and pure. This demands an almost total relinquishment of interest in other activities of life except the chosen path. The mind is fluid and runs after sensual pleasures. Art demands total undivided focal attention. Hence Patañjali succinctly explains that the mind must be controlled and then sublimated to serve the artistic nature of yoga to its highest potency. Yoga or any art requires acute sharpness of intellect and alert organs of perception. In yoga there is no competition, but it requires freedom to think and reconstruct with a desire to perform better. Then it brings to the yogi the most exalted enlightenment. From now on, wherever the yogi and whatever he does, his thoughts are rooted in spiritual communion, which takes him to the zenith of spiritual life.

Before practising the Yoga systems, it is required that the person must spend his study period in the first state of the four Āśramas. The first is called the Brahmcārya Āśrama. The Atharva Vedā confirms this as follows:

"A Brahmacārī wields radiant Vedic knowledge. All noble traits reside in him. He creates and absorbes in himself, Prāṇa, Apāna, Vyāna, elocution, mental force, heart, knowledge and wisdom. O Brahmacārī bestows on us the power of sight and hearing, glory and food, seed for progeny, pure blood and strong belly. Having mastered the above mentioned forces, the Brahmacārī, exercising austerity in the Brahm Āshrama, deep like an ocean, exerts to bathe in the water of knowledge. After graduation (Sanātaka) being glorious and vigorous. He shines exceedingly on earth." [AV 11.6.24-26, 3115-3117].

A Brahmacārī is the lord of breaths [AV 5.25.14, 1192]. This means that he is graduate in the Yoga system of breath and his body (the prāṇas) and mind (the 'I' and 'you') are under control. When this state is achieved, it is possible to become a real Yogi or Yogini. In this state a Yogi finishes his journey with the force of knowledge, and never turns his thought aside. Thereby he does not withhold from the learned, the enjoyment of food.[5] Food must be read as spiritual knowledge for the soul.

The powerful world that stands through its innate strength, the motivating force of the Veda, the all-creating Ten (the ten prānas), and the forces of Nature (Sat-Raja-Tama), like the Sun, Moon etc. are fixed round God, like a wheel about the nave.

---

[5] The Art of Yoga; B.K.S Iyengar; Harper Collins Publishers India Pvt Ltd; New Delhi; 1985.

Experience consists in the absence of the notion of distinction between the Puruṣa and Objective Essence, which are really quite distinct-from-each-other, because it exists for another. By Samyama on his own object, comes the knowledge of the Puruṣa.The essence of the Will-to-be is of the nature of illumination; and when it overpowers the qualities of disturbing energy (Rajas) and inertia (Tamas), which are equally related to it by co-existence, it takes up the form of the notion of the distinction between the Puruṣa and Objective Essence. Widely different from that changing objective existence also in characteristic is the Puruṣa who appears as pure consciousness. They are quite distinct from each other. Experience consists in the notions of the two not being taken as distinct, because the objects are shown to him. The notion of enjoyment is the knowable, because the essence of matter exists for another. There is another notion, however, the notion of the Puruṣa, which is quite distinct from this, and which appears as pure consciousness.

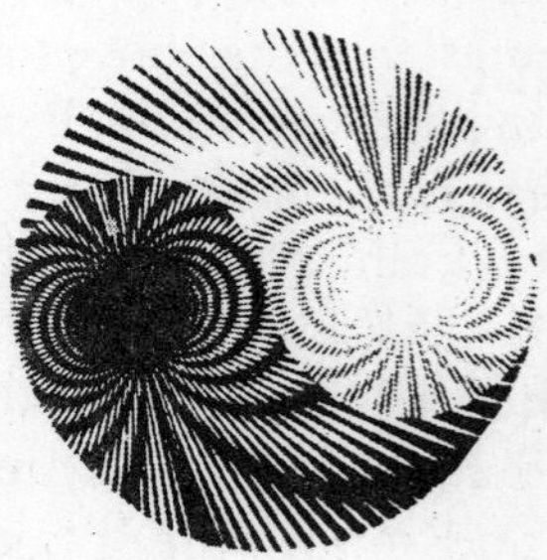

Figure 8: Heart Centre

The important wheel turns in the heart center in the body (see figure 8). The heart (Hṛdaya), centre is the knowledge of the mind. In the lotus-like cavity, the temple in the city of Brahmā lives the Intelligence. By performing Samyama with reference to that, comes the power of knowing, the citta. The self is called Brahmā, being largest of all. His city is that in which he is living, knowing it as he does to be his own. Cavity means hollow. The same is the lotus too with its face downwards. The same is the temple. Here the mind knows the mind (the

Manas knowing the Citta): Intelligence lives there. By Samyama over that, the Yogi knows the Citta with its modifications.

The essence of the Will-to-be means not only possessing the nature of illumination, but modified too at the same time as the discriminative knowledge, and therefore extremely pure and luminous, it therefore bears extreme resemblance to consciousness. This would mean confusion. The Will-to-be is of the nature of the quiescent, the disturbed, or the forgetful notions. When consciousness is reflected into it, then the quiescence, the disturbance and the forgetfulness are fastened on to the consciousness. This happens in the same way as the moon reflected into pares water, looks as if it is trembling on account of the unsteadiness of the water.

Consisting of enjoyment is of the Objective Essence. It may be said that experience is the feeling of pleasure and pain as being in consonance or dissonance with the prevailing mental trend at any time. We should know that the self is the enjoyer; the knowable is that which he enjoys.

The Wheel of Life

The above-mentioned wheel (see figure of the cakra) about the nave (nābhi) in the Atharva Veda (11.7. 4, 3144) explains that the wheel of life moves on. It has the understanding for its strength; the mind for the pole (on which it rests); the group of senses for its bonds, the five great elements for its nave, and home for its circumference. Home is called the circumference because, as the circumference limits the wheel, even so home (wife and children) limits the affections and acts of life. Decrepitude and grief overwhelm it, and it has diseases and calamities for its progeny. That wheel relates in time and place. It has toil and exercise for its noise. Day and night are the rotations of that wheel. Heat and cold encircle it. Pleasure and pain are its joints, and hunger and thirst are the nails fixed into it. Sunshine and shade are the ruts (it causes). It is capable of being agitated during even such a short space of time as is taken up by the opening and the closing of the eyelid. It is enveloped in the terrible waters of delusion. It is ever revolving and void of consciousness. Months and half months measure it. It is not uniform (being ever changing), and moves through all the worlds. Penances and vows we its mud. Passion's force is its mover. It is illuminated by the great egoism, and is sustained by the qualities. Vexations (caused by the non-acquisition of what is desired) are the fastenings that bind it around. It revolves in the midst of grief and destruction. It is endued with actions and the instruments of action. It is large and is extended by attachments. It is rendered unsteady by cupidity and desire. It is produced by variegated Ignorance. It is attended upon by fear and delusion, and is the cause of the delusion of all beings. It moves towards joy and pleasure, and has desire and wrath for its possession. It is made up of entities beginning with Mahat and ending with the gross elements. It is characterised by production and destruction going on ceaselessly. Its speed is like that of the mind, and it has the mind for its boundary.

This wheel of life that is associated with pairs of opposites and devoid of consciousness, the universe with the very immortals should cast away, abridge, and check.[6] That man who always understands accurately the motion and stoppage of this wheel of life, is never seen to be deluded, among all creatures. Freed from all impressions, divested of all pairs of opposites, released from all sins, he attains to the highest goal.

As mentioned above the wheel's mover is the force of passion and desire: the power of Kāma Deva. This power is difficult to stop. Even Kāma Deva confirms his own power in the Mahābhārata as follows: "No creature is able to destroy me without resorting to the proper methods (viz., subjugation of all desires and practice of Yoga etc.). If a man knowing my power, strives to destroy me by muttering prayers etc. I prevail over him with the belief that I am the subjective ego within him. If he wishes to destroy me by means of sacrifices with many presents, I deceive him by appearing in his mind as a most virtuous creature amongst the mobile creation, and if he wishes to annihilate me by mastering the Vedās and Vedāṅgas (branches of the Vedās), I over reach him by

[6] Mahābhārata; Aswamedha Parva; Section XLV; Sri Kisori Mohan Ganguli

seeming to his mind to be the soul of virtue amongst the immobile creation. And if the man whose strength lies in truth, desires to overcome me by patience, I appear to him as his mind, and thus he does not perceive my existence, and if the man of austere religious practices, desires to destroy me by means of asceticism, I appear in the guise of asceticism in his mind, and thus he is prevented from knowing me, and the man of learning, who with the object of attaining salvation desires to destroy me, I frolic and laugh in the face of such a man intent on salvation. I am the everlasting one without a compeer, whom no creature can kill or destroy. For this reason thou too, O prince, divert thy desires (Kāma) to virtue, so that, by this means, thou mayest attain what is well for thee."

The saintly yogi enjoys all the fruits of his karmās with indifference and remaining untouched by them. The Sāṁkhya sūtra says: "The body is like the potter's wheel" (3.82). The potter revolves with his stick the wheel and then leaves it alone but the wheel keeps on running for a long time because of its accumulated force or momentum. Even so, the human body goes on enjoying the fruits of the 'prārabdha' (already operative) karmās and performing actions. The yogi does not, however, perform karmās like the ignorant but karmās he does do, though wise. There is never the absence of karma and knowledge so long as there is life. Karmās do not become the cause of bondage for them. He does them naturally like the actions of attending to sleep, hunger, thirst, nature's call, etc.

The wise yogi's goal is towards the omnipresent, sentient Brahm. According to his understanding, just as in prakṛti all the actions are performed simply by the proximity of God and God is unattached, unconcerned and indifferent, free from joy and sorrow, love and hate, even so, in spite of possessing the physical body, the yogi is a mere witness, unattached and unconcerned, to the karmās and declares that his relation with his body is like that of Brahmā with prakṛti, of mere proximity. Whatever actions and activities are taking place in the body and in the psychic apparatus are due merely to the proximity of the sentient soul. It should be the ideal of all yogis and the learned and the wise that like God they remain unconcerned and unattached to the body.

Yoga, Science and Art

The term Science is known as Śāstra or Vidyā. Art is known as Kalā. Śāstra means order, command, precept, rule, religious or scientific treatise, any sacred book or composition of divine authority. Vidyā means knowledge, science, learning, and Kalā means any practical, mechanical or fine art. The Atharva Veda adds in both that the practice of both is with dedication and sacrifice. The learned is Scientific and Divine Objects is the Art. "O God, Thou art Foremost amongst the learned and all divine objects, exhibit Thyself in our heart. Thou art the Eye of men and the forces of nature. May the noble sacrificers, in the company of men of mature Knowledge, performing the yajnas, living together happily, attain to God and prosperity (AV 4.14.6.: 697).

Science is an acquired knowledge and it is objective. Art is experienced knowledge. Its intelligence is decisive and hence subjective. Some arts are well known in Hinduism. Music is known as Saṅgīta Śāstra and Saṅgīta Kalā, dance as Nātya Śāstra and Nāyā Kalā, sculpture as Śilpa Śāstra and Śilpa Kalā; yoga, too, is known as Yoga Śāstra as well as Yoga Kalā. Like all other arts, yoga is also a science and it is a philosophy too. That is why it is called Yoga Śāstra as well as yoga Darśana. Yoga analyses the turbulent mind and shows the ways and means of reaching the ultimate goal of freedom, this is science (Śāstra). As science, Yoga conveys truth. On the practical level, Yoga keeps the body healthy, the mind quiet and pure, and the self in beatitude. It is therefore a darśana and this means vision, seeing, acting, showing, exhibiting, teaching, an aspect or semblance, a doctrine, a system of philosophy. The practical aspect of Yoga Darśana conveys the artistic aspect of Yoga with its precision and beauty.

We can divide art in two types. One is the art of pleasure (Bhoga Kalā)and the other of abiding divine ecstasy (Yoga Kalā). The art of pleasure brings transient comfort and contentment to the viewers. Being pleasure-prone, it attracts the masses and has their support, bringing the artist in close contact with them. It has a quality, which excites and distracts and may end up in desire and lust as Kāma Kalā. Single-minded adherence in reaching the pinnacle of art without being caught by excitements and distractions is Yoga Kalā, which requires intensity of purpose and concentration with deep penetration. The artist is not caught in the web of the senses but heads towards spiritual bliss. This Kalā integrates him the very core of his being.

A blend of Bhoga Kalā and Yoga Kalā is essential for an artist of calibre. Mastery of Bhoga Kalā alone makes one a slave of the senses, while mastery of Yoga Kalā alone would make a person useless and non-fruitful to society. A judicious blend of both Bhoga Kalā and Yoga Kalā will enable the artist to present his art with self-respect, character, good judgment and an even balance. The Sāma Veda denotes that Agni has beloved forms wherefrom desires originate (Kāma) and that Agni is Wise by making his body beautiful, exalted by sages (Yoga) (SV 1710 and 1711). Agni is represented as a corpulent man, red in colour, with two faces, and eyes, eyebrows, and hair of a reddish tawny hue. He has three legs and seven arms. He rides a ram and has that animal emblazoned on his banner. From his mouth forked tongues or flames emit, by means of which he licks up the butter used in sacrifices. These characteristics each have their special significance. The two faces represent the two fires, solar and terrestrial, or creative heat and destructive fire. The three legs probably refer to the three sacred fires of the Brahms-the nuptial, the ceremonial or funeral, and the sacrificial; or they may denote his power over the three portions of the universe the celestial, terrestrial, and infernal regions, which is manifested by the three forms he takes, sup., lightning, and sacrificial fire. His seven arms, like the seven heads of Sūrya's horse, are originally derived from the prismatic divisibility of a ray of light, or may denote the universal power of the all-pervading nature of fire.The expression of art is filled with spiritual passion and feeling, and can be at the same time humorous, elegant, graceful, excellent and beautiful.

The Rīg Vedā (10.90.12) denotes that Candramā is the woman who gives body to every creation and belongs to the lineage (family) of the Sun or Sūrya. This is in the sense of the priority. The Agni of the Candramā goes first as in the society: Ladies first! Before starting a sacrifice we pray for Candramā first with lightening the flame or Batti. The next is the incense or wisdom. Agni is cleaning the mind to absorb the wisdom. This is comparable with cleaning the blackboard before writing. And according to this principle in yoga, we purify the mind first; before the pūjā we take a bath or before eating washing our hands. Woman is the symbol of aesthetics and beauty. She pertains to the sense of the aesthetics, characterised by a love of beauty. This concerns with pure emotion and sensation as opposed to pure intellectuality.

Yoga Kalā belongs to the field of emotions, instincts, intuitions and insights (Antaḥkaraṇa). It is guided by the application of principles, which are brought to the surface by practices and experiences so that analytical knowledge and factual knowledge are synchronised and felt. This synchronisation or harmony is the aim of all art; so it is with yoga. It is an education, which refines man mentally and spiritually. Then the practitioner is elevated to a state of excellence, full of flavour, elegance and grace.

The purpose of yoga is to develop the body, discipline the mind and stabilise the emotions in order to refine man as a whole. It brings into perfect accord the disparate forces of the body, the muscles, joints, limbs, and the circulatory, respiratory, digestive, glandular and genito-excretory systems. It also integrates the senses of perception, the mind, intelligence, will-power and consciousness with the self, making them work in harmony (RV 5.81.1). It puts an end to the division of body, mind and soul. In the words of the Yoga Sūtras, no opposites remain. The end of yoga, as of art, is the attainment and expression of happiness, contentment, fulfilment, freedom and beatitude in order to reach the summit of indivisible existence. Yoga is a psycho-spiritual subject connecting man with the object of contemplation. Lord Kṛṣṇa calls it a means of achieving equanimity, harmony and balance in man's power of thinking and acting. Patañjali speaks of single-minded effort and uninterrupted flow of contemplation. The yogi controls and blends the movements of the body and integrates them with his consciousness, moving on towards the path of the Supreme. Yoga, according to the Gītā, also helps one to develop proficiency in performing actions and virtuosity in the presentation of art. The aim of life is to become one with nature,

In the domestic mode of life, those who are of pious conduct, who desire the fruits of virtuous course of behaviour with spouses in their company, have this mode of life ordained for them. In it Virtue, Wealth and Pleasure may be obtained. It is thus suited to the cultivation of the triple aggregate. Śrī Bhrigu said in the Mahābhārata[7] that in the domestic mode of life the following are allowed, viz., the use and enjoyments of floral garlands, ornaments, robes, perfumed oils and unguents. Enjoyment of pleasures derived from dancing and music, both vocal and instrumental, and all sights and scenes that are agreeable to the sight. The enjoyments of various kinds of viands and drinks belonging to the principal orders of edibles, viz., those that are swallowed, those that are lapped, those that are quaffed and those that are sucked. And the enjoyment of pleasures derivable from sports and every kind of amusement and gratification of desires. Bhimsena continues what the importance is, of desire "One without desire never wishes for wealth. One without desire never wishes for virtue. One who is destitute of desire can never feel any wish. Without desire diverse kinds of action that are seen in the world would never have been seen. For these reasons, desire is seen to be the foremost of the triple aggregate of virtue, wealth and desire." The Kalā tattva mentions several types of nidhis or wealth that people can achieve through yoga. Nine of these are the highest. All these forms of secret powers are based on desires of people. For more detail, we refer to chapter 2, Understanding the Spiritual World in this book.

Kāma, Pleasure and the Erotic

The third aim of life to be discussed is Kāma, which means

---

[7] Mahābhārata, Śānti Parva, Section CXCI.

pleasure or desire. Kāma also means work and in this context, the work of desire. Kāma is the mental inclination toward the pleasures of the senses and is particularly connected to the erotic. Sexual behaviour may be learnt with the aid of this text and the counsel of worthy experts in the arts of pleasure (SV 13.6.3). Nevertheless, Vatsyayana (author of the Kāma Śūtra) acknowledged that money and social success are more important than love. And that virtue is more important than success and fortune. The ideas, on erotic techniques and methods, were passed down through an oral tradition from the ancients. The legendary founder is Nandi, Siva's companion, and about the eighth century B.C. Shvetaketu known to us from the Bṛhadāraṇyaka and Chāndogya Upaniṣads, is said to have summarised them. Between the third and first centuries B.C. several authors wrote shorter works on different aspects of eroticism, including Suvarnanabha on erotic approaches, Ghotakamukhā on the art of seducing girls, Gonārdiya on the wife's duties and rights, Gonikapūtra on relations with other men's women, Kuchamara on occult practices, and Dattaka who wrote on courtesans with the help of a famous courtesan of Pātalipūtra.

These were combined together in the oldest text we have today, the Kāma Sūtra, who probably lived in the fourth century C.E. In style and language the Kāma Sūtra is considered quite similar to Kautilya's Artha Śāstra. Famous as the world's oldest and the most detailed sex manual prior to our century, the Kāma Sūtra reveals the life-style and sexual morals of ancient India. Vatsyāyana declared that everyone in life must pursue three aims successively. Childhood is dedicated to acquiring knowledge and is a celibate phase; the erotic predominates in adulthood; and old age is dedicated to the practice of virtue (dharma) and spiritual liberation (mokṣa). Vatsyāyana defined artha as material goods

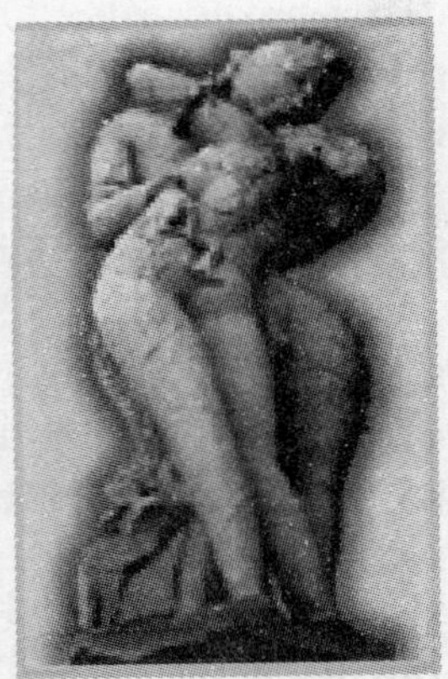

Figure No. 9

or wealth and said that it "consists of acquiring and increasing, within the limits of dharma, knowledge, land, gold, cattle, patrimony, crockery, furniture, friends, clothing, etc.

Since sex is natural to all animals why does it need to be studied? The preliminary acts between a man and a woman can benefit from rules of conduct. Among animals the female is driven by instinct with little consciousness during the sexual season. Although Vatsyāyana said he is a fatalist, he recognized that success depends on human effort. The pursuit of pleasure must be coordinated with virtue and material goods. The man who is incited to lust is excessively proud or concerned about his own appearance, qualities and achievements (SV 4.3.2). And he also has a strong feeling of disapproval and aversion toward what seems base, mean, or worthless. An abnormally enlarged emphasis on the sexual life can be self-destructive as well as ruin others. Nevertheless sexuality is essential to human survival. The one accomplished in wealth, love, and virtue attains the greatest happiness in this world and the next. The art of loving so pleasing to women, which allows children to be born, has been described by sages in sacred books.

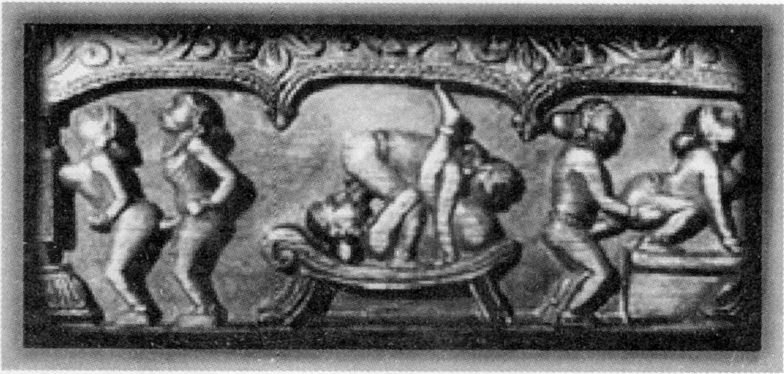

Figure No. 10

Yoga can recondition tone and develop the sexual powers of the individual to a greater degree than any tonic or stimulant, and can do it on a sounder and more lasting basis (SV 15.1.2). The misery and anguish experienced by people because of sexual frustration are not so easily handled, and often baffle both the physician and the psychiatrist. A sexually weak person is often jealous by nature, and jealousy can contaminate the entire fabric of his life. He can become a victim of persecutory hallucinations or of monomania's, suspicious of conspiracies against him between his wife and friends, or in the case of a woman, between her husband and his female acquaintances. This can result in other unpleasant physical and mental symptoms. Tranquillisers worsen the basic condition by lowering the threshold of mental and physical tolerance, apart from causing unpleasant side-effects.[8]

Here, Yoga can step in as a super-tranquillizer, replacing the harmful side-effects with exhilarating benefits. Yoga's contribution to the brain, or to be more accurate, the mind, is greater than that of drugs. It is sound, real and enduring. The Yoga-tempered urge deepens finer feelings of consideration and love. There is conscious pleasure in giving, and in the realm of sex you will experience gratification in proportion to the pleasure that you learn to give.

The benefits of sexual intercourse are manifold tranquillity, forgiveness, tolerance, love, consideration are but a few. An unsatisfied sex urge can lead to frustration, vindictiveness, nervousness, perversions, misanthropy, mental disorders and physical diseases. Efforts to completely suppress sex are never truly successful.

No man should think of sexual intercourse as the supreme test of his manliness, nor the woman of her femininity. This can destroy the naturalness of a perfectly normal situation and may turn the sex act into a failure. Look upon it as a wonderful and integral part of a healthy and complete life, and never as a competition or a test. While Yoga tones up sex, it is giving you control over it.

This control grows and is akin to an efficient switch which you can turn on or off at will instead of letting your energy dissipate wastefully. The science of yoga teaches the art of

---

[8] Yoga and Sex; Pandit Shiv Sharma, Kailash Nath Sharma; B.I. Publications Pvt Ltd; New Delhi; 1973.

living. It helps and guides us in daily life, in every sphere of action and in improvement of human relationship, irrespective of one's belief and profession. This control over sex energy, is an exclusive gift of Yoga. No other technique known to the physician or the psychiatrist offers this mastery to the individual. This cakra can delay orgasm when Praṇāyāma is applied. When making love, one can also deduce the degree of willingness of the other party from the breathing. A heavy breathing mostly implies consent.

The Kāmāsanas (different sexual postures, see subsequent figures) are analogous to the Yogasanas. Some physicians advise middle-aged couples to avoid attempting different sexual positions as they may lead to spraining of muscles, but this problem would not arise in the case of people already accustomed to Yogic positions. Yoga stabilises the mind. A practitioner of Yoga will not tremble with fear when approaching sex. A path illuminated by the light of Yoga will remain pure and bright, even when it leads to the fulfilment of Kāma. To condemn knowledge of sex as a sin, and to glorify ignorance as bliss, merely promotes unnecessary misery, incompetence, fear and damage to the psyche. People inculcating this psychology may have good intentions, but their results are evil. Sex is often a victim of politics. Sects are trying to increase their members. Fundamentalism today is exploring sex to multiply their forces. They have a hidden agenda to become a majority in the world. Sex becomes a high industry and is the fuel of the factories.

It is the induced psychological reaction of the participant in the sex act, and not the natural physical or psychic reaction following it, that depresses or exhausts a person. The sufferer may have been led to believe that the love of God, or perhaps of a country, necessitates a hatred for sex. It is for these reasons that the very same sexual acts which gave the Greeks energy and inspiration can today depress devout followers of religions which denigrate sex and range themselves against the natural expression of a powerful physical and psychic demand and need. Sex should be recognised as an irrepressible natural urge and treated as an art and a science, which can lend colour, beauty, refinement and clean enjoyment to man's existence. Love is sex as sex is love.

Those suffering from heart disease are advised to follow their doctor advice on the frequency and method of sexual intercourse. Generally, coitus should take place after a period of physical and mental rest. The active role should mainly be taken over by the healthier partner in a position particularly comfortable to the heart patient. The act should be performed in the nude or, at very least, no tight-fitting garments should be worn. Relaxing Yogāsanas such as Vajrāsana and Śavāsana, with regulated Prāṇayāma, will help to keep away further recurrence of the disease. The Ayurvedic dictum, "Stop your exercise (including sexual) before you become breathless", should be meticulously followed.

Erotica

The issue of erotica was misunderstood for a long period. The answer became clearer as galleries all over the country started to display contemporary works that presented nude figures of unmistakable gender, usually in sexual attitudes. The participating artists were heedless of existing taboos. We have been raised to fear the 'yes' within ourselves, our deepest cravings: endured feeling of displeasure or indignation. This can also be the cause of a lack of sexual desire. Low sexual desire is a lack of interest in sexual activity. Discrepant sexual desire refers to a condition in which partners have considerably different levels of sexual interest. These dysfunctions may be caused by physical problems such as fatigue or illness; the use of prescription medications, other drugs, or alcohol. Psychological factors, including learned inhibition of sexual response, anxiety, interfering thoughts have a contra productive influence. Observing and judging one's own sexual performance, lack of communication between partners, insufficient or ineffective

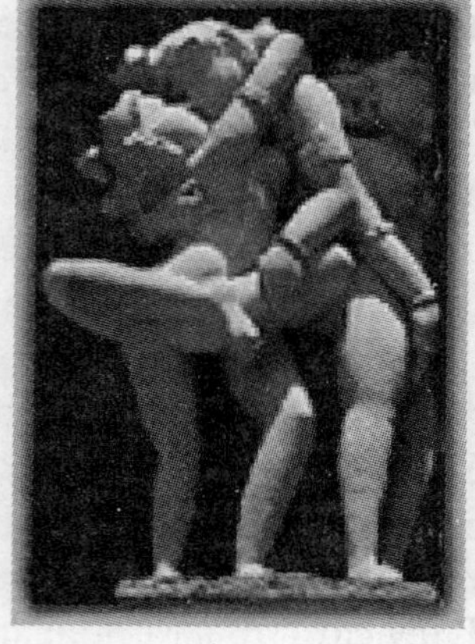

sexual stimulation, and relationship conflicts are also factors for decreasing of attitude. In such cases, a qualified sex therapist can work with a physician, if necessary, to determine the cause and best options for testament.

Indians writing about erotica is a perfectly respectable function of medicine, and about the ways to make the person enjoy sex. These are an important part of reproductive physiology. Erotic practices have been diversified. Sex used to be single-crop farming, like cotton or wheat, now people raise all sorts of things.

The most famous collection of such stanzas, that of Bhartṛhari, perhaps the greatest poet of India next to Kālidāsa, consists of lyric, didactic, and erotic poems. Considered the second great master of the erotic stanza is Amaru, who is probably of a later date than Bhartṛhari. His collection is known as Amaruśataka. The difference between erotica and pornography is that erotica is about sexuality and pornography about power and sex-as-weapon. In the same way we have come to understand that rape is about violence, and not really about sex at all. Eroticism has its own moral justification because it says that pleasure is enough for a person. It is a statement of the individual's sovereignty.

Even the dance style of the north of India, the Kaṭhak, is a subtle dance that emphasises footwork and speed. Kaṭhak is decorative rather than interpretive and often the themes of the Kaṭhak style are erotic. The relationship between Rādhā and Kṛṣṇa had long been celebrated in often highly erotic art and literature, notably in the Sanskrit poem Gita Govinda (The Song of the Lord), composed by Indian poet Jayadeva in the 12th century. Caitanya's teaching drew on this tradition, in which the union of the divine pair was acknowledged in their joint worship as Radha-Kṛṣṇa

The 64 Arts

Erotic science should be studied along with other subjects even before adolescence and after marriage with one's mate. Young people must educate about this important part of life. They can learn from those who have had sexual experience.

Vatsyayana listed 64 arts, which include music, dance, drawing, and carpets, flower bouquets, etc.

Even in the ancient times there were prostitutes with high standards and arts (Bh.T. 6.1.58-65). Prostitutes who were beautiful, intelligent, and well educated in these arts were honoured in society and called courtesans. A man who is expert in the 64 arts is much appreciated by women. It is recommended that sexuality be satisfying to a virgin gained a good reputation, though Gandharva marriages based on mutual affection and love were generally considered the happiest. Exceptions made for prostitutes or widows provided that it was only for pleasure in income. Young girls were also considered suitable for love affairs. Vatsyayana declared that passion knows no rules nor place nor time, and variety fosters mutual attraction. "Whether they continue having sexual relations, or live chastely together, true love never decreases, even after one hundred years." He asked rhetorically, "Practiced according to his fantasy and in secret, who can know who, when, how, and why he does it?" After making love one should be affectionate so that a solid attachment may be established through friendly conversation. Those who gain each other's trust end up becoming attached to one another out of habit. The totally trusting wife considers her husband a god and is completely devoted to him. She takes responsibility for the household. Widows may remarry and begin a new existence, and according to the ancient tradition an unsatisfied woman may leave her husband and choose another to her taste. Vatsyayana recognised the ethical marriage as the best and said that some men do not pursue adulterous relationships for reasons of ethics: He said: "Reasonable people aware of the importance of virtue, money, and pleasure, as well as social convention, will not let themselves be led astray by passion."

The English poet and playwright William Shakespeare said in his performance Twelfth Night (Act 1, Scene 1)

"ORSINO If music be the food of love, play on,
Give me excess of it, that, surfeiting,

The appetite may sicken and so die."

In this atmosphere we can continue:

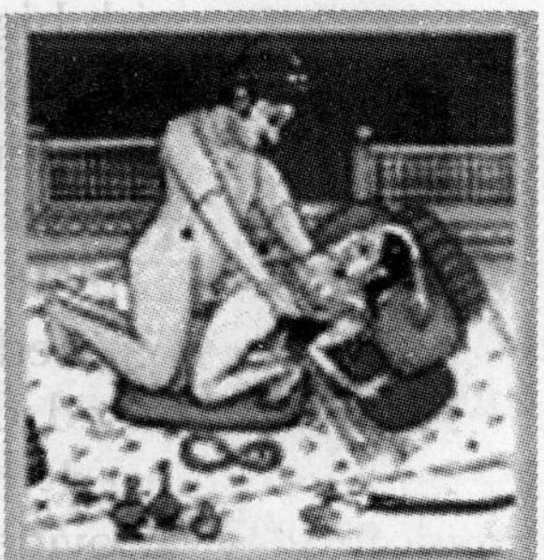

"let me become high, in the sense of love, instead to die."

What is refreshing in this treatise is the openness to sexual pleasure and its naturalness without the shame and puritanical guilt so well developed in other cultures that have invaded modern India as well. The erotic is treated as an important aspect of human life and as the sacrament of marriage that unites the couple more than anything else can. Instead of being burdened by inhibitions in ancient India people were encouraged to learn about their sexuality and develop the art of loving through education and practice. Only now in the late twentieth century does the world seem to be acknowledging the wisdom of these techniques and this highly skilled art. The hunger for sex can be huge, love becomes never ever a sandwich!

Women and Mokṣa

How delicious is a woman when artfully played upon, how capable could she be of producing the most exquisite harmony; of executing the most complicated variations and of giving the divinest pleasures. Women must be divided into four classes of temperament. These are: Padmini, Chatrini, Śaṁkhini and Hastini. The same correspond with the four different phases of Mokṣa, or Release from further Transmigration. It depends on the highest level of attraction, love and beauty. The first and the highest is Sāyujyatā, or absorption into the essence of the Deity; the second is Sāmipyatā, nearness to the Deity, the being born in the Divine Presence; the third is Sārūpatā, or resemblance to the Deity in limbs and material body; the fourth and last is Sālokatā, or residence in the heaven of some especial god.

For the name of woman is Nāri which means 'Na Ari or no enemy (resistance) and such is Mokśa or absorption, because all love it and it loves all (mankind).

- Padmini means Sāyūjyatā, also called Khadgini-Mokśa (Sword-release), the absorption of man into the Nārāyaṇa (Viṣṇu), who lives in the Kṣīrabdi or Milk-sea, one of the Śeven Oceans, and from whose naval sprang the Padma or Lotus-flower. On this flower the Creator created all.
- Chatrini is Sāmipyatā-Mokśa, like those who having been incarnated as gods who perform manifold and wonderful works. These are assistants, demigods or parts.
- Śaṁkhini is Sārupatā-Mokśa, even as the man, who takes the form of Viṣṇu, bears upon His body the Śāṁkha (conch shell), the Cakra or discus, the super energy source of all cakras, and other emblems of that god.
- The Hastini is Sālokatā-Mokṣa, for she is what residence in Viṣṇu's heaven is to those of the fourth class who have attributes and properties, shape and form, hands and feet. Also the Bible of the Christians mentions that God creates people according to His image. Due to the aspects shape en form, hands and feet learned people changes. Some time to sequence of the Sārupyā and Sālokyā. My opinion in this matter is that the identity becomes first and then you can enter the area or Sālokyā as Dr Prem Acārya has quoted (before). We have to identify our Self to the Super Self.

As mentioned above we have different kinds of ladies. The choice of a life partner depends on a number of conditions for both men and women. These conditions are concerned mainly with internal and external qualities. The inner qualities of a woman remain in the shadow during this era because of beauty. Not everything that shines is gold! When feelings or emotions become stronger and go beyond the mind the chances of divorce or failure in a family can be larger. Beauty, character, (fundamental) attitude, knowledge (life consideration) wealth and status are ideal aspects which every human dreams of, this is especially applicable to the youth. To establish a good future, character and knowledge are very important, even for the next family generations. A man or woman is like a tree if he or she cannot move. That's why act and tact of the Kāmaśāstra or Science of Love are prescriptions of Dhanvantari for a good marriage. A household is known to be correct and behaved. Every member should be social and cultural, wise and learned, prudent and patient.

Tantric sexuality

In the area of sex and erotica the Kaulavali Nirnaya Tantra is the most influential and greatest. The Kaula tantra is the parameter. According to tradition we can divide the practitioners into three classes: Divya (sattva or divine), Vīra (strong, heroic or rajas) and Paśu (tamas or beastlike). Yet the Vīra, or heroic Sādhanā, is only a part of the Kaula tradition and is only for a certain category of practitioners. The Sādhakas are males and Sādhvinis females who can benefit from the practice of the Kaul Tantra. It is prohibited for the Paśu, who is likely to misunderstand both and its inner significance on a superficial level because only humans can use and produce Ānanda or happiness. This is the highest level within creation according to the koṣas or sheaths. For Paśu or animal minded is not competent to practise this rite, it is poisonous. The rīte of the game of happiness and beauty needs a prologue. Ejaculation is often considered the most important event, particularly for both individuals. Ejaculating contains two aspects. The first is the discharge. During this time of sexual revolution the discharge becomes subjective. The physical and mental satisfaction overrules the beauty of this art. To express the ratio regard to the speed of movements, the acceleration determines the quality and the height of feeling. The ability of an emulsion in the sexual game is important. In this process the brightness values of their true proportion to one another depend on the brilliant electric spark discharged in the inner atmosphere. This is the rainbow or Indraprastha (the arrow of seven colours of the king Indra of heaven) that become visible in heaven during the time of rain. Tuned to, be tuned and to be united become music in life. The scale or grades of the finishing depend on the release with or without a sound. During the discharge there is a flash (or flashes) of lightning. That's the core within this score. One or both emit a shrill cry and silence becomes the happy end.

Western changes

Progress in modern science is remarkable due to the exchanges of law in several countries. In 1986 we had changes on the field of civil liberties and civil rights. Traditional concerns of civil libertarians over such issues as free speech, separation of church and state, equality, and rights of the accused were somewhat muted in 1986 as the United States focused on a social agenda filled with civil-liberties overtones involving such issues as affirmative action, gay rights, abortion, pornography, and testing for use of illicit drugs. The Reagan administration, unusually active in promoting social policy changes, filed a record number of briefs before the Supreme Court but was rebuffed in many important decisions bearing on social issues.

Classification and experience

The first class (divine) undergoes the process of intercourse, as the realisation of the Gods just like wine-nectar. The second or Vīra undergoes this interaction as alcohol, comparable with the business class in the aircraft, while for the Paśu it is prohibited as it is done without understanding. As per the traditions of today (mostly in the west) this Tamas technique is the Slave and Master (SM) combination of this field. A Vīra, who wants to be liberated, uses the Five M's or Makārs. The Kaula Tantra explains that these five Makārs form a part of a rite, performed by the Viras. To activate and stimulate the sexual game the group uses the principle of the five M's. The Paīcha-Makārs are Maithuna (intercourse), Madya (liquor), Mudra (bean), Māṁsa (flesh) and Matsya (fish).

In terms of spirituality we translate the above experience of the five-M's in the heaven as follows. The Kularnava Tantra says that the divine person, or Divya, realises the flows from the 1,000-petal lotus (Sahasrār cakra) as the nectar of the body (liquor). Flesh is the sense of duality. Fish is the disordering of the senses and sexual intercourse is the union of Kuṇḍalini with supreme Śiva. Indeed, true sexual intercourse is union with the goddess within. This is the bridge or rainbow between the earth and heaven.

Intercourse with any other woman is adultery. That may be true for the Divya, but not for the Vīra. In this time of lack of dharma, such are daily practice.

These considerations make it clear that far from Tantra being synonymous with sex, sexuality is a part of the Sādhanā (work on oneself) and the tradition is only at a certain stage and for a certain time. The human being is the highest form of creation and their sex is not dependent on any seasons. The sex of the animal is based on seasons. If someone practises Tantrik rites, uses a mantra or Yantra from books, without being competent (Adhikāra), not only is there no success, but, on the contrary, he or she is cursed by the goddess. The Kularnava Tantra (chapter II, 116-118) confirms this as follows: "Beguiled by false knowledge as propagated, certain persons, deprived of the Guru-Śiṣya tradition, imagine the nature of the Kuladharma according to their own intellect. If merely by drinking wine, men were to attain fulfilment, all addicted to liquor would reach perfection. If mere partaking of flesh were to lead to the high state, all the carnivores in the world would become eligible to immense merit. If liberation were to be ensured by sexual intercourse with a Śakti or Power, all creatures would become liberated by female companionship." The possibility exists that it was comparatively late that the Tantric schools went "underground." Judging from texts like the Kālikā Purāna, it seems that Tantric sexuality was a part of everyday life.

The Guru-Śiṣya (master-student) tradition or relation is based on knowledge. Knowledge has come through Saṁkalpa. A new consideration of yoga is based on this Saṁkalpā, a science of creation. This yoga does not belong to anyone in particular just like everything in nature. It belongs to all those who want to practise it. There is no one to command you and there is no market for it to be sold in. There is no bondage and there are no milestones. You have to walk away from the bridge, away from the master. It means that the student, researcher or devotee has to go on what he or she has learned from the master or Guru. The spiritual quest is a thorny path that ultimately must be walked alone. Every path of yoga must have been blessed by the firm, compassionate, and boundless wisdom of the master. A master or Guru is a comprehensive guide and an acclaimed teacher who shares the unique and holistic approach to a healthy life for his dedicated student.

The Devi's Desire

Kāmeśvaṛī

The Lady of Desire is Kāmeśvaṛī. She is the first Lady or Nitya in the cycle. We denote her secret formula or vidyā (mantrā) according to the Tantrarājatantra:
Aiṁ Hriṁ Śrīṁ Aṁ Aiṁ Sakala Hriṁ Nityaklinne Madadrave Sauh Aṁ Kāmeśvarī Nitya Sṛī Pādukaṁ Pujayāmi Tarpayāmi Namah.
The same Tantra gives her Dhyāna or meditation image as red in the centre like 10 million dawn suns, having a diadem of rubies, wearing throat ornaments, necklaces, waist chains and rings. This first Lady is the red Lady. She has six arms and three eyes. She bears a crescent Moon and smiles softly. She holds a bow of sugar cane, flowering arrows, noose, goad, and a nectar-filled begrimed cup. She shows the mudra of bestowing boons. The five arrows of desire (Kāma} are Longing, Maddening, Kindling, Enchanting and Wasting. These five Kāmas are five forms of Kāmadeva.

In this context of knowledge Lalitā stimulates the power of the brain. She is the Mother of knowledge and changes her form in Kṛṣṇa. Kṛṣṇa is described here as the five forms of the Kāmadeva. These are Kāmarāja (Hriṁ), Manmatha (Kliṁ), Kandarpa (Aiṁ), Makara (Bluṁ) and Manobhāva (Śṛiṁ). They correspond with five colours: yellow, white, red, purple and blue, a majority in the colour dispersion of the rainbow. Each of the Kāmadevas has two eyes and two arms, the hands holding the sugar cane bow and flowering arrows, the very form of the five elements (earth, water, fire, air and ether).

Nityaklinna Nitya

This is the Devī or Power of the Liquid. Her name means Always Wet. Her secret formula or mantra is:
Aiṁ Hriṁ Śriṁ Nityaklinne Madadrave Svāhā Iṁ Nityaklinna Nitya Śrī Pādukaṁ Pūjayāmi Tarpayāmi Namaḥ

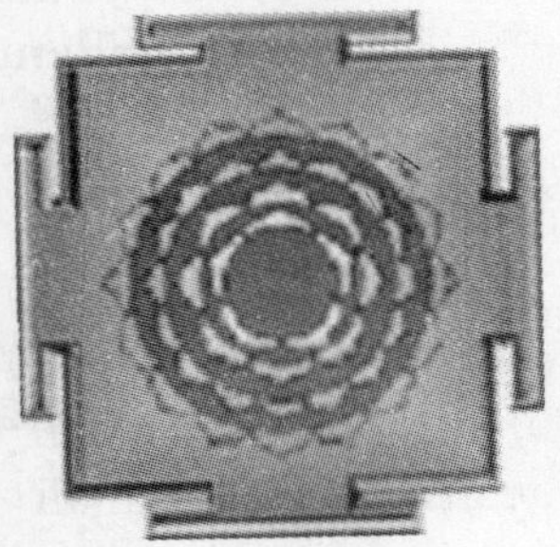

Figure No. 11: Nityāklinna

She bestows enjoyment and liberation and subdues the three worlds (physical, astral and carnal) for one siddha (successful) in her vidyā(mantrā).

The Nityaklinna herself is restless with desire, smeared with red sandal paste, wears red clothes, smiles, has a half moon on her head, and holds a lasso or noose, a cattle stick or goad, a cup and makes the mudra dispelling fear.

Metaphysical Thoughts of Patañjali

The Yoga of Patañjali is based on the metaphysics of Sāṁkhya, but it differs from Sāṁkhya in one important point. It was realised that it was not possible to get on with these two utterly different principles Puruṣa and Prakṛti. The difficulty is obvious, as was mentioned. How could anyone think of these two things, unless there is a thinker of the two things? The person, the element, or the principle, that is aware of the existence of Prakṛti on this side, and Puruṣa on the other, remains as a third thing altogether. Such a witnessing principle cannot belong to either Puruṣa, or to Prakṛti. But the Sāṁkhya says that there cannot be a third thing. For it, there are only two things. The Sāṁkhya defeats itself by positing two utterly different principles.

The metaphysical aspect of Yoga as propounded by Patañjali, felt the difficulty, and, so, there was an introduction of a deity called Īśvara in the Yoga philosophy. This word Īśvara should not be associated with any devotional systems, or the God of the religions. Patañjali's Īśvara is quite a different thing altogether. It is a pure '*deus ex machina*', a contrivance that has been made necessary to explain the relationship between one

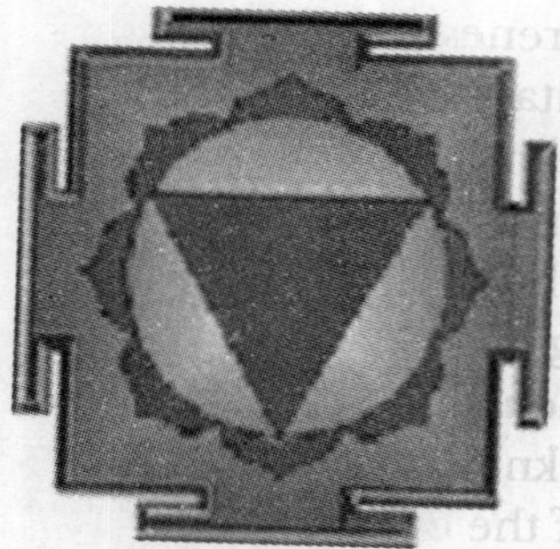

Figure No. 12: Thoughts of Patāñjali

thing and another. Patañjali had his own arguments for positing the existence of Īśvara. It was felt that there cannot be only two parties in a case. If there are two camps opposing each other, who will decide the case? People do good, people do bad. There is a reaction set up to every action, good or bad. Now, who will dispense justice in the form of a nemesis that is set up by actions, good or bad? A client cannot be a judiciary. It cannot be Puruṣa; it cannot be Prakṛti. There is a third element necessary, a judge in a court. Patañjali introduced this judge, and he called this judge Īśvara.

Yoga and Vedānta

Vedānta is one of the six darshans or philosophies of Hinduism. Advaita Vedānta is the school of thought within Vedānta. It's a philosophy to bridge the gulf between the secular and the sacred, action and contemplation, in human life, through a comprehensive and lofty spirituality. It is the flower that makes the vase become valuable. Yoga teaches us how to colour your life and to get control of the vase, the body. As soon as the flower is there, water comes automatically in the vase. This is the sequence between theoretical and practical knowledge. This school believes that everything in the universe shares a single soul, including you, God and me. Vedānta philosophy uses the word "Sat-Cit" (Soul and God; Jīva and Śiva), which means Existence-Consciousness (AV 8.9.1: 2231).

The most common means, which are often practised conjointly to reach spiritual enlightenment, are Jñāna- and Rājayoga, mental Sādhana or meditation in silent and Haṭha or 'physical' yoga, which literally means 'effort'. Jñāna Yoga means wisdom or knowledge in Sanskrit. Jñāna Yoga is a technique for seeking liberation. The identification with the real Self (rather than with the body or ego) is developed in this Yoga by a steady effort to discern or discriminate between pure awareness and the objects of awareness. This branch of science is closely associated with Advaita Vedānta.

The difficulty of language is such that no word can be used at all to designate what Sat-Cit means. They are not two different things or states. It is Being which is Consciousness, or Consciousness which is Being. Being is Consciousness, and Consciousness is Being. So the hyphen is used, Existence-Consciousness, because no other way is known to write it down. Existence which is Consciousness is of the character of Bliss. Why is it Bliss? All suffering and finitude, every difficulty and penury of any kind, is the result of the finitude of one's nature. When one has become the infinite, all desires are fulfilled. Thus, essentially, the Self is Sat-Cit-Ānanda; Existence-Consciousness-Bliss. Here Infinity and Eternity get blended into All-Being.

The essential nature of Man is divine, the awareness of which he has lost. The causes are his animal propensities and the veil of ignorance. Man, in his ignorance, identifies himself with the body, mind, Prāṇa (life elixir) and the senses. Transcending these, he becomes one with Brahmā or the Absolute, Who is pure bliss. Brahmā or the Absolute is the fullest reality, the completest consciousness. That beyond which there is nothing that is the innermost Self of all is Ātmā or Brahmā.

Jīvas are different from *Braha* in the state of bondage, but become one with Him in the state of liberation. This is expressed by the 'mahāvākya's' or great verses in the scriptures, 'tat-tvamasi' (you are the absolute (tat/Brahmā); "That thou art!" and "aham brahmāsmi" (I am Brahm). "Know thyself" is the oracle of Delphi; 'Tat-tvamasi' is the proclamation of the Upaniṣad. The Upaniṣads explain that the knowledge of the self is the knowledge of the cosmos, is a universally accepted doctrine of all philosophies and religions today.

The Upaniṣads say, "Sarvaṁ Khalvidaṁ Brahmā", which means the whole universe is the Absolute appearing, as, if it is external to itself. The objects of the world, the things that are before everyone, are facets of consciousness. God Himself is in front of man, as it were. The Puruṣa Śūkta of the Veda tells us that all these things that are seen are the limbs of the One

Puruṣa, the All-Being. Every atom, every ingredient, every location or point of objectivity is the head of the Cosmic Being. The Absolute is the only reality. This is the conclusion that metaphysical idealism draws, which do not mean those external objects, do not exist. Only, the objects are not isolated material entities. Things are not what they seem. Modern science has tended to come to a similar conclusion. Extremes meet at the same point. The outermost probe of science has coincided with the innermost probe of the philosophers. The deepest self of man is identical with the outermost reality: the universe. The Ātmā is Brahmā Thou art That; Tat Tvamasi. Here is the metaphysical or, as it is sometimes called, the ontological conclusion of the epistemological predicament, the knowledge process. Jñāna Yoga, the process of knowledge has led to a grand discovery that there is One Being in the universe.

Our goal of life is God-realisation, which means merger of our soul or Jīva ātmā into the Ātmā (the Jīva into Śiva). The Jīva experiences itself to be a part of the Eternal Brahm or Universal Consciousness. This consciousness or indwelling Spirit in every individual remains as a mere witness of all his actions (BG 13:22,31), so long as, he is not willing to listen to it. In Vedās, this spirit and the soul (Jīva) are compared to two birds perched on a tree or a body (Mn. Up. 3.1.1-2; RV 1.164.20).

Etymology of the Term YOGA

According to the supernatural part of the wisdom which is mentioned above, the super perceptibility of the senses, and the functions and the composition of the term 'yoga' can be translated as follows:

The 'Y' of this word indicates action or vibration. The soul of a creature is also a part of the vibrating Energy. Death or Yama, a larger energy, keeps supervision of the souls in the cosmos. The highest soul or Ātmā is God or Puruṣa.

The 'O' of this word indicates a sound-or detonation funnel, the sky. It also indicates "coming into the open air" through the path of salvation or sāmadhī (mokṣa). It also has the shape of the cosmos after the Big—Bang. Within the hymns of the Vedā one must articulate this sound from the throat or from the nose. This is the I-icon in Sanskrit, similar with the Omega; I am the alpha and the Omega, the first and the last, the beginning and end, the eternal (in the bible: Revelations 1:8, 11; 21:6; 22.13). The sounds, which imitate the Big—Bang, are nasal in which both the solar and the lunar energy are produced. This is the reason why we have two nose breaches. There breath is a constant process in life, the body grows continuously just like the universe. Expanding is just like the breath of people as long as the Creator exists. Lord Śiva, the highest energy, creates the universe in meditation and the Great Mother energy, here as Kuṣmāṇḍā makes an end product-the cosmos.

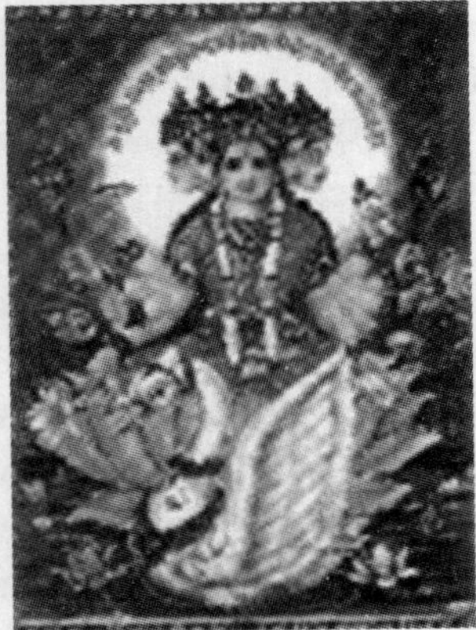

Figure No. 12: Mother Gāyatrī

Mother Gāyatrī is the energy of salvation, which causes the Big—Bang of this product. We can talk about the cosmic trias politica, the three state powers, namely legislative, executive and legal power. This macrocosmic state is similar with fecundation, growth and delivery of a baby. This triad is established in the heart of people and in the sun in the cosmos. Pregnancy lasts approximately nine months and each month of the growth of the child corresponds with a planet in the cosmos. Whereas Mother Kuṣmāṇḍā stands to the cradle of the cosmos for people, she indicates the Kua (read: Kuṣa grass or hair of Lord Viṣṇu) as a symbol for Ānanda or blessing during the dead ceremonies. The dead ritual executes with the Kuṣa grass. The Kuṣa grass symbolises the connections between souls within a pedigree. This grass breaks the attraction of the earth and frees energy so that she can move upward into heaven. We retrieve Kuṣa as a symbol in the Devanāgarī (Sanskrit, Hindi, Marāthi etc.) as the line or link that is drawn above the characters; entirely inherent to glow for each other and for the lineage or Gotra (pedigree). Each pronouncement is a minuscule copy of the Big—Bang because they contain ultrasounds. There are proportionally eleven gotra's to the eleven aspects of god Śiva.

Śiva, the father of all souls or Jīva's (Śiva-Jīva-principle) has eleven types of vibrations in His body which needs Śānti and rest, to establish peace and love within the cosmos. This harmony brings music in our life and that of others which characterise themselves by friendship, charity and domesticity.

The 'G' in this word indicates fire or spirit (Āgni). Fire heats all the things that are radiated slightly with dark red to white. In short, Yoga makes the soul glow and melts the substances on the soul so that she's able to glitter as pure. At this heating process the hidden energy Kuṇḍalini awakens in people and she rises up as a tortuous snake around the backbone. Thereby she activates the backbone with a strict of 32 couples of nerves. At this process of awakening all energy wheels or cakra's in the body, work optimally. The Lālanā cakra in the pharynx keeps the jaws together with the 32 (2x16) cogs twisted on each other. The Lālanā cakra provides here supernatural capacities to people (semi-Siddhi's). With these particular capacities one can easily achieve wealth, celebrity etc. Lālanā cakra is activated by the energy of food, which means the ātma-pūjā. Food must be chewed minimum 32 (2x16) times. This sacrifice is both for people and for god. The Jīva itself dwells in the larynx (voice box) and the Śiva in the forehead triangle where the Third Eye is located in wisdom. The mouth is therefore a sacrificial well (Havankuṇḍa), as mentioned in the Rīg Vedā (I.1). The voice or the Śabda is a detonation product, which is by the soul in the larynx germinated and implemented by the tongue in the pharynx. This is the sound-or the detonation funnel is formed or deformed characterises the person.

The Human Body

The human body as stated in our ancient Hindu literature is composed of five gross elements—Pāthivi (earth), Āpah (water), Tejas (as fire) Vāyu (gaseous material) and Ākāśa (ether). Muscles, bones, glands, hair, nail and skin form the earthly element, are the various secretions with the body. Blood is the watery element. Impulses moving to and from along the nerves, which are concerned in the receiving of impressions from the organs of sense and discharging them to organs of action, make up the gaseous element in the body. The emotional activities of the body arise from the ethereal element; while desires make up the fiery element of the body. Of these five elements of which the body is composed, Ākāśa and Vāyu remain as germinal spots in the embryonic life. Light in the form of cosmic energy enters the body at birth and excites the gaseous element to activity which is then transferred to the Gandharva region. Gandharva is the power or the region which holds, sustains and enlivens our body and on which are, dependent the growth and decay of everything in our physical form.

The Ātmā

The Ātmā is the common Consciousness as a part of God in all beings. A central fact is his inherent divinity. There is apparent, fictitious difference in bodies and minds only. There are differences in colours and opinions. But, the Ātmā is the same in all. A thief, a prostitute, a scavenger, a king, a rogue, a saint, a dog, a cat, a rat-all have the same common Ātmā.

The Ātmā is the one amidst the many. It is constant amidst the forms, which come and go. It is the pure, absolute, essential Consciousness of all the conscious beings. Liberation or Mokṣa implies oneness of Self. Oneness of Existence is Reality, and the realisation of this Reality is Mokṣa.

Mokṣa is the breaking down of the barriers that constitute separate existence. Mokṣa is the absolute state of Being. There is the unity of all-pervading and all-permeating consciousness, realised with certainty, like that of an orange, which we see in our palm. Mokṣa is not an attainment of liberation from an actual state of bondage, but the realisation of the liberation which already exists. It is freedom from the false notion of bondage. The individual soul feels itself to be in bondage on account of ignorance caused by the power of Avidyā. When the false belief caused by delusion is removed by Knowledge of Ātmā, the state of Mokṣa is realised in this very life. It is not to follow after death. Wisdom or knowledge is not restricted. The source of our life, the source of all knowledge is the Jīva ātmā, the innermost self.

The realization of the Self is the destiny of each soul, attainable through renunciation, sustained meditation and frying the seeds of karmās yet to germinate. It is the gateway to mokṣa, iberation from rebirth. The Self lies beyond the thinking mind beyond natural feeling, beyond action or any movement of even the highest state of consciousness. The Self-God is more solid than a neutron star, more elusive than empty space, more intimate than thought and feeling. It is ultimate reality itself. The innermost Truth, all seekers seek. It is well worth striving for. It is well worth struggling to bring the mind under the dominion of the will. After the Self is realized, the mind is seen for the unreality that it truly is. Because Self-Realisation must be experienced in a physical body, the soul cycles back again and again into flesh to dance with Śiva, live with Śiva and ultimately merge with Śiva in undifferentiated oneness. Jīva is actually Śiva. Just as water poured into water, milk poured into milk, ghee into ghee become one without differentiation. Even so the individual soul and the Supreme Self become one.

The Self is hidden in all beings like butter in milk. Subtle seers who are endowed with pure, sharp see it and subtle intellect and who practise constant deep meditation regularly.[9] Just as you extract butter from buttermilk by the process of churning, even so you will have to take out the Ātmā from the Koṣas by the churning of constant meditation with the help of the churning of the energy wheels or cakra's.

In the practice of the contemplation the frequency range of the interaction is 11 dimensional between the person and the higher power in the cosmos. This is called the unity of Jīva to Śiva. Śiva is the higher strength, which consists of 11 forms of happiness, rest, peace and harmony radiate among other things on the earth and within which we can focus ours place. This irradiation is expressed in the pūjā with the Dikapālas. Jñāna yoga (knowledge and practical experience) contain the total process of pūjā, yoga and everything around,

---

[9] Ten Upanisads; Swami Sivananda; A Divine Life Society Publication; Tehri- Garhwal; U.P. Himalaya's; 1993 (page 34); Vedānta-sāra Upaniśad, mantra 3.

concerning language, sign, wisdom and insight. In spiritual sense, yoga and pūjā, are the two hands of people which become the cosmic underlying icons, which are able to witness and understand. Pūjā is the right hand of life, in living and also after life. Mainly of the vedā's concerning the concentration and meditation in and during the pūjā.

Concerning the karma of people we talk about of a higher form of energy. This energy is based on the current state or the person's karma. As mentioned above we called these energies demigods and Ṛṣis, super visions and seers (bookkeepers) in people who are in service of humanity. Both have also ended up by means of a human body at a high spiritual level and are now in astral form. This astral form is also a body by which they fulfil their cosmic duty as a donor or an ăccountant. All energy or gods (devi's or deva's) that are active in our body operate with astral strength such as an e-mail. They are in super microform. We can't deny that we are becoming stronger or intelligent both in our body and in cosmos the basic principle applies give and take just the way we usually do in common life.

Number 16 in Yoga

Writers down the ages have expressed their admiration for hidden meanings behind numbers. Take for instance the number sixteen. It is encountered in various places in nature, in the universe and within us. Both the upper and the lower jaw of human beings have 16 teeth. Teeth must mill the food (sacrifice) before it can pass through. The cheeks are being moved both by the powers of Viśuddha (Throat) and of the Ājñā (third eye) to mill it. This process is called Svāhā just as in a Homa or sacrificial ceremony. The number 16 can also be traced in the human body. For instance the Viśuddha-cakra where the soul, as part of God, resides has 16 lotus leaves.

In this connection we see the correlation between the Yajña and the Ājñā. First the food passes the Viśuddha where man is central, the so called ātmā-Pūjā. The ātmā or Jīva resides in the throat. Then it goes in Ojas in essence form throughout the Ājñā to the brains where the godly energies of Daivic-śaktiyān originate.

The planet Jupiter or Bṛhaspati, which stands as a symbol of God, has 16 moons. The compilers of the Vedās were aware of this. Only recently were they proven right.[10] Bṛhaspati by the way, is his shape as Paṇḍit, the biggest Guru; the original Paṇḍit who teaches ceremonies to human beings and leaves behind a prototype. At every ritual ceremony Bṛhaspati is honoured as the first one in the section Svastivācana (introduction or invocation). This goes as follows: 'May the Master of vast knowledge, may Mighty God prosper us. May the Nourisher of all, the Author of all the Vedās prosper us. May He, the Giver of all comforts like the horse, prosper us. May God, the Lord of all the elements of Nature, vouchsafe us prosperity.

The 16 moons of Jupiter symbolize the 16 qualities (kalā's) of God who is not manifested and impenetrable. The secret of the creation has been revealed by the Puruṣa Sūkta. It contains 16 hymns and occurs in all four Vedā's. Jupiter as Bṛhaspati is in the Third Eye in a micro shape, which makes a link at sufficient devotion with the mother planet Jupiter in the cosmos. In this way a balance arises both inside and outside the body. As a result, the soul is able to travel outside the body, where the zero-point in the forehead cakra (Ājñā) is focussed like a flashlight on the fontanel. This astral connection in the yoga practitioner is identical to those of the sun on the neutral points (to the blue of the sky), two points on both sides of the sun in which the polarisation of the sky decreases to a minimum. The rest is the zero point in the brain at the fontanel. At rest the length of exhaled air is 16 inches (Angulam).[11] The breathing exercise or Prānāyāma is for a healthy and long life indispensable. The breath brings energy in people who innovate structures in society.

The awakening of the Kuṇḍalini is the end aim of yoga. Kuṇḍalini is the Cosmic Power in the Cakra in our body.

---

[10] The illustrated guide to Astronomy; Bill Yenne; Ars Scribendi BV; Harmelen; Belgium; 1995 (page 181).

[11] Secret Power or Tantrik Breathing; Swami Sivapriyananda; Abhinav publications; New Delhi; 1996.

Because God is Energy, this energy is also Goddess. With this energy the soul merges with the Super Soul. For more detail, see below. Once awoken, it purifies and harmonises this cosmic energy in the body and as a result of which a human being becomes One with the creation. Humans should aim at Awakening and mastering the Kuṇḍalini. It especially concerns the state of mind that all inclinations and desires are in balance. One becomes calm and peaceful. The implications of yoga and spiritual teachings are also considered for the problem of war and peace. What is even more important, yoga offers a programme of personal commitment to real peace. This practice of yoga gives practices and contemplations that will help those working for peace to cultivate peace within which eliminating all seeds of violence. The limbs as well as the systems of yoga are tools to reduce violence in and outside our body, and to create a turning point between violence and non-violence. This separation automatically becomes a merging between the mind and body.

In the world library Encarta we find that in the state of harmonisation in music sound assumes 16 harmonics as most important. Modern science declares that in the state of harmonisation, sound (music) assumes 16 harmonics. The frequencies of these harmonics are multiples of the frequency of the fundamentals. Young, healthy persons hear sounds between 16 kHz to 20 kHz; sounds under 16 Hz we hear as disturbance, and we can't hear sounds above 16 to 20 kHz. In old age a fall of up to 9 kHz is normal.[12]

The voice of a boy changes at the age of 16. He develops a beard. This is called the milk beard. According to developmental psychology the adolescent years (between 16-20 years), is when sexual maturity is reached, but mental maturity is still incomplete. The body develops like a neutral line or a magnet and is free for possible (unfavourable) influence as soon as the Larynx or throat cakra is activated by the Kuṇḍalini. Here we find the 16 vowels or svaras of the Sanskrit alphabet. This alphabet is a compilation of energy

[12] Encarta 2005 and www.hku.nl/usa/central/index.html.

sources. The signs are photographs of energy types that hide behind these characters. In the central part of those characters the Śakti—or energy conscience of the individual remains. The female energy or Yoni-divisions in the cosmos are also indicated as 16 Kalā's or qualities of the moon. Fifteen of these represent the change of the positions of the moon in all circumstances (see figures 14 and 15), whereas the 16th is Lalita-Tripurasundari or the Śakti-consciousness. Lalitā has her own (Gāyatrī) mantra, which is as follows: Oṃ Tripurasundaryai Vidmahe Kameśvaryai Dhimahi Tanno Klinne Pracodayāt.

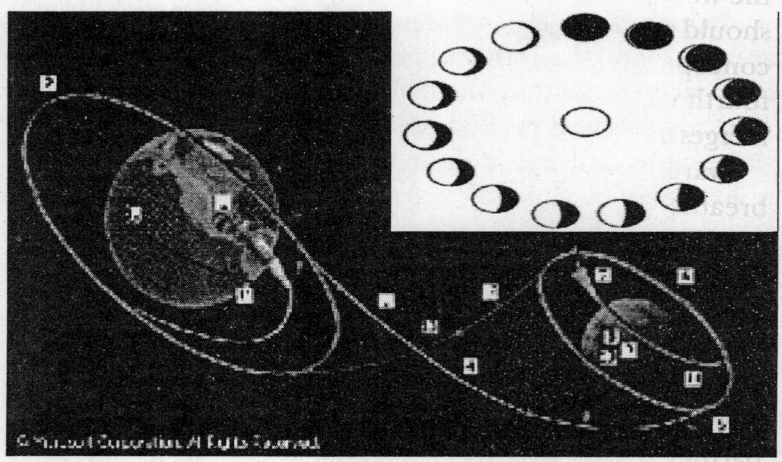

Figures 14 and 15 The exchange in the positions of the moon

She is the Devi (Angle) of the sounds within the cosmic knowledge (svara's) whereas Śiva (Īśvara) has control of the consonances. This is the link between the soul with the All-soul (Jīva-Śiva; Svara-Īśvara). The combination of Śiva-Śakti feeds knowledge, wisdom and spirituality, and develops harmony. These 16 characters connect the energy of the body by means of the Third Eye in the astral body. In this matter the 16 sacraments are indispensable in life.

Yoga and Svara (Sound)

The immaterial processes in the human being are coordinated by the Kuṇḍalini Power. Kuṇḍalini is described as a Devi or goddess luminous as lightning, who lies asleep in the root cakra coiled like a serpent three and a half times round the Svayambhūliṅga which is there, and closing the entrance to the Śuṣuṁṇā or the centre of the backbone with her head. Nothing is said as to the outer layer of the force being active in all persons, but this fact is indicated in the statement that even as she sleeps she maintains all breathing creatures. Breathing means life. And she is spoken of as the Śabda Brahmā, the Energy or voices for wisdom, in the human body. Śabda means word or sound. In the process of the creation of the world this sound was issued in four stages. We probably should not be far wrong in associating these with the Western conceptions of the three states of body, soul and spirit, and a fourth which is union with the Divine or All-spirit. And Yoga merges the "union between the human soul and the Divine soul."

Svarodya-vijñāna, is the science of prediction about the breather's health, his future and auspicious, or inauspicious possibilities in various steps of life through the rise of breathing in one or the other nostril. Due to a causal relationship the Prāña vāyu and the Manas are one. Although, due to the diversity of the sūkṣma-Śakti (Subtle Power) the activities and fruits of Svarodaya are infinite, yet a little of it is being described here for the benefit of the Yogis. There is no better partner in life than the Svara-vijñāna. This wealth is a secret in our life. Destruction of enemies, meeting with members of the fraternity, achievement of wealth, fame and bride, interview with kings, and even subjugation of kings-all these can be achieved through Svara-vijñana. All the Puranās, Smṛtis, Vedāṅgas and Tantras, holy books and formulas, have originated from Svara. This science of Svarodaya is superior to all other sciences. Just as one needs torchlight in order to see the things in a house, so for self- enlightenment one needs the knowledge of Svarodaya to get insight in the inner self.

The Vāyu or air is composed with. We breathe only and the breath is called: Svara. The air of our breath carries several kinds of energies for production to keep the body alive. Our body is a huge factory that fabricates, transports and exerts products internally. There are ten kinds of Vāyus (Airs) residing in the body, viz., Prāṇa, Apāna, Samāna, Udāna,Vyāna, Nāga, Kūrma, Kṛkara, Devadatta and Dhanañjaya. All these Vāyus keep roaming in the various vessels of the body. A person adept in the science of Svarodaya experiences the activities of these Vāyus through the three most important Nādis or transport channels—the Piṅgala, Iḍa, and Śuṣuṁṇā.

Yoga and Devanāgarī

The importance of happiness and for the pleasure of this world we find in the following quotation in the Veda (AV 4.14.4: 696):

"Emancipated souls, in their march to salvation, the abode of happiness, don't aspire for the pleasures of this world. Transgressing both the Earth and Heaven, they continue their progress till they reach the world of light. The learned aspirants after salvation, do realise, the nature of soul and God, the showerers of happiness" (see also YV 17.69: 919).

Yoga is impossible without happiness. The characters of Sanskrit are indicated on the leaves of the lotus of the cakras or energy wheels as potentials. Happiness is a product of the energy driven up by the cakras and which becomes visible on the face of people, viz. a yogi. This is why happiness has been mentioned as the red thread in yoga and pūjā or sacrificial ceremony. On the one hand these ceremonies in daily life serve as cooling and on the other hand are loading or filling fresh energy products of the cosmos by means of the way of concentration and meditation. This literally means: it is on the one hand making the body passive (neutral situation) and on the other hand removing dust or noise from the soul through sound or ultrasound.

Devanāgarī is a cosmic alphabet, a "group photograph" of sources, which transmit positive energy, and is expressed in our voice. These are vowels and consonances of energies. Besides this group we still have uncountable energy types in the cosmos with other sorts of effects. The Devanāgrī is therefore a compilation of icons that improve rest, happiness and positive thinking. Both yoga and pūjā use mantras or hymns to join ideas. 'Mantra' literally means "that which liberates the mind." Mantra is often a word or words in Sanskrit. The soul is like an active moving mantra. She is our real identity and the body is the vehicle of identity or soul. Regarding the study of sound and language, the first and foremost question that stands is, how when and where the language originated. Among the hosts of theories on the origin of speech is one contended by almost all the scholars, both at home and abroad, that the Vedās are the profounder of the divine origin of speech (RV. 8.100.11)

According to the Kularnava Tantra[13] as mentioned before, Sanskrit characters are images of energy in the cosmos. The Kularnava is the Devanāgarī, which also presents the Sanskrit alphabet. This is a cosmic route map of spiritual parameters in the eternal cosmic sphere, which has at least 9 supernatural qualities or koṣas. These koṣas are helpful to people in daily life. Devanāgarīes can be compared with cosmonauts, medical students and doctors who perform their practices and or services under supervision of their superiors. This logical formation sector in the cosmos with relation to people turns Hinduism into a philosophy of life instead of a religion. Planets are therefore gods or higher strengths. People are already visiting planets in the universe. For instant: people are already walks on the moon.

Devanāgarī means a "village or dwelling" of deva's (devi's) or energy donors. For computer science they produce 'bites' with ... 1 and 0. Each number represents cosmic energy (devi or deva) and the cosmos itself. The capacity is a plural of this combination. As we have already mentioned in the Introductory chapter, Cosmic capacities are obtained by means of meditation. These higher energies were former masters of the universe. By contact with the Kulā or Gotra at the pūjā time we make direct link with these spiritual predecessors with the result; the devotee obtains blessings from the highest representatives or agents of god in heaven.

[13] Kulah is the dynasty with energies of the 9th koṣa (Nava means 9) or spiritual qualities and treatises on ritual, meditation, discipline. In the Sanskrit grammar we see that the Visarga is changing, the consonance Ha, in a half character of the consonance Ra, the so-called Ardha or half Rudra: RV 10.90.2.

These are the celestial gurus which people turn to for help on a daily base. The 52 selected icons of Devanāgarī are a force of cosmic diplomats in the sky where higher strengths accompany daily persuits. These are positive icons which carry out the good presentation and ambiance. These 52 are ever changing and multiply in 20x50 to produce the optimum spiritual strength for the yogi in the Sahasrāra cakra. At this stage he multiplies its spiritual capacity with Sahasrāra (means 1,000 or 50x20). This is the sum total of all the lotus leafs with Sanskrit characters in 6 underlying cakras. Devanāgarī is a larger society of the devi's and deva's then just the 52 characters of the Sanskrit alphabet. This society has a larger enforcement in the cosmos for or remaining activities. These so-called "armies of gods" are the guards of the cosmos and humanity. Of course there are demonic strengths as a contra army, which we avoid, in daily contact and or in language use.

Yoga and Havan (fire sacrifice)

The term 'Havan' has been described as follow. Ha is Śakti or energy and Va is rhythm or vibration; time or age. The Rīg Vedā confirms this process in the first mantra. By means of the Purohita Agni the essence of sacrifice transfers to god. The Purohita filters the sacrifice by means of the Veda mantras with their appropriate gestures and rituals. Fire sacrifice is a mass energy as oil for the maintenance of the cosmos, particularly the ozone layer. This happens by the acquired characteristic of oxygen in which the molecules from three atoms exist with a strongly oxidising and disinfecting capacity; it arises from ordinary oxygen. The cosmos is a part within God himself. This part is our house that needs maintenance. The Vedā's contain cosmic mysteries, which are required for this maintenance. This keeps up in the cosmos and improves physical condition and purifies the soul. There are modifications of our properties with influence of changed life conditions. One is here for giving, whereas one works daily to deserve. Life exists from a balance between two acquired characteristics, namely giving and taking.

In the Vārāha Upaniṣad the term jewel (ratna) of the first mantra of the Rīg Vedā is clarified. This Upaniṣad's talk of ratna pūritā dhātu-blood filled with pearls, i.e. jewels of life force. In today's language it is called hormones. When blood is filled with jewels of life force, then there is buoyancy of life, benevolence of the heart and hence peace (RV 1.1):

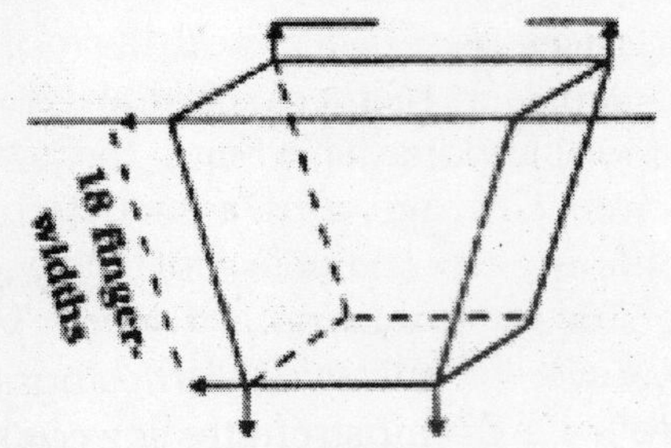

12 finger-widths

Figure 16 The shape of a Havan Kuṇḍa

18 finger-widths

A Havan is always performed in a Kuṇḍa (firepit). The kuṇḍa is usually like an inverted pyramid, narrow at the bottom and broad on the top. The bottom should be a square of about twelve finger-widths of the one performing the Homa. The top should be one and a half times the bottom, which makes it eighteen finger-widths. The height of the Kuṇḍa should be about the same size as of the top. Digging an inverted pyramid like opening in the ground, keeping the bottom narrow and the top broad, as shown in the figure makes the Kuṇḍa.

The term 'deva' means give, what is also confirmed in this mantra. Through sacrifice the foundation is laid for a higher sort of creature which can also be reached by yoga. A spiritual aspirant tries to discriminate and control all the urges of the bodily senses as well as the mind, and it is this self-control (Sv. Up. 1:15; 2:2) which enables him to submit himself to the inner voice or controller or consciousness, to reach Self-realisation (Bh.G. 5:21-26; 10:11,20,22; Kaṭha Up. 3.3-12).

The well-known donor in our body is the celestial god, Indra, who has the management of our mind system and has provided us with knowledge and wisdom. That is why during the pūjā we sacrifice to him as a generous donor. In meditation he appears in our conscience and awakes the mind until we are cosmically aware of our identity. This astral god is beyond the cycle of reincarnation. This is the training period where we reach the zero point or turning point, which is in the third eye and is the resting-place. It is in following intensive prayer that one experiences rest, peace, and harmony. In a yoga-session, in this stage, tears begin to roll down the face and the nose becomes moist and may also begin to flow. This is as an indicator for joy, courage and a healthy, long life. A spontaneous smile appears on the face of the yogi as becoming a symbol of the link and interaction of energy between inner and external nature. One lives on with happiness and this becomes alive in love. Then happiness flows to its source, the heart. That's the result of good meditation which ends in a glorious smile. This smile is not seen in the material world. Smile therefore is certainly no pocket piece.

Yoga of idols or anionic forms of deities is probably the most common and important ritual performed by followers of contemporary Hinduism. Compared to the sacrificial ceremonies of Vedic religion which still take place occasionally but which are relics of a religion that can no longer be considered as living, Yoga is performed daily.

Cakras are activated energy from a bigger nature to breathe, to filter the inner self and to give much more energy to the micro organisms in the body. This purification process is called Prāṇāyāma. Prāṇāyāma is a part both of the pūjā and the yoga. The lighting mechanism has therefore an ambiguous aim. This ambiguous aim retrieves in the term spirituality, foundation of the energy processes and spirit (inner) and rituality (inner and external). Spirituality reinforces the inner will and increases methodically. This means that yoga is pūjā or the other way around, also because each form of yoga acknowledges the merger of the soul with the Super soul.

Yoga and Mantras

Both yoga and pūjā occur by mantras. Especially in pūjā we

use a lot of mantras. Mantras change and heal our brain. Our brain forms the dwelling of the gods. From our larynx to the head we called this the heaven and below the larynx till the legs is called the hell. Ojas (eightfold extract of the body juices) and mantras have the same impact for achieving salvation. The quantity ojas stipulates the enlightening process of the person. There are a lot of mantras. They are classified as Vedic mantras, Tantrika mantras and Purānic mantras. A subdivision is in: sātvic mantras, which are recited for enlightenment, wisdom, divine love, compassion etc; rājesic mantras, which are recited for offspring and prosperity; and tāmasic mantrās to appease bad spirits, to do harm upon others or to commit evil deeds. If the mantra is used to commit evil, it is called vāma-mārga or black magic. The conclusion: Mantras are keys for liberation.[14]

Just as milk pervading the entire body of a cow comes out only through her udder, so also the Supreme Ātmā, though all pervasive, develops only in the Divya-deśas (divine places). A Sādhaka is instructed to worship in any of these Divya-deśas according to his qualifications. All these are extremely helpful in obtaining Yoga-siddhi. With the help of Dhāraṇā the Iṣṭadevata, the favorite God, manifests in the Divya-deśas. Divya-desaśevāna is extremely beneficial in Mantrayoga.[15]

Yoga and Physical Exercises

The aim of Yogic exercises is to activate the cakras found in the body. For a better understanding of the treatment in this chapter, I will give below a summary of the discussion. Cakras form the ganglions (nerve junctions) or centres of strength and consciousness in the human body. The frequencies of vibration of the cakras correspond with the planets in the universe in and with which they are connected. This connection takes care of the exchange of power between the individual and his environment e.g. the universe. To that purpose the human body contains nerve junctions and glands. The seven

---

[14] Yogacārya Astadala Yogamala; B.K.S. Iyengar; Allied Publishers Limited; New Delhi; 2000.

[15] Mantra-Yoga Samhita; Dr. Ramkumar Rai; Chaukhambha Orientalia; A house of Oriental and Antiquarian Books; Delhi; 1982 (pag.71).

main cakras can clearly be perceived as colourful multi-bladed wheels or lotuses. They are found along the spinal cord from the base up to the skull. For this, see the survey 'cakras'. There are seven cakras under the spine which are hardly visible. These are seats of instinctive consciousness, the source of jealousy, hatred, envy, guilt, grief, etc. They form the lower or infernal world, better known as Naraka or Hell. Thus there are altogether 14 important cakras. The cakras, arranged according to their position and quality of interactions, can be divided into two groups of seven cakras each (RV 1.154.1).

The seven higher cakras are:

- Mūlādhāra (at the base of the spine): controls memory, time and space;
- Svādhiṣṭhāna (under the navel): controls reason;
- Maṇipūra (solar plexus): controls the will;
- Anāhata (centre of the heart): immediate and conscious knowing;
- Viśuddha (throat): divine love, seat of the soul;
- Ājñā (third eye): divine insight;
- Sahasrāra (crown): enlightenment, divinity.

The seven lower cakras are:

- Atala (hips): fear and lust;
- Vitala (thighs): white rage;
- Sutala (knees): jealousy and revenge;
- Talātala (calves): constant mental confusion;
- Rasātala (ankles): selfishness;
- Mahātala (feet): lack of scruples;
- Pātāla (soles): murder and malice (to trample).

For people with a busy working schedule at the office, there is a simple and safe technique, called the Office Yoga. This yoga is a practice of simple movements which one can do a few minutes at a time throughout the day. These practices relieve the tensions and stress of sedentary working life. It contains stretching, breathing exercises. These are simple, safe and fun to do, most of which can be done sitting in your chair at your desk.

Respiration

Air is of vital importance for human existence. Through air, breath comes into our lungs and further into our body. Without air and breath man and all life on earth would die. Breath played a role in the coming into existence of man as we read in Genesis (2:7): "And the Lord God formed man from dust of off the ground, and breathed into his nostrils the breath of life; and man became a living soul."

If God withdraws the supply of air, life on our planet will come to an end. In this section I therefore intend to elaborate on this matter.

Cells that control our respiration are called "respiratory cells." They are situated behind the brains on the area called medulla oblongata. The nerves in this centre are connected with the nerves in the higher centres of the brains and the spine and therefore the emotional state of our mind can influence our breathing. Emotional stress can increase the frequency of breathing, whereas emotional calmness can decrease it. Man long before modern science already knew the close connection between the frequency of our breathing and the emotional state of our mind. The earliest civilisations, for example those of India and China, developed methods to control breathing and to bring about a change in emotions and the state of consciousness by means of breathing. In Taoism there is a breathing exercise which is known as T-ai-si or embryonic breathing. The Chinese practise this breathing exercise with a view to longevity. The Sufis also practised control of breathing.

The Dhikr technique of the Moslems is similar to some of the Hindu breathing exercises. Thousands of years ago the seers discovered that there is a vital cycle in the body which is called 'Prāṇa'. They also discovered that there is a close connection between breathing and Prāṇa, between Prāṇa and thinking and thoughts and mind. To put it briefly, they discovered that Prāṇa is related to the whole mechanism of the body and they developed a training system which is called Prāṇāyāma. Etymologically Prāṇa means "life force" or "elixir of life". Yama is 'death'. The life force which thwarts death e.g. which consciously and constructively seeks out death, but now in the form of mokṣa, in which death is controlled by breathing rhythms. Breathing slowly and quietly results in deep relaxation and extends our lifespan, whereas the effect is the other way round when breathing rapidly. At birth a being (including plants and insects) is not allotted a lifespan but a fixed number of bṛeaths. The one that breaths rapidly will die sooner (e.g. the frog) whereas one that breaths slowly will live very long, like the elephant. There are many trees that live longer than people. In the programme Heaven's Breath of 02-11-1997 from the English television network Discovery, scientists disclosed that at birth, a baby is given a supply of 600 million breathings. Harish Johari indicates that the number of breaths for a human being has been set at 946.080.000, at 15 breaths per minute.[16] The corresponding age is set at 120 years. With this every human being's life is determined.

At birth man is not supplied with years of life but with a supply of Prāṇa or 'breath'. The breath gives life force, the most essential and indispensable nourishment for the body. Life force enables the body as well as the mind to function and to react to inward and outward impressions and/or incentives. If, at a given moment, the body does not function anymore to work out its karma because breathing has stopped, the soul will leave this physical body because it has become worthless. We then speak of death. Hence Prāṇāyāma is a system, not only for living a long life, but also for living a life of harmony in which one's ideal of life can be realised. Even in Christianity there is evidence that breath was used for spiritual enlightenment.

Fast and deep breathing for a longer period of time results in losing CO_2 (Carbon Dioxide) too rapidly. This leads to inelasticity of the muscles, stupor (coma, apathy) and cataleptic coma (Y). Many religions use incessant reciting, song and dance to get into a trance. A method to increase the CO_2

[16] Breath, Mind and Consciousness; Harish Johari; Rochester; Vermont; Destiny Books; U.S.A.; 1989 (page 15).

percentage in the blood is by breathing slowly. Increasing the percentage of CO_2 in the blood means a decrease of the percentage of oxygen (O_2), which results in anoxia, a feeling of lightness in the head and a trance-like feeling, which sometimes can lead to mystic experiences. Meditation and yoga try to influence the CO_2 percentage in the blood via the Prāṇāyāma method, in order to attain a mystic state.

By controlling the movement of the lungs and the respiratory organs one can indirectly control the Prāṇa, which vibrates within all of us. Some people practise a sort of Prāṇāyāma which is called Pūraka(to fill up). Others practise a sort of Prāṇāyāma which is called Recaka (to empty). Others again practise Kumbhaka, in which breath is arrested in the body. Usually the practice of Prāṇāyāma is a combination of Pūraka, Kumbhaka and Recaka. Pūraka or to inhale. Inhale through the left nostril. Now think of the navel, plus Viṣṇu. Kumbhaka or to hold back. Now the second nostril is pinched. Now think of the Heart, plus Brahmā. Recaka or to exhale. Now exhale slowly through the right nostril. Now think of the Forehead, plus Śiva.

There are several sorts of Prāṇāyāma. They are divided in Adhama, Madhyama and Uttama. This division is the result of the time difference in the Pūraka (to inhale) period. The time gap between Pūraka, Kumbhaka and Recaka is in each of the three methods 1:4:2.

In literature it is pointed out that a person's health and character are, to a large extent, reflected in his breathing pattern. In general, people who breathe short are weak, nervous and very unreliable; whereas those who breathe long and deeply are mostly reliable and happy people. When someone gets excited, his breathing pattern changes rapidly because he gradually breathes shorter. When someone develops exalted thoughts within himself, he will gradually breathe more slowly.

In the Vedās it is stated that man needs 21.600 breathings in a twenty-four hour period in order to live a wholesome life. This means that one should aim at a breathing pattern of an average of 15 breathings per minute. According to the data of the Vedās the number of breathings for a lifetime of one hundred years can be estimated at about 700 million. This number correlates with the number of the male's sperm cells per ejaculation.

Relation of respiration with age

Ordinarily a human being breathes about 13 to 15 times per minute. Thus, in a full day and night (24 hours) the total number of respirations reaches to about 21,000. It is an established fact that lesser is the number of respirations of an organism per minute, the greater is his life-span. In other words if we control and minimise the number of our respirations we can increase our life-span.

Svara and its Rise: Many people may not have noticed this but it is a fact that the continuous act of Inspiration and Expiration instead of being performed simultaneously through both the nostrils is performed with a fixed periodic rhythm through left and right nostrils alternately. That is, when the period of one nostril is over breathing automatically passes in to the other nostril for almost the same period. This act of breathing is called Svara, and passing of this act from one nostril to the other is called Udaya or Rise of breath on that nostril. This Svara + Udaya = Svarodaya, is thus a Science of Divination from the rise of breathing in one or the other nostril. Duration of respiration in one Nostril: After the rise of breathing in any nostril it continues through it for 2 Ghaṭakas or one hour. This means that breathing alternates from one to the other nostril after every one hour in a rhythmic manner.

Name of the Svaras: The left Nasal passage is called Iḍā and right the Piṅgalā. The middle passage is called Śūṣuṁṇā. When the Svara is flowing through the left nostril it is called Īśvara and when it is flowing through the right nostril it is called Piṅgalā-svara. When however, the Svara is flowing through both nostrils simultaneously or alternates erratically in both nostrils, it is called Śuṣuṁṇā-svara.

The Idā is representative of Moon and the Piṅgalā of Sun. Therefore, the Iḍā-svara is called Moon-svara and the Piṅgalā-svara the Sun-svara.

In order to follow the subsequent descriptions these various names of the three Svaras must be kept in mind. Method of knowing the Svara: Press one nostril and note if breathing is going on in the other unobstructed. In case there is obstruction then the former nostril should be left and this one is pressed. Now if the breathing is going on completely unobstructed in the former then it is that nostril through which the Svara is flowing. For example, press the left nostril first, if the right is breathing completely unobstructed. If there is obstruction then leave the left and now press the right nostril and see if the left is breathing smoothly and in an unobstructed manner. If there is no obstruction then it should be presumed that the left Svara is flowing.[17] However, if there is no obstruction in either, or there is some obstructions in both then it should be presumed that the Śuṣuṁṇā-Svara is flowing. Thus the nature of the Svara should first be determined before proceeding to any prognostic inference.

Method of changing the Svara from one Nostril to another: Whenever there may be a necessity or desire to change the respiration from one nostril to another, one should lie down for a while sideways on the side of which the nostril is breathing at the moment. Soon the breathing would change over to the other nostril. For example, if one is breathing from the left nostril, and wants to change it to the right, he should lie sideways pressing the left side. This will automatically change his breathing to the right nostril. In other words, one should lie to the opposite side of the nostril of which he wants his breathing to change over. Lying on the left side will induce breathing through the right nostril, and vice versa.

Kuṇḍalini Yoga

Haṭha Yoga prepares the body for the spiritual path via physical and breathing exercises. It is the most superficial component of Tantra Yoga for it merely prepares and conditions the body so that the individual can practise meditation with fewer obstacles. Patañjali has given a list of thirteen distractions:

[17] Sivasvarodaya; Ram Kumar Rai; Prachya Prakashan Varanasi; Second Edition 1987.

Vyādhi (physical disease), styāna (langour, mental laziness, sluggishness, lack of interest), saṁśaya (doubt, disbelief, indecision), pramāda (negligence, carelessness), ālasya (physical laziness, idleness), avirati (self-indulgence, sensual gratification), bhrāntidarśana (living in the world of illusion, mistaken notion, erroneous views), alabdhabhūmikatva (missing the point, failure to reach the aim), anavasthitatva (backsliding, inability to maintain the progress achieved, inability to maintain steadiness in the practice). These are the causes of mental distractions (citta vikṣepa). Pain (dukha), dejection (daurmanasya), tremor of the body (aṅgamejayatva) and irregular, laboured or heavy inbreaths and outbreaths (śvāsa-praśvāsa) are the companions (sahabhuva) of mental distractions (PYS 1.30 en 31).

These are the obstacles enumerated by Patañjali, from physical disease to tremors of the body (today we call this Parkinson's disease), heaviness of breath and cardiac diseases. If there is rheumatism in any part of the body, the intelligence cannot flow in these areas. For this reason the yogis traced different āsanas so that the trillions of cells in the body, which are born in a split second and die in a split second, may have fresh blood brought to them so that they are fully activated. Today these are lifeless stillborn cells because we do not use them.

The main components in Yoga are the postures or āsanas. The word 'āsana' means 'comfortable, stable poise'. The aim of the āsanas is for the meditator to learn to control his or her breathing. A particular āsana, the 'lotus', is considered to be the best posture for meditation. In lotus, the spine locks in a straight position and the posture can be maintained for a long time without breaks in concentration. Maintaining a straight spine is important for meditation since the poise permits the rising of kuṇḍalini (see figure below), or 'spiritual energy,' from the lowest cakra at the base of the spine to the highest at the crown of the head. According to tantrik teachings, 'cakras' are energy centres located in various parts of the body, through which spiritual energy can flow. The rising of kuṇḍalini during meditation marks the onset of a mystical experience (see figure 17).

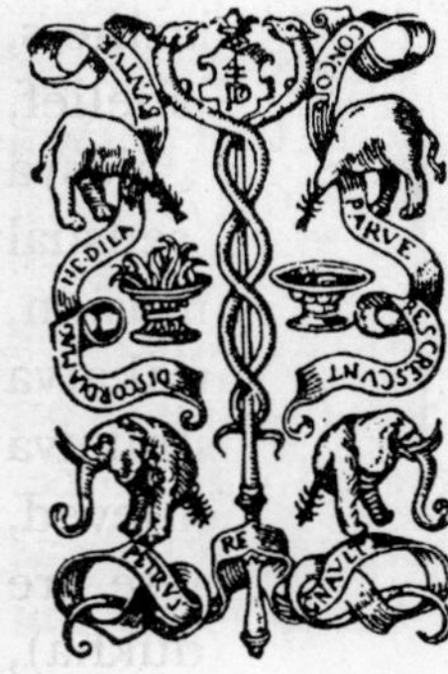

Figure 17
Aesculapius, the rising Kuṇḍalini

'Sādhana' or tantrika meditation involves concentrating on a particular object or thought, such as a candle flame, image of a deity or a mantra, for a stretch of time, which can take from less than 30 minutes to long hours. One of the commonest forms of meditation, which is also used by meditators studied in this dissertation, is focusing on a 'mantra'. 'Mantra' literally means "that which liberates the mind." The mantra is often a word in Sanskrit, which is used in the Pūjā, the offer ceremony, or given in secret by a spiritual master to a disciple. Each meditator has his or her particular mantra to concentrate upon during meditation. Meditation almost invariably induces relaxation, and a feeling of inner peace, as it reduces the stream of thoughts coming to mind. These characteristics are inherent to the pathway to a mystical experience.

According to Tantric literature, there is a very mysterious and powerful force in the human body, which bears the name of Kuṇḍalini-force or 'Snake-force'. It lies, as a snake in a coiled up and inactive position, at the base of the spine, at the Mūlādhāra-cakra. As, according to the Tantras, this immense force remains in a dormant state during a person's life, most people are not aware of its existence. It is assumed that if someone develops himself spiritually through meditation or Prāṇāyāma, this force slowly rises through the Śūṣaṁṇā nerve (spinal marrow). This ascending of the Kuṇḍalini-force is known as the awakening of the Kuṇḍalini (see figure 19).

This force rises slowly and steadily and does not shoot up in a straight line. When it passes through each of the psychic centres (Cakras), the person is given complete control of one of his senses. When, for example, it reaches the Maṇipura-Cakra, opposite the navel, the person gets complete control of his eyesight. Without the awakening of this force a samādhi (union with God) is not possible. It is described, that the

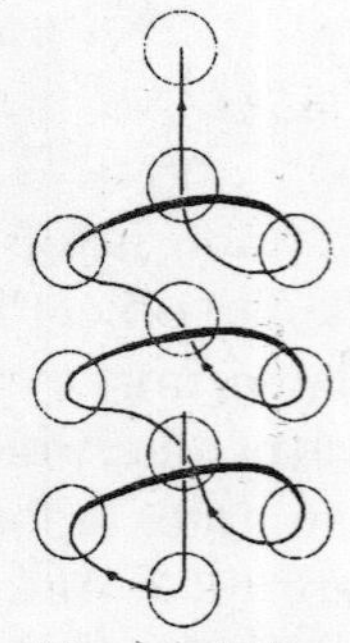

Figure 18 The awakening of the Kuṇḍalini

kuṇḍalini-force passes through all six Cakras and might be united with Sahasrāra at the top of the head. If this happens, that person obtains cosmic consciousness, the highest form of realisation.

By activating the cakras and by meditating on Sadā Śiva (Śiva in trance) on the crown one tries to get into a trance. Here Mā Durgā plays an important role as Siddhidātrī (Śakti) and Pārvatī (as the spouse of Śiva).

Yoga and Śāntikāla

The zero point is also compared with a radar system (explained in the Introduction) which rotates in the Ājñā-or fore head Cakra and where the third eye awakens. It is the point or place where reality becomes enlightened and the illusory energy disappears. In this centre arises unity with the cosmos and in astral form we move through the cosmos from one centre planet to another (planets). As soon as we reach this point, tension, stress and other kind of mental diseases are removed. The rest and peace in this center serves as a medicine and has been confessed as Śāntikāla. Śāntikāla is the "sphere or peace", the level within Śuddha māyā where forms are made of inner sounds and colours and where great energies reside. These energies confessed as devas and Ṛṣis (seers), smaller than an atom, help an aspirant or student to concentrate in his study or research.

Yoga reduces the passive status of the soul and raises her frequency or acceleration, as a car, which accelerates from neutral into the first acceleration. Interaction takes place between people and its energy source (functioning in the cosmos as a clerk), the engine becomes effective which multiplies the energy in people. This is necessary to be able to absorb the values in the cosmos and to communicate with the higher power. Change in cosmos is a constant. Due to this a combination arises between rest (0, zero) and action (1, one). The invention of the computer is a large step in the development of people. Nowadays everything is controlled by the computer, both in the world of peace and in the world of disorder (war and weapons). In computer language 0 and 1 become one bit. Human mind is the largest computer in the world. Yoga here has been defined as the connection between the human and cosmic computer. The various paths of Yoga are considered to be the different files in the hardware system. We can download knowledge in the field of sport, commerce, policy etc. and exploit them. The connection that arises in that relation between people and cosmos, is happiness, love and piety.

Yoga as Software

This software is necessary for everyone on earth to understand and to get an insight of the cosmos. These three pillars are the basis of yoga. People have already developed techniques at a rather high level. Supersonic planes which are in use for a long time. They have a speed above that of sound. Telephone, computer, fax, Internet, e-mail, digital photograph, digital camera etc. are digital instruments which are invisible, but are used by people for important aims. This is called the Internet Technology (IT) which applies in this time and is indispensable. One who can't handle the computer, can't keep up longer with market developments and is not in accordance with market systems. These processes take place in the astral part as a light source of our universe. In the astral body, the aura field, of the cosmos there are a lot of energy sources which are invisible. These are cosmic energy sources or icons. Hinduism knows a lot of large and small icons or energy donors (devas). They give strength and offer space to enter in the film-or sky layers of the universe. Arousing the strength of the dam is mostly translated by many as adoring a god whereas it concerns a relation and or connection based on love and piety.

Some call these energy forms gods who are in service of the large architect of the cosmos. They find their legitimacy to adore them in favour of strength and blessing. A spiritual or yoga approach of this relation is a link with a higher source of energy similar to that between people and the light of the sun.

A yogi downloads the cosmic energy or fundamental tones from nature. The body as an instrument is brought concentration on the correct tone just like a musician handles his instrument. According to yogic science receiving the energies or sounds is just like a range of diatonic tones and the other following tones of an octave.

The yogi is able to increase the speed or capacity by meditation. The speed can be faster than the largest computer and the fastest e-mail in the world. It depends on the density in his yoga programme, which has been carried out consciously and constructively. For this reason it's not strange that the masters from the east can wander around infinitely in the cosmos and solve large mysteries of the cosmos for humanity. It is indicated that the relation between the people and the cosmos can be eternal when spirituality increases in the human being. The increase of this capacity in pūjā-and yogic science is indicated with Nidhi and that of the spirituality as Siddhi (supernatural capacity). People are a part of and within the cosmos. For the materialist who wants to remain wrapped in wealth and richness, yoga offers perspectives to him or her. As mentioned above people have a higher capacity to think and feel with the practice of meditation because a person rises in meditation, 11 dimensions of higher happiness, peace, rest and harmony. To master this, increased physical and mental strength is required. With those strengths the practitioner can anticipate a higher echelon, to download, to receive energies in the body and to implement the same. It is possible to make a lot of things more transparent and to continue meditation and he is able to bundle the cumulated energies hence work toward the next level.

The yogi lengthens his tongue until it reaches the space between the eyebrows and then introduces it in a reversed position into the mouth searching for nectar in the Soma channel where the nectar for immortality flows (RV 6.58; SV 1574; YV 33.97). The yogi attains silence with closed eyes until he hears nāda (primal sound). This sound varies0 in strength from that of the cricket's chirp to that of the large kettledrum.

Sound, is knowledge, knowledge produces sound. This is the essence of our body.

This is the appreciation, which a yogi absorbs from the cosmos; the divine dew, the saved up result of the night. This is spiritual energy mist, which condenses especially at night, particularly against the end in the blue hour (04.00-08.00 hours), for devoted people. By means of systematic breathing this mist or elixir (prāṇa) from the air is inhaled. Other creatures do this too. The hummingbird for example, a splendid coloured elegant bird (Trochilidae), with a long tail and a very long awl form its nozzle, which sucks honey from the core of a flower with short intermittencies. The number or colour of the flowers is not important but the honey. This colour which forms the rainbow is characteristic of the link in and with the cosmos in the state of spirituality. Honey is important in ritual ceremonies. Collected cream of milk is converted to essence (butter or ghī) that also has the colour of honey, which the devotee sacrifices to the gods (Brhd. Up. 2.5: mantra 1-14). The vibration of the interaction of the hummingbird is similar with the ultrasounds of our voice and of the soul. We must remain stable to do our best in society.

However, a critical note can be placed in meditation: meditation is a pleasant rest exercise, but must be practised within your own limits. At exceeding the limit, one can cause damage to the mental and cognitive system in the brain, as a result of which one is unable to do something in life. In short: a fallen tree is not counted to the forest.

Chapter 4

Āsana

The Meaning of Āsana

Mere materialistic prosperity does not make us happy. It is an art to organise our life in such a way that we experience inward joy in everything we do. It is not the physical comforts, which one gets in abundance in this age of science and technology, but a state of mind, which gives us a sense of fulfilment and satisfaction. It is strange that doctors now advise their patients to try alternative therapies and avoid taking recourse to medicines. They say that more than medicines what a patient needs today is faith in his ability to recover and resolute determination to survive. We see Yoga Centres flourishing in all parts of the world, which aim at making people physically, mentally and emotionally fit. Negative feelings like greed, desire to grab resources at the cost of others, intolerance, arrogance, ethnic and religious prejudices, cruelty and apathetic attitude towards the difficulties of others need to be curbed (YV 3.45: 110). It is also not necessary for us to believe in God but of course we need to have faith in ourselves and in the system which ensures survival of collective life. All forms of life on this planet are bound together. One who does not believe in coexistence, non-violence and tolerance cannot be spiritual. Unless we realise that every life form on this planet has a part to play and has a right to live, the seed of compassion does not sprout within us.

The Western reader may be surprised at the recurring reference to the Universal Spirit, to mythology and even philosophical and moral principles. He must not forget that in ancient times all the higher achievements of man, in knowledge, art and power, were part of religion and were assumed to belong to God and to His priestly servants on earth. The Catholic Pope is the last such embodiment of divine knowledge and power in the West. But formerly, even in the Western world, music, painting, architecture, philosophy and medicine, as well as wars were always in the service of God. These arts and sciences have begun to be emancipated from the Divine for the emancipation of man's will, as distinct from the Divine will. We continue to value the purity of purpose, the humility of discipline and the selflessness that is the legacy of our long bondage with God. I consider it important as well as interesting that the reader should know the origin of Āsanas and the knowledge of the Cakras.

Āsana means balancing your body structure from head to toe, making you aware of the needs of the posture and correcting any defect, which may arise due to poor posture. The development of the feeling of stillness, balance and comfort, in normal physical activities is also an aspect of yogic discipline.[1]

Formerly it was assumed that there must be 8.400.000 sitting positions, corresponding with the number of reincarnations one has to undergo before reaching *samādhī.* Of course it would be impossible to describe them all. That's why in the treatises on the subject only a few hundred are described. And for those that practise yoga solely for purposes of health improvement only a few dozen postures are described. Remarkable results have been and can be achieved for mental and physical well being of a person with their practise. According to Sāṁkhya Yoga, our mental states become conscious only because they happen with reference to a Puruṣa from whom they catch reflection.[2]

In the performance of Āsanas, two avenues or paths are involved. One is the evolutionary, expressive or exhibitive path, taking the self towards the body, towards the pores of

---

[1] Yoga Darshan: Vision on the Yoga Upanishads; Paramhansa Satyananda; Ganga Darshan; India; 1993.

[2] Yoga Philosophy: In relation to other systems of Indian Thought; S.N. Dasgupta; Motilal Banarsidass Publishers Pvt. Ltd.; Delhi; 1996.

the skin, towards the periphery. The other is the involuntary, intuitive or inhibitive path, where the vehicles of the body are driven towards the self. The union of these two paths is the divine marriage of the body with the soul and the soul with the body. We must learn in our performance of Āsanas to express the outer form and beauty of the pose without losing our inner attention. Skin is an organ of perception. It does not act. It receives. The skin receives all actions, but if your flesh overstretches when you are performing an āsana, the skin loses its sensitivity and sends no message to the brain. You want to get something. You want to do it quickly. You want to succeed in doing the pose, but you don't feel the reaction. The flesh extends so much that it makes the organ of perception insensitive, and because it has become insensitive, the reflection from the action to the mind is not felt.

Medical science speaks of efferent and afferent nerves. The efferent nerves send messages from the brain to the organs of action for them to act. The afferent nerves send messages

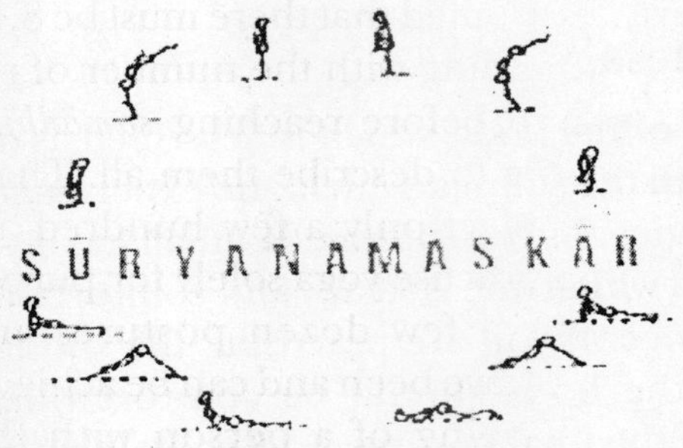

Figure: 19 The Positions of Sūryanamaskār

from the organs of perception to the brain about what they perceive. Yogis also speak of the same, but use different words. The efferent nerves are known as fibers of the flesh or nerves of action (Karmā-nāḍi) and the afferent nerves are called fibers of the skin or nerves of knowledge. Perfect understanding between the nerves of action and the nerves of knowledge, working together in concord, is yoga in the physical sense.

Non-traditional, dynamic posture refers to āsana, performed as fast movement, which does not allow the practitioner to remain quiet and comfortable due to the involvement in continuous movement. Sūrya Namaskāra (Greetings to the Sun god) is an example of a dynamic āsana in which one is constantly moving from one posture to the next. However, this actually represents one stage of āsana practice, and there are five stages which should be understood. The body has to undergo different kinds of changes; it is not static or stable by nature.[3] First, from the normal state in which we use the movements of our body in a limited way, it moves into the second playful, dynamic state where we run, jump and stretch. From there it moves into the third state where we are able to touch our toes or to bend backward without straining any part of the body. Then the fourth state follows, where we are able to maintain our physical balance, in the balancing posture. The fifth stage is, where we can adopt a body posture for an extended period of time during which the body remains perfectly still, motionless and at ease, without feeling any type of discomfort or pain. So, these are the five stages of āsana practice.

Body Stillness

The stillness of the body, which is described as dehasāmya, is different from the stillness which one experiences at the time of āsana practice. In Yoga Sūtras, Patañjali has described āsana as postures in which one is steady and comfortable at the time of performance. If you are practising the shoulder stand or headstand, the body should be comfortable, steady and immobile, in the final posture. So Patañjali has incorporated the concept of steadiness of the body in the practice of āsana. But apart from that, even when we are not practising āsana, there should be comfort and steadiness in the body that is the concept of dehasāmya.

Dehasāmya develops the awareness of our physical posture in different conditions. There are many people who sit for a long time on chairs and have lower back problems and shoulder problems. In dehasāmya, automatically, no matter what you are doing, even if you are working in the garden, in

[3] Chakra's Energy Centers of Transformation; Harish Johari; Destiny Books; U.S.A; 1994.

some industry, or in the office, the body awareness is there. It is balancing your body structure from top to bottom, making you aware of the needs of the posture and correcting any defect, which may arise due to poor posture. So, development of the feeling of stillness, balance and comfort, in normal physical activities is also an aspect of yogic discipline.

Below you can see the simple and easy way to sit and to start your meditation. The first figure shows the Sukhāsana, and the second the Ardha Padmāsana.[4]

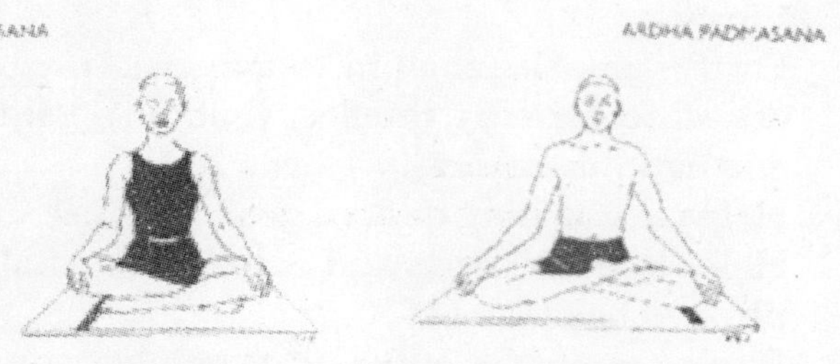

Figure 20: Āsanas Figure 21: Āsanas

Stillness of Vision

Stillness of vision is called dṛṣṭisāmya. dṛṣṭi means 'vision' or 'eyesight', and sāmya means 'stillness'. Vision is an activity of the eyes. Vision is also an activity of the receptive power of the mind, and vision is also awareness. Becoming more and more aware is developing a broader vision in abstract terms. Vision also means distraction and dissipation of the senses and of the mind (RV 6.9.6). So, fixing the senses and mind on one point of concentration is dṛṣṭisāmya. When working, when reading, when enjoying anything in life, when involved in any activity, the mind has to be firm and focused.

Āsana, Seat Materials

The word āsana as used here, doesn't refer to a posture but to the material, used for sitting. A person who's doing Mantra Sādhana (meditation with prayer) should not use an āsana

[4] Āsana Pranayama Mudra Bandha; Swami Satyananda Saraswati; Bihar Yoga Bharati; India; 1997.

that has been used by somebody else, unless that person is the teacher, a holy man, or one who is spiritually evolved and to whom the Sādhaka has an emotional attachment.[5]

Good Āsanas

The following are prescribed as good Āsanas: Kuśāsana (āsana made of kuśa grass) is supposed to be very auspicious and can be used for any kind of mantra jāpa or worship (RV 3.24.3). Kuśa has been praised in the Vedās. The effects of Kuśāsana are as follows:

- Purifies antahkaraṇa (the four internal organs). These are mind (manas), intellect (buddhi), being (citta), and ego (ahaṁkārā).
- Helps in attaining desired goal.
- Helps in purification and enhances mental and physical health.
- Cleans impurities of the place and environment.
- Conserves energy of the aspirant.

The skin of a black deer (YV 4.30: 158) gives Siddhis (secret powers), liberates the aspirant from bondage, and ensures that the aspirant is never short of money.

Any kind of deer skin or antelope skin helps. We mention this as follow:

- Conserves energy of the aspirant.
- Subjugation of the senses.
- Sublimation of sensuality.
- Achieving realisation or a state of total awareness.
- Acquisition of spiritual powers.
- Curing disease caused by aggravation of mind and curing bile and blood diseases.
- Increasing individual magnetism.

Tiger or 'leopard skin' (AV 4.8.4.7) is suitable only for aspirants of Rājasic(dominated by rajas) temperament. It brings luxuries suitable for a king, creates anger, and keeps the aspirant away from snakes, scorpions, and other insects. It protects the aspirant from environmental disturbances and

---

[5] Tools for Tantra; Harish Johari; Distiny Books; Rochester; Vermont; 1986.

obstacles. It is purifying, like Kuśa or deerskin, and helps tame the tiger of the mind through the subjugation of the senses.

Wool and silk both help in the attainment of desired objects (YV 2.5: 36). A red wool āsana is especially beneficial in attaining objects of desire. These materials also conserve the individual's energy and purify the mind.

Haṭha Yoga

You all think that dress is important. But dress beautifies only the outer body, whereas yoga postures tone and beautify the inner body, making each and every part tidy, neat and clean. Then you need not dress up for external display. If dress beautifies the external personality, yoga beautifies the inner personality. By yoga you enjoy yourself by feeling the beauty of control and action without division. By the practice of Haṭha Yoga, the various vestments of the Self-are uncovered one by one till the Ātmā reveals himself as naked as the body. That is the essence of Haṭha Yoga.

The essence of haṭha Yoga is being explained with three examples of awareness from the *Haṭha Yoga Pradipika*, chapter IV.[6]

- First of this is water and salt: Take a glass of water and mix in some salt. Stir the water. When it has been stirred, taste the water from the bottom, middle or top; the salty taste is the same at all levels. Similarly, by the mastery of Haṭha Yoga the body appears as Self, the consciousness appears as Self, Self appears as Self and the whole being appears as Self. The same Self is tasted everywhere (HYP 4.5).
- Second is vessel and sea: Take a vessel and put it on the sea. If it is empty, it floats. We say it is empty, but the Haṭha Yoga Pradipika says it is filled with air. If you press the vessel into the sea, it is filled with water - so whether it is empty or full, know that it is always full either with air or with water. Similar is the case with yoga practice. When the body and consciousness come in contact with the Self, they

[6] Haṭha Yoga Pradipika; Swami Vishnu Devananda; Om Lotus Publications; Motilal Banarsidass Publishers Pvt. Ltd.; New Delhi; 1987.

together become the Self. Self penetrates the body like the water or air of the vessel. The rivers of the body and mind, and the rivers of intelligence and consciousness, join the sea of the Self (HYP 4.56).

- Third is camphor and flame: Camphor and flame are separate. Strike a matchstick and bring it to the camphor; the camphor and flame become one, the camphor dissolves. In the practice of āsanas, the camphor of the body is burnt by the flame of intelligence so that it dissolves and becomes one with the flame of the soul (HYP 4.59).

The aim of the exercises in Haṭha yoga is to stimulate the Cakras and to distribute the generated *Kuṇḍaliṇi* energy throughout the body. The Kuṇḍaliṇi is the microcosmic form of universal energy or more simply, a vast storehouse of static, potential psychic energy, which exists in latent form in every being. It is the most powerful manifestation of creative force in the human body.[7] Below in the figure you can see the location of the subtle body and the flow of the Kuṇḍaliṇi, going up to the Sahasrār Cakra.[8]

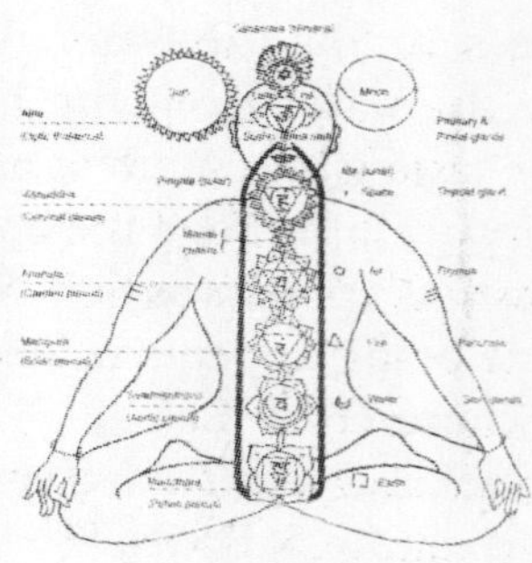

Figure 22 Location of the subtle bodies

The body is dull, Tāmsic. Āsanas are given to bring the body to the level of the vibrant mind (manas), which is Rajo Guṇa. From the inertia of the body should the body be as vibrant as

---

[7] The Tantric Way; Ajit Mookerjee and Madhu Khanna; Thames and Hudson; London; 1977.

[8] Secret Power of Tantrik Breathing; Swami Sivapriyananda; Abhinav Publications; Delhi; 1996.

the mind. Then practice further to change the vibrant body, mind, intelligence and consciousness to become Sāttvic so that one joins the unfading light of the Self, which is beyond the Guṇa. This is the effect of Āsana. Peace has to come from this. If the essence of yoga is lost, peace is lost. Each cell of the body has to have peace for it to be experienced in consciousness.

Remark

The author of the book describes the Lālanā Cakra as follows: "Between the viśṇuddha and the higher ājñā is a secret cakra called the lālanā (female energy or the tongue). It is also known as the tālu cakra because it is situated at the base of the palate (tālu) region just behind the uvula. Meditation and visualisation of this cakra is a secret to be learnt from a guru. Some ancient Tantric texts say that the rising kuṇḍaliṇi energy should be made to pass through the Lālanā centre on its way to the ājñā cakra. This can be accomplished with the help of the 'haṁsa' mantra.' There are more writers who denote this Cakra between the Viśṇuddha and the Ājñā Cakra. The above figure of this book quotes this chakra between the Ājñā- and the Sahasrāra Cakra.

Āsana and Prāṇāyāma

According to the yoga theory, the body takes in Prāṇa or life energy via breathing or directly through the working of the Cakras. Subsequently it is transported by the Nādis to all parts of the body, during which it is converted into various forms of Prāna energy, suitable for various organs and tissues. A good āsana for this aspect of yoga is important. It is usually assumed that there are five main sorts of Prāna or Vāyu ('wind'): Prāna (i.e. a sort of Prāna which is associated with respiration), Āpana, Samāna, Udāna and Vyāna. They function as follows:

- Prāna: is active between the throat and the diaphragm. Regulates the functions of breathing, speech and heart. It is the elixir of life, the life-giving ions (atoms). It creates love, passion and spirituality, the higher energy impact.

- Āpana: is active in the region under the navel. Regulates the function of the large intestine, the kidneys, bladder, genitals and rectum; activates in particular the bowels. This energy pours the pit etc. out of the body and is rolling the lower part of our body (pātālas).
- Samāna: is active in the region of the navel and regulates the digestive process and the process of assimilation. This is the fuel for the fabric in the digestion area.
- Udāna: penetrates the region above the throat and the four limbs. It is assumed that it regulates the five senses and brain function. It also controls the upward flow of life energy in the body. Hyperactive Udāna causes dizziness and over heating in the head.
- Vyāna: penetrates the entire body, spreads vitality and maintains a balanced flow of energy.

This immortal Soul, which is the source and support for all the Prāṇas, mind, intellect, senses and the body, abides in the chambers of your heart. This Ātmā is in the heart where there are a hundred and one arteries. Every one of these has seventy two thousand branches. Vyāna, which does the circulation of blood, moves in these arteries. Udāna, which goes up through one of these, leads you to the higher worlds by means of your meritorious actions, to the evil worlds by means of your evil deeds and to the world of men by a mixture of both deeds.

In the case of Jīvanmuktas or liberated sages who have nothing more by way of births or worlds to live in, their minds and Prānas get absorbed in Brahmā. The individual soul merges itself in the Supreme Soul or PāraBrahmā. In the Jīvanmukta there is no question of any forerunner like the Udāna Vāyu. The liberated sages with their minds purified by renunciation and with knowledge of the imperishable Ātmā are completely absorbed at the time of death, there is no return to this world for them.

Apart from the Prāṇas, the upa-Prāṇas or secondary Prāṇas are also known. These are Nāga, Kūrma, Kṛlikara, Devadatta and Dhanañjaya. The Textbook of Yoga says that the Nāga or 'snake' regulates the secretion of saliva by the salivary glands, hiccups, and causes vomiting. The Kūrma or 'tortoise' causes the closing e.g. fluttering of the eyelids etc. The Kṛikara causes sneezing and hunger. The Devadatta or 'given by God' causes yawning (relaxation) and sleep and the Dhanañjaya or "conqueror of wealth" penetrates the whole body and is responsible for decomposition of the dead organisms.[9]

The following mantra shows the way as to how to meditate by Vaidika Prāṇāyāma :[10]
Oṃ Bhūḥ Oṃ Bhūvaḥ Oṃ Svaḥ Oṃ Mahaḥ Oṃ Janaḥ Oṃ Tapaḥ Oṃ Satyaṁ. Oṃ Tat Savitur Vareṇyaṁ Bhargo Devasya Dhīmahī Brahṁ Bhūr Bhuvaḥ Svaroṃ
(Taittiriya Aranyaka 10.27)

Health and Harmonic

Scholars assume that the energy breathed in, is indispensable for life.[11] This is therefore the most important reason why they have thought out breathing exercises that enable us to control our breath, which is important for having a healthy and long life. With a longer life, the bandwidth liberation is wider. The table below shows the normal life span in relation to the breaths per minute. A man would live a 100 years based on 14 to 16 breaths per minute.

Table 3: Breath and normal life span compared with animals

Name of animal	Breathe per minute	Normal Life Span
Dog	50	14 years
Horse	35	30 years
Elephant	20	100 years
Tortoise	5	400 years
Snake	2.3	500 years
Man	14-16	100 years

Source: Kaul (1994)

[9] The Textbook of Yoga; George Feuerstein; Ank-Hermes bv; Deventer; 1978.

[10] First steps to Higher Yoga; Shri Yogeshwarananda Parmahans; Yoga Niketan Trust; New Delhi; 1987.

[11] Aspects of Yoga; Kaul; H. Kumar; B.R. Publishing Corporation; Delhi; 1994.

Swāmi Satyananda Sarasvati states that it is written in the Ayur Veda (a branch of the Atharva Veda) that the human body is controlled by three 'vital juices': phlegm (Kapha), wind (Vāyu), and acid or bile (Pitta). The movement these three function irregularly, the metabolism of the body becomes disturbed and ultimately all sorts of ailments develop.[12] The term Ayu means long life.

The most important objective of the postures and physical exercises, such as the Pavanmukta-or farting/belching exercise, is the improvement of an unimpeded flow of air through the canals or Nāḍis, especially through the coming off of the impediments in the joints or knots. This knot or Granthi is the Mūlādhāra or base (the knot of Brahmā), the Anāhata or heart (the knot of Viṣṇu), and the Ājñā or eyebrow (the knot of Śiva), to reach the Sahasrāra. The knots are described in the chapter cakras. The secondary objective is to activate the esoteric system of the cakras and the canals and to consciously control their flow of energy.

Maintaining a certain posture for a couple of minutes or longer, while breathing quietly carries out static āsanas. They give a soft massage to the internal organs, the endocrine glands, the muscular system and the nervous system, and are a good preliminary exercise to meditation because of their calming effect on the mind. Concentrating oneself mentally on a part of one's body carries out these āsanas. The exercises are, among other things, good for the hamstring muscles, which are stretched by them, and the joints of the hip, the sacral bone and the lumbar vertebra which are loosened. Flatulence, constipation, back pain and also excessive fat in the abdominal region are remedied in an effective way. All the organs in the abdomen are brought into harmony and intestinal disorders, such as diabetes can gradually show an improvement. The kidneys, liver, pancreas and adrenal glands are activated. As the organs in the pelvis are also brought into harmony, the postures and exercises are especially useful to

[12] Theories of the Chakra's; Bridge to Higher Consciousness; The Hiroshi Motoyama; Theosophical Publishing House; USA; 1978.

remedy gynaecological complaints. They also improve the flow of fresh blood to the nerves and muscles of the spine and give spiritual consciousness. Nothing in the universe (bodies and celestial bodies) can do without the Prāṇa or air e.g. energy. Prāṇa controls everything and everyone. By yawning, parts of the body are pulled together and apart; a periodical screening of the law of nature. The urge to yawn, however, must not be suppressed. The Vāyu Tattva is the principle and the composition of air, which is also dealt with in the Bṛhadārānyaka Upaniṣad, Taittiṛiya Upaniṣad and Chāndogya Upaniṣad.

Pratyāhāra

After Prāṇāyāma comes Pratyāhāra, the withdrawal of consciousness from the senses. The seer Patañjali (PYS 105) says: "Abstraction (Pratyāhāra) is the process by which the senses do not come in contact with their objects and follow as it were the nature of the mind." The mind is withdrawn from the objects of the senses. The mind is by nature unsteady, for it is at every moment being affected by sight, sounds, and so forth, of external objects which Manas through the agency of the senses (Indriyās) perceives. It must therefore be detached from the objects of the senses, withdrawn from whatsoever direction it may happen to tend, freed from all distraction, and kept under the control of the dominant self. Steadiness (Dhairya) therefore is the aim and result of Pratyāhāra.

Senses are restrained, like the mind, when the mind is restrained. They do not stand in need of other means like the control of the other organs. Just as bees fly, as the queen flies; and sit as the queen sits; so the sense becomes restrained, as the mind is restrained. This is Pratyāhāra. The meaning is that inasmuch as the mind does not come into contact with objective sounds. This, as cause of forgetfulness, attachment and aversion, the senses of sight, too do not, on account of the absence of that contact, incline toward their objects. This is the imitation of the mind by the senses. Patañjali says, the aim of Pratyāhāra is the highest control of the senses (PYS 106). Some say that the conquest of the senses is their non-attachment to sound, etc. Attachment is a defect, which draws them away from the good. Others say that inasmuch as the enjoyment of unprohibited objects is proper, it should be said that contact with sound, subject to one's wishes, is the conquest of the senses. Others again say that the conquest of the senses is the obtaining of knowledge of sound, without their causing pleasure and pain, in the absence of attachment and aversion. It is only the want of action of the senses, on account of the single-pointedness of the mind. It is for this reason that this control is the very highest.

Concentration

Concentration is focusing the mind on a concrete object, the image of an object, or on abstract matters, such as mercy or tolerance. In the beginning, it is very difficult for an untrained mind to concentrate on an object. Śrī Swami Śivananda advises in his book Concentration and Meditation to sit down in a room and to meditate on the colour, the form, the various parts of a rose, such as the leaves, the stem and pollen.[13] Also on the different sorts of roses, such as white roses, yellow roses, red roses, on the various preparations of roses, such as rose water, rose syrup, scents, rose extract, jam. On the various applications of the rose, such as rose water for the cleansing of the eyes in ophthalmology, as a purgative with constipation is also possible. As flowers and garlands for the worship of God and for wearing. On the different qualities, such as the cooling effect on the body system, its wholesome effect with flatulence. The price of roses and rose garlands, the places where they can be found in abundance and various other things which are associated with the rose. With this, every thought, which is associated with other objects, must be shut out. Through this concrete method the mind is trained for abstract meditation. This method is suitable for extrovert people. Practise daily, during a month, every morning at 5 o'clock for half an hour. In an advanced state it is done in the

---

[13] Concentration and Meditation; Śrī Swami Śivānanda; The Divine Life Society; Tehri-Garhwal; U.P.; 1997.

reversed method of tallying up the things that enter the thoughts, so that the inner viewing screen is freed for the mind.

Meditation follows after concentration. Meditation makes ones experience happiness, whatever the circumstances. Happiness is always present in anyone. It is up to a person to draw from the source of Ānanda (happiness). Mantra is also a way to become aware of that source of Ānanda in oneself. That source is also called Paramātmā or the unconditional consciousness, the kingdom of God. And Śivananda says that meditation is in fact unravelling death,[14] as the final purpose is nothing more than leaving the body in constructive awareness and attaining a liberated state: mokṣa.' The number of objects or abstract matters that can be meditated on, are nearly limitless. The Swami advises to meditate daily on virtues for ten minutes. Trained Yogis use Mudrās and Bandhas to withhold cosmic energy.

Mudrās and Bandhas

Mudrās are gestures, which retain cosmic energy in a certain form and return it in support of the spiritual driving force at concentration. The latent supernatural energy in nature is immediately recognised by the Mudrā and manifests itself via this conception in the practitioner and supports him/her during the exercise or effort to gain health and well being. It is comparable to a hitchhiker asking for a ride, the V-sign for Victory, the protruded middle finger to offend someone, etc. Mudrā acts of course, take place in the higher spheres. Scholars have developed a great number of gestures in support of the various inner processes. For more particulars, I refer to any good treatise on yoga. In *Kuṇḍalini Yoga, Mudrās* however do not play any role.

The word *Bandhas* literally means 'locks.' It is a specific exercise in which certain parts of the body or organs are locked or tied, coupled with holding the breath. The purpose is to realise a better concentration for more compact meditation and absolute self-control.

---

[14] The Science of Pranayama; Swami Sivananda; The Divine Life Society; Tehri-Garhwal; U.P.; 1997.

Jalandhar bandha is one of the three important Bandhas, which are essentially performed during Kumbhaka in Prāṇāyāma. Excessive pressure is developed in the lungs during Kumbhaka, which elevates blood pressure. Hence it is interesting to know the effect of Jalandhar Bandha on blood pressure (Systolic and Diastolic). It is observed that blood pressure increases during the practice of Kumbhaka as there is excessive pressure developed in the lungs during the Kumbhaka. The position and the description of the Jalandhar Bandha indicate that there is some relation between increased blood pressure and Jalandhar Bandha. Jalandhar Bandha creates the pressure on the Carotial Sinus, which in turn reduces blood pressure. Measurement of blood pressure can be done by checking the rhythm of breathing during Kumbhaka, but with a proper Jalandhar Bandha i.e. by contracting the muscles of the neck from all sides and then bending the neck little forward.

Chapter 5

Cakras and Powers

Cakras and Health

The concept of Cakra is vital in Hinduism. Cakra means wheel. They are the nerve plexus or centres of force and consciousness within the inner bodies of humans. In the body there are the nerve plexuses, ganglia and glands connected with the planets in the universe with which their vibrations correspond. They effectuate the interaction between the human being and the universe. The energy for our health is a mixture of inner powers and the surplus from the atmosphere. There are seven principal Cakras, which can be seen psychically as colourful with a multi-petal or a lotus structure. These are wheels or lotus situated along the spinal cord from the base to the cranial chamber. Seven barely visible lower Cakras exist below the spine. These are seats of instinctive consciousness, the origin of jealousy, hatred, envy, guilt, sorrow etc. and constitute the lower orders of evolution and diabolical (hellish) forces, called Naraka or Pātāla.

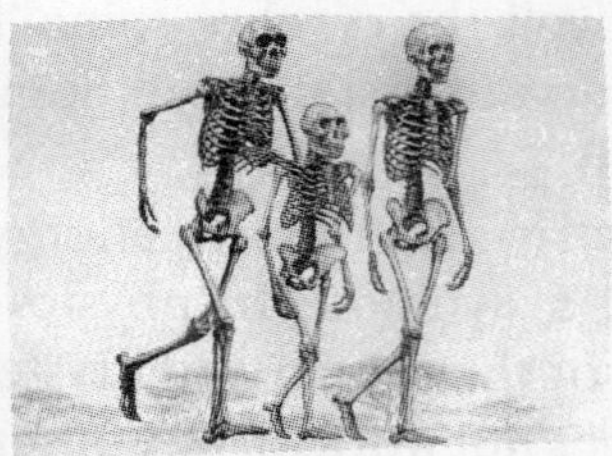

Figure 23: Naraka or Pātāla

The figure indicates that all species of organisms originate through the process of biological evolution. In this process, new species arise from a series of natural changes. In animals that reproduce sexually, including humans, the term species refers to a group, whose adult members regularly interbreed, resulting in fertile offspring-that is, offspring themselves capable of reproducing. Scientists classify each species with a unique, two-part (Androgyne or Ardhanāri) scientific name. In the evolution theory humans are defined as Homo sapiens, and in the vedic hymns they are called "*the divinities*". "He who knows the three cognisable (worlds); the sage (who knows) the mysterious birth of the *divinities* (abiding in them); he who is beholding the good and evil acts of mortals, he, the sun, the lord, makes manifest their intentions; the Divinities abiding in them - of the Vasus on earth, the Rudras in the firmament, the Adityas in heaven (RV 6.51.2).Not devoted people in the theology and particularly in Hinduism are inclined to define the sources of strength as gods. Also when less developed people can't understand powers then they appoint these powers as god. Due to this situation a way of life will be translated as a religion. Not everyone is religious and that's why we should divide the energy fields in an internal and an external section within the creation and the creatures. All beings are under the impact of cosmic energy. This energy takes two forms, viz. Light and Oxygen The Rīg Vedā named the two forms Mitra (the Sun) and Varuna (the ocean) that have a wider field of activity, as they together rule over the whole world (RV 5.63.8). They are even said to encompass the two worlds (RV 7.61.4). They, by their power can exert their influence anywhere and force. In our body, Mitra and Varuna are respectively the cerebro-spinal fluid surrounding the whole of the nervous system, and Soma, as the cerebro-spinal fluid within it.

A cakra is an electric generator or energy wheel, especially for direct current: a dynamo. In physics we quote this as capacity to do work or the property of a system that diminishes when the system does not work on any other system, potential energy. The generator and its potentials are found in the term 'Savitra and Pūṣaṇa. Savitra in his abstract form is the efferent impulse moving along the fibres of the nervous system. The

Rīg Vedā denotes some qualities of Savitra. "He illumines every nook and corner of the world (RV 1.13.5, 7). His golden arm, he stretches aloft to the heaven and downwards to the end of the earth (RV 11.38.2). He moves in a golden car regarding all creatures in the Vedic world on a downward and upward path" (RV 1.35.2,3). The godly energy Pūṣaṇa is the holder of the Universe. "He moves onwards, holding the Universe and takes his abode in heaven. Being the best of charioteers, he drives the wheel of Sūrya downwards." (RV 6.53-55). It is considered the source of energy or consciousness.

The cakra is a small 'planet' in our inner body that also orbits like a planet in the cosmos (upwards) and satellites a Pātāla or semi cakra (downwards). These are small dynamos started from the hips to the feet and comparable with asteroids or planetoids. Comparable with the water household in the body in which several sizes of pumps are operating and are dependent on tasks. Each cakra contains several kinds of energy waves, linked with the radiation of several energies of planets in the cosmos. Each planet in the cosmos supplies energy or medicine (bliss) to our body via a cakra. We have mentioned earlier that all the energies are comparable to drops of the ocean (God). We find this process follows in the Rīg Vedā: 'They bore up from the ocean waters, by the winged horses (potentials)attached to their car, anothor hymn refers to Indra as the generator and this manifestratives (or houses)as his proberitials. 'Indra, the prototype, has assumed various forms, and such is his form as that which (he adopts) for his manifestation: Indra, multiform by his illusions, proceeds (to his many worshippers), for the horses, yoked to his car are a thousand. Indra has assumed various forms. He presents himself as Agni, Viṣṇu, or Rudra, or any other deity who is the actual object of worship, and is really the deity to be adored: he is identifiable with each. The horses yoked to his car are a thousand. His chariots and horses are multiplied according to the forms in which he manifests himself: agreeably to the Vedāntic interpretation of the stanza, Indra is here identified with Parameśvara, the supreme first cause, identical with creation' (RV 6.47.18). Many hymns will confirm that the gods and goddesses are 'born' from one source. Due to their duty and actions they take several names and forms, while the 'person' or the power is the same. Focusing on our society we have many soldiers and captains but not every soldier is a captain, and not every captain has to be a soldier. We have even the Captain of the Industry that has nothing to do with the army. This assumes the principle of All in One and One in all.

Yoga as Doctor

The seven cakras have their own source for cosmic power and are linked to a particular planet. This hyperlink is constantly in process for our psychical and mental progress. The medicines for daily use we can achieve in few seconds on the natural way for a natural healing. Rīg Vedā mentions in this case the following: "One (Rudra) brilliant and fierce, (yet) the distributor of healing medicines holds his *sharp weapon* in his hand (RV 8.29.5). In principle, yoga is our doctor for health, beauty, pleasure, rust, peace, harmony etc.This sharp weapon is yoga under control. The Veda proceeds with the result of that control called the Soma-medicine. "Mitra and Varuṇa, I take the Soma when the sun is risen; it is medicine to the sick (RV 8.73.17). Soma and Sun are both related to space, energy, light and mind stability. These four are given in the following hymns "Borne by his steeds, may the divine Savitā, who is possessed of precious treasure, and filling the firmament (with radiance or light), come hither, holding in his hands many things good for man, and (both) tranquillising and animating living beings. May the outspread, vast, and golden arms of Savitā extend to the ends of the sky (Space) (verily) we glorify his greatness: may the sun impart energy unto him (energy) May the divine Savitā, who is endowed with energy, the lord of treasure, bestow treasures upon us concentrating infinite lustre(mind stability)" (RV 7.45.1-3). These four elements activate the cakra's that can treat disease in their location and control the healing process as soon we make the hyperlink through meditation. Medical science also confirms this process.

Medical science is teaching about yoga and meditation. There are several interesting results in the field of yoga due to experiments based on methods of breathing. Jalandhar Bandh is one of the three important exercises for our body, which are essentially required to be performed during Kumbhaka (holding the breath) in Prāṇāyāma. The effect of Jalandhar Bandha issued to control blood pressure (Systolic and Diastolic).

Control and upgrading of our energy are mostly done by yoga sessions. It is good for our health, wealth and peace and that of our society to practise yoga, due to the multiple effects on inner and outer nature. In this chapter we will draw methods how to increase quickly and efficiently inner power and health with the explanation of each cakra. Meditation is here medication for free!

Durgās and Kinis

Energy is coordinated by several sources or groups in our body, viz. Durgā's, Kini's and gods and demigods. In the process of creation Durgā is manifested as the goddesses Rādhā, Lakṣmī and Sarasvatī. Besides different manifestations in form of goddesses She impacts the cakra energies upwards. Associated with divine power in the cosmos we refer to a mantra in Sāma Veda 'From you a bull but newly born, O Āgni, ... the kindled everlasting flames rise upward ... (SV 1221). Durgā is also sometimes elevated to supreme status. Depending on a duty She appears with her respective identity and name. In spite of the duties She has several forms, viz. Śailputrī (the firmness of the earth, seated on the Himalaya), Brahmacārini (radiates light and purity), Candraghaṇṭā (sound and waves), Kuṣmāṇḍā (architecture and construction), Skandamātā (five-fold knowledge), Kātyāyanī (bliss of meditation), Kālarātrī (time and rhythm), Mahāgaurī (tolerance and non-violence in creations) and Siddhidātrī (liberation).

The diversity of these powers of the Goddess makes Her the most adored goddess among all the female manifestations. In fact, barring a few goddesses all others are believed to be a form of Goddess Durgā. Every woman who becomes a mother achieves the level of a demigoddess, because a Mother is the highest status.

In the same perspective we have another scene of goddesses with a lower power or density. Dākinī, Rākinī, Cākinī, Kākinī, Lākini, Sākini, Hākini and Yākini, are the queens of the eight respective Lotuses. These goddesses are linked with the energies in the lower creation of the cosmos known as the Pātālas. Due to the abundant materialistic powers all these aspects are formed by a Kini. So we have Dākinī (emotional desires, fear of death; who strikes terror into the hearts of unbelievers), Rākinī (personality, fantasies, furious materialistic desires), Cākinī (scientific and erotic desires), Lākinī (radiation of electric energy, heat), Kākinī (art, worldly expressions), Sākinī (cosmic and secret knowledge, light), Hākinī (unconditional truth), Yākinī (action of salvation). In the Rīg Vedā you will find a hymn which refers to the multi-headed Kini's "Come with your shining and well-guided chariot, having a leader, a driver, (fitted). With excellent wheels to our dwelling, (to bestow upon us) male offspring: cut off with secret indignation the heads of those obstructing (the adoration) of the mortal (who worships you) (RV 6.62.10).

Human is God

Human is god if he can distinguish human and divine. There are eight sheats or koṣas in the body as parameter for the nomination of the power and the super power. After the fifth quality or koṣa a human being is capable enough to be called a godly person and is indicated as an angel, devi or deva. They enjoy the Ānanda or happiness, unlimited wealth and success in life and business. This is charging the battery with free of charge. "Fierce, vigorous, strong-armed, they need not exert (the energy of their) persons: bows and arrows are leady in your chariots; the glory (of conquest) over (hostile) armies is yours. The energy (or battery) is not unknown as quoted in the Rīg Vedā (8.20.12, 13). The Veda declares clearly about young and long-life in the following hymn: "Youthful (Maruts), approaching us with benevolent hearts, grant prosperity to those liberal men who worship you, who zealously healthy heart, youth and prosperity.

When we examine all the cakras in the parts and subparts of our body, we understand that there are powers, which can not be understood through ordinary mind. As mentioned above there would be gods, but they are functioning as energy sources or powerhouses in our body. We need these energies to increase the frequency from high to low and vice versa. It is based on the need within the access and volume of that part of the body. Yogic science mentions that we have seven main cakras as dynamo in our body and also in each substantive part of the body such as the elbow, arms, hand palm, finger, phalange etc. They all operate as independent components just like the main seven cakras. These operational components are in minuscule form. This theory reflects in the ideas of the secular person that there are uncountable gods in people and or in the cosmos. It is a fact that Internet technology is one of these potentials, but still not godly. We use astral energy fields in the cosmos for our communication, pleasure, relaxation, etc., today. A similar instrument is a battery, which can be charged. The voltage, limit of time and size is dependent on factors, which can increase and reinforce the energy fields. In spite of that astral strengths are invisible but almost accepted in society. We can compare these compact energy forms with the above-mentioned form of deities. There is One God with several kinds and forms of energies. The strength fields are routes or devas which make themselves available for human beings, the creation and other creatures. For this reason it is not wise to declare a life consideration as a religion with multiple gods without having insight into the matter. The Big Bang has been monotonous from which a lot of consonances resound in all of creation and in the cosmos. The same is similar with a fire explosion from which a lot of sparkle arise with their own (volume and heat) burning capacity. It would be judicious to declare the consonances to gods and to place the alphabet on a furnace bridge in the church. The language must be kept alive and dynamic by and for the people. Look before you leap to express critical thoughts because people are gods and gods in heaven are looking for opportunities to become human. Human only can pass through the orbit toward salvation.

How to become a human

A natural death of a cow is like a breeding place for at least 330 millions angels or devas. The devas stay in the cow in microform as like chips in a computer. A cow has four stomachs, which classify the quality of knowledge just like a catalyst. This quality, impulse to donate, is the most important aspect in the human being. After this surplus a creature becomes a human. Gau or cow also means tolerant. For this reason it is not astonishing that within the reincarnation theory people use the cow as a link class. Humans can reach this altitude by giving at least one cow in a ritual to a priest or saint. A highly-qualified human is a yogi. The yogi is a Gau and is prepared to sacrifice everything for salvation, the end of the circle of birth and death.

AUM, the Big Bang

As mentioned in previous chapters, creation started with the Big Bang and that is simply the AUM sound in Hinduism.[1] The first character of this word is 'A'. 'A' vibrates within the Mūlādhāracakra at the base of the spine. The second sound 'U' vibrates within the Viśuddha- or throat Cakra. The third sound 'M' vibrates within the Ājñā and Sahasrāra Cakras, the seat of the highest God. The spot above called Anusvāra represents the soundless sound Parānanda. The Upaniṣads explain AUM as standing for the whole universe and its parts, for its past, present and future. From this original vibration originated all manifestations. "God is only one who is hidden in all living beings. He is all pervading and is the inner self of all creatures. He presides over all actions and all beings abide in Him. He is the witness, pure consciousness and devoid of all qualities." (Sv. Up. 6.11). The first mantra of the Īśopaniṣad indicates that "Brahman is perfect and everything that comes from Brahman, is also perfect."

As the soul is the life of the body, which without it would be a carcass, so is the Supreme Spirit the essence of the

---

[1] The cosmic vibration *AUM,* OM, Ashima Kaul Bhatia, Aravali Books International, New Delhi, 1998.

individual soul's being. And yet, even as the soul is 'lost' in the body, the Supreme Spirit, functioning as the Soul of the individual soul, loses cognisance of its real Divine nature. It is the Supreme Spirit that moves, though in reality there is no motion, It being the one Reality. There can be no motion when there is nought else. It is far away, because we fail to realize it. It is near, because it is immanent in everything and is in recess of one's own heart.

A body is a combination of five elements (Pañca-mahābhūta), known as ether, air, fire, water and earth (Puruṣa Sūkta 2: Yadbhutam). These came forth from the subtle objects. These produced in turn Śabda (sound), Sparśa (feeling), Rūpa (shape), Rasa (taste) and Gandha (smell). Sound is first and foremost. From this can be deduced that the world came out of sound.[2] Aum orOṃis the original sound. This is the name of Brahman or God. Aum stands for the creator, Viṣṇu the preserver and üiva the destroyer. It stands before the whole universe that is made up of Trigunas or the triple manifestation of nature (Puruṣa Sūkta 15: Paridhayastrih). Those are Sattva or calmness, Rajas or passionate activity, and Tamas or inactivity. Esoterically seen Aum stands for our physical, astral and causal bodies. A is a throat sound, U a middle sound and M is formed with the lips or the end of the vocal cords. In short Aum stands for everything what is and is not manifested. It is the word out of which everything originated.

Seven Principal Cakras

The Lord took so many Avatāras just as Śrī Rāma, Śrī Kṛṣṇa Śaṅkara, Hanumāna, Buddha, Jesus, Mohammed, Zoroaster etc. but they all had to go to others without any exception for treading the divine path. Because as soon as a person is placed in the womb, he is imprisoned in the Mahāmāyā with most vigilant guards just before and after his birth. (The discharges called maul instead of Māyā before and after the birth of a

---

[2] Meditation onOṃand Mandukya Upaniṣad, Śri Swami Śivānanda, The Devine Life Society, U.P., India, 1997.

child) that bag in the womb is cut and comes out only after the child's disconnection with it.

As long as the child is in the womb it is quite intact and it is attached to the child in its subtle form, and so unless that is cut, a sunder in his future life by a person already crossed over it, that child can not overcome it. Only a practical and powerful Sādhaka, Preceptor of Karana Satguru is able to maintain that capacity to cut that bag and its assistants as Hridaya Granthi, the Heart-knot, the Saṁskāras and the false imaginations of an ignorant Jīva. The intellect sharpens the knowledge, which flashes like the-lightning (RV 8.15.7). For as long as this is not done, one has to follow his own intelligence which puts him most miraculously once showing a line to be genuine.

Every seven years we pass through a cakra. These are the characteristics, which determine the theme of our life in that period. Every period can be divided in seven additional major themes that have a one-year duration. After seven by seven years we terminate a cycle of 49 years.[3] Then a new cycle starts. We get the chance to start a new on a higher level of development with new learning processes. In the next paragraph we will describe the cakras in order. The seven principal cakras are (Puruṣa Sūkta 15, Saptasyāsana):

- Mūlādhāra (at the base of the spine): controls memory, time and space;
- Svādhiṣṭhāna (under the navel): controls matter;
- Maṇipūra (solar plexus): controls the will;
- Anāhata (centre of the heart): immediate and consciousness
- Viśuddha (throat): divine love, seat of the soul;
- Ājñā (third eye): divine insight;
- Sahasrāra (crown): enlightenment, divinity.

Yoga and Nadis

Haṭha Yoga is described in the Yoga Upaniṣads as a means to attain physical and mental purification and balance. Haṭha is

[3] Theories of the Chakra's, Bridge to Higher Consiousness, Hiroshi Motoyama, Uitgeverij Ank-Hermes bv, Deventer, 1990.

generally translated as 'force', whereas in yogic literature the word Haṭha is made by the combining of two mantras, Ham and Tham. These mantras correspond with ṭhe Iḍa and Pingalā Nadis. In this context the term means the yoga through which these two forces are balanced. Iḍa, a major Prānic channel within the body, represents the passive aspect of Prāṇa which is manifested and experienced as mental force or Cit Śakti. Piṅgala is related with the solar, vital energy or the dynamic force or Prāṇa which is manifested and experienced in the physical dimension as Prāṇa Śakti. According to the description above, Haṭ̃ha yoga is the yoga of channeling the Prāṇas in the body.

Below follows a description of the cakras with an indication about how they might be stimulated. Figure 24 gives the location of the cakras and figure 25 the Nadis, Iḍa and Piṅgala.

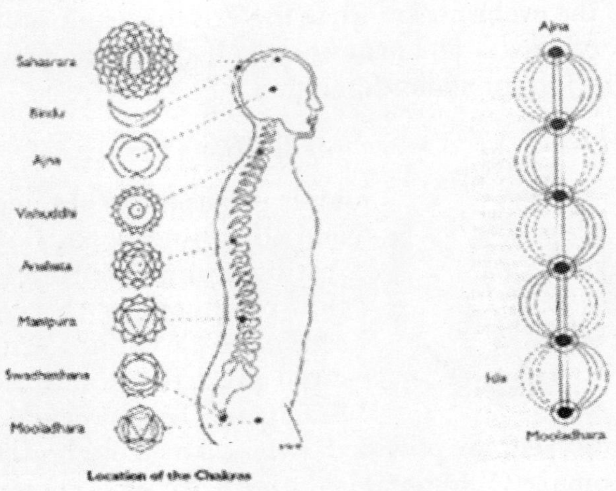

Figure 24 Figure 25

Source: Asana Pranayama Mudra Bandha, Swami Satyananda Saraswati, Bihar Yoga Bharati, India, 1997.

The Iḍa, Piṅgala and Śuṣuṁṇā are the three main Nadis. The Iḍa is the Nadi situated on the left side of the Śuṣuṁṇā. It is white in colour, corresponds to the lunar principle and ends in the left nostril. The Iḍa stretches in the form of a bent bow from under the left nostril to below the left kidney. The Piṅgalā is situated on the right side of the Śuṣuṁṇā. It is red in colour, corresponds to the solar principle and ends in the right nostril. Like the Iḍa it is bow-shaped.

The Śuṣuṁṇā which is enclosed within the Brahmaqaṇḍa or spinal column corresponds to the principles of the sun, moon and fire. It proceeds from the Kandayoni Cakra just above the sex organs, to the Brahmarāndhra or principal aperture at the base of the skull. In general practice it may be said to correspond to the central channel of the spinal cord. Inside this enclosing channel is a finer channel called the Vajrini, and inside that another channel called the Citrini. The latter is as thin as the thousandth part of a hair and it is on this that the Cakras are based, and along it the awakened Kuṇḍalini proceeds.

The Iḍa is referred to as the Gaṅgā of the subtle body, the Piṅgalā as the Yamunā, and the Śuṣuṁṇā as the Sarasvatī.[4] These three rivers meet at a certain point above the middle of the eyebrows known as the Triveṇī, 'triple braid', the triple confluence. The man who can bathe by the power of yoga in the Triveṇī attains liberation.

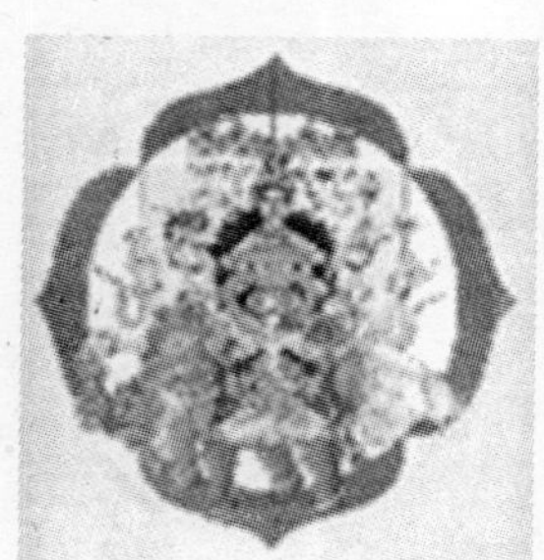

Mūlādhārā Cakra

Mūla means the beginning or the root and Ādhāra means basis (also called the first button). Mūlādhāra is the central flow of energy or the central nerve scheme of the cosmos. Within this area dwell the cosmos and the creatures. Brainpower, willpower and guts, healing power, etc. are provided by this cakra in our body by the Moon (Soma or Candramā) in the form of cosmic energy. The visible results in life are i.e. wealth, beauty, rest, peace, harmony etc. (also referred to Rudra Sūkta 2).

Both God and the creatures have the capacity to create. Gaṇeṣa (problem solver as Lam), Durgā or Śailaputrī in her first form, icon for earth, and Ka, the first consonant of the Sanskrit alphabet (as mentioned above) are the most

[4] Chakra's, energy Centers of Transformation, Harish Johari, Distiny Books, USA, 1987.

important elements in this cakra. This cakra is located in the pelvis, between the anus and the genitals nearby the perineum (anal cleft). It is connected with the tailbone at the base of the spine. It is the foundation based in earth (flesh) and is connected with the first three vertebrae. It opens downwards and from there coordinates everything that is fixed, such as the spinal column, bones, teeth, nails, legs, anus, rectum, large intestine and prostate.

In the Mūlādhāra lies the source of the three most important nerve channels: Iḍa (female), Piṅgalā (male) and Śuṣuṁṇā (neutral). They surround the spine and are in connection with the physical, the astral and the carnal body ending in the crown, the forehead, and the throat.

The slumbering female cosmic energy Śakti or Kuṇḍalini lies here in the tailbone and when released, it rises to the Sahasrāra or the fontanel, to her spouse Śiva. By keeping the male and female sources of energy separate, vitality is created in the bodies of creatures.

The Mūladhāra cakra represents the manifestation of the individual consciousness in a human form, viz. the physical birth of the body. Stimulating it is the starting point of yoga. The rise of this force is known as the awakening of the Kuṇḍalini. When he passes each of these psychic centres, a person gets complete control of one of his senses. Meditating on the tip of the nose leads to a beginning of consciousness, freedom from illness, lightness, inspiration, vitality, power, endurance, insight into the inner purity, a soft tone in the voice, and an inner melody.

The process of liberation starts only with the awakening of this force (HYP 3.108). Peculiar about this energy is that when someone falls on his tailbone, he can go blind or become clairvoyant because then, some of this force is released. Central to this cakra is the sense of smell. The cakra is physically activated while sitting by moving the buttocks to the left and to the right and subsequently clockwise and anti-clockwise. While one is sitting in the tailor or lotus position with a straight back, the cakra is mentally activated by folding one's hands, keeping them underneath the navel, resting the pulses on the thighs, closing the eyes and concentrating on the tip of the nose. Then open the eyes slightly, while you keep on concentrating. When the eyes get tired, close them for a while and keep concentrating in thought. When the eyes have come to rest again, open them and keep concentrating. This process should go on for ten to twenty minutes. One should constantly have the tailbone in mind, reciting the bīja or primal sound Oṃ Laṁ Oṃ. This combination of posture and sound is the method to stir up the Mūlādhāracakra. This method applies to all cakras, each with its own primeval sound.

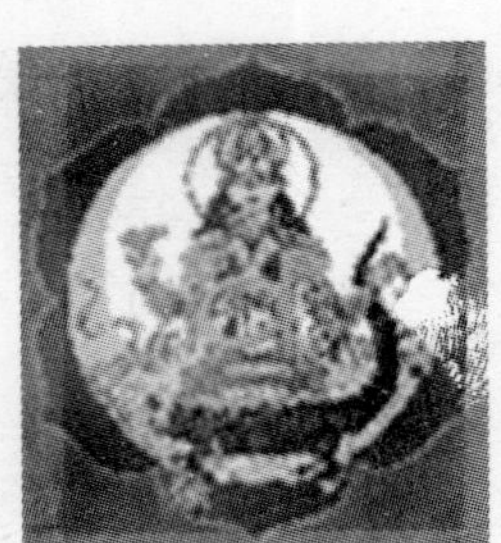

Svādhiṣṭhāna Cakra

The Svādhiṣṭhāna-or spleen cakra is located at the plexus genitalis on the upper part of the sacral bone, approximately at the pubic hairline. This chakra opens to the front and is controlled by the element water. Brainpower, willpower and guts, healing power, etc. are provided by this cakra in our body by the Mercury (Budha) in the form of cosmic energy. The visible results in life are i.e. wealth, beauty, rest, peace, harmony etc.

From its position it controls the pelvic region, reproductive organs, kidneys, bladder, all bodily fluids such as blood, lymph, digestive fluids and sperm. It is connected with the glands, the ovaries, the prostate and the testicles. The name means 'Abode of the Self'. It is also denoted as the sex cakra.[5] This cakra can delay orgasm when Prāṇāyāma is applied. When making love, one can also deduce the degree of willingness of the other party from the breath. Heavy breathing mostly implies consent.

The earth of the Mūlādhāra cakra dissolves in the water of this cakra and serves as an inspiration for creative work. We know that the sperm cells can only move when they meet with the sperm fluid (during ejaculation).The purpose of the exercise is to clear impediments in the abdomen so that the

[5] Yoga & Sex, Pandit Shiv Sharma & Kailash Nath Sharma, B.I. Publications Pvt Ltd., New Delhi, 1973.

energy there can flow freely. The second purpose is to train the lungs to draw maximum energy from the breath for a long and healthy life.[6] Through the left nostril the breath covers the female left half of the body, which is cool, and then it carries the cool air to the male right half, which is warm, and the other way round. In this way a balance is brought about between temperature and temperament of everything, also in the universe (with the moon and the sun energy). With this cakra taste is central.

The power of creation is carried out in this second cakra. Brahmā did this in His quarter part and as a result Brahmā (the female Mā) arose. In this part He produces that motherly aspect that's comparable with the ovum of the woman. Mā-Śakti or Brahmacārini (second Durgā) is therefore the creating energy which penetrated in all cosmos and takes its place in the second cakra, coupled with planet Mercury. The original principle or Dharma of God Himself has been expressed in the character Sa of the Svādhiṣṭhāna cakra (RV 10.90.2, Sarvam Yadbhūtam Yacca Bhāvyam; all that is, and all that is to be). This character Sa indicates Sanātan, the original or the first cosmic discipline, which starts from the Supreme and then applies it for each soul. This Sa adds energy in the body, the biorhythm and the seed of the 'knowledge tree' (hidden in water) which will be developed in the next six cakras. Sa stands also for the beginning of the human being. Below we give the idea of modern science on this field.

The figure shows fossil evidence that the first humans evolved from ape ancestors at least 6 million years ago. Many species of humans followed but only some left descendants on the branch leading to Homo sapiens. In this slide show, white skulls represent species that lived during the time period indicated; gray skulls represent extinct human species.

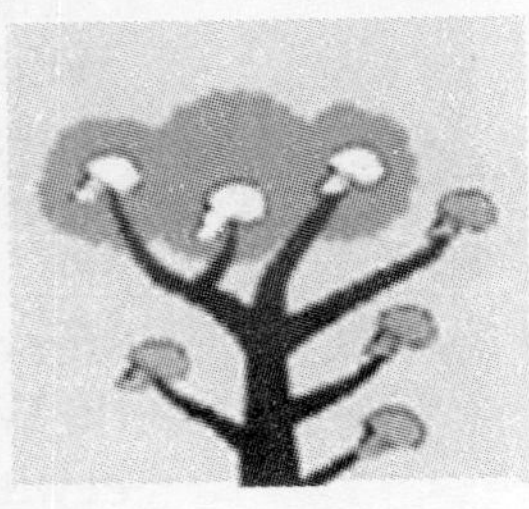

Figure 26 Three white and four gray skulls

[6] Breath, Mind, and Consciousness, Harish Johari, Destiny Books, U.S.A., 1989.

What is remarkable is that the figure shows the three skulls for the past, three for the future and one for the present. This is equal to the seven main cakras in the three knots. Within these knots we have our biorhythm. The biorhythm is ẕalso stipulated in these cakra. The two devi's Rākinī and Cākinī (heads) are established here. Also Gaṅgā and Varuṇa (female and male water - milk - god), Brahmā, Brahmacārini (the third), Gaṅga and Vāruṇa are sort of energies that stipulate the further development of the mind in this cakra. The consonant Kha, icon for water, has a great meaning in this cakra, viz.OṃKhaṁ Brahmā (YV 1975).

Moving the buttocks to and from, and subsequently by retracting and releasing the rectum physically activates the cakra. The genitals are also practised in the same manner. Next to the physical exercise the breathing has to be regulated. In this way: inhale (Lūm or Pūraka), hold the breath (Antar Kumbhaka), exhale (Anlūm or Recaka) and then stop breathing for a while c.q. put in a breathing space (Bāhir Kumbhaka).

In actual practice this can be done as follows: Pinch the right nostril with the thumb and inhale slowly. Keep the breath for a while. Then pinch the left nostril with the middle and ring finger and let the air escape slowly through the right nostril. Slowing down 'improves' the energy. The cakra is mentally activated as denoted in the discussion of the Mūlādhāracakra, now with the primeval sound Oṃ Vaṁ Oṃ. When producing this sound, one must mainly concentrate on the genitals.

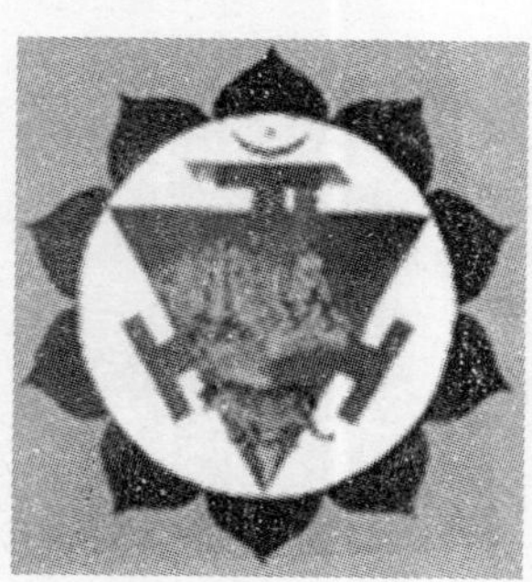

Maṇipura Cakra

Maṇipur means 'the city of the jewels.' This cakra is situated in the abdomen, two fingers above the navel, and opens to the front. Brain power, will power and guts, healing power, etc. are provided by this cakra in our body by Venus (Śukra as Brāhmaṇa, the secretary of Viṣṇu and the Guru of all demons) in the form of cosmic energy. The visible results in life are i.e. wealth, beauty, rest, peace, harmony etc. It attends to will power, supplies energy for the spleen, the stomach and the liver, the gall bladder and the Neuro vegetative system. In short, the giving of meaning to one's existence. It is connected with the pancreas (liver). Eyesight is central here. It is also known as the solar plexus that is controlled by the element fire which stimulates digestion and the intake of food so that the entire body can get the energy, necessary for survival.

Cosmic Doctor and Teacher

This cakra is also of significance in mythology. It is indicated in the Rīg Vedā (10.90.13; Nābhya Asidantarikṣam; from His navel came the firmament) how important this conjunction literally is, due to the usefulness of vegetative sacrifice as nourishment or Prasādam, and the role of the air as part of the digestive process (Ācamaniyam). The child is a visible result of the sacrifice of love. Due to the demonic principles (Śukra) sometimes a child adds demonic characters. The atmosphere originated from His navel. And because the baby's navel is connected with that of the mother, this navel is connected with this atmosphere as well. In this way, even the smallest creatures are in contact with the larger ones within the line of creation. And did not Lord Brahmā, who brought about all creation, come from the umbilical cord of Lord Viṣṇu (the God of Preservation)? From this network the ten Prāṇas or essential breathings are governed as Rudras (archetypes of Śiva). The original energy (divine) added with Dharma retrieves in this cakra, the creator in the quality of Viṣṇu (Sattva). One is here able to feed and to accompany the embryo which has already arisen in the second cakra. The factor A (from AUM) is in the first and second cakra to the order. You are the manager and or doctor who deliver the baby from the "golden egg" or Hiranyagarbha to lead an independent life. This management includes that on the one hand the umbilical cord of the mother, which is coupled with the cosmos and on the other hand with the umbilical cord of the baby. With this link a trinity arises within the link between god, people and the unborn child. Cosmos is a product of the umbilical point of Viṣṇu. From this umbilical point the first lotus arises, Brahmā who created the cosmos. From the source, Viṣṇu (Maha Viṣṇu or Brahmā), arises the element of creation gradually in name and conformation will change from man to woman. The creating energy remains unchanged and it is coupled to the moon. The Atharva Veda compares the unity with the unity of husband and wife. "Let thy soul and mind be knit together. Embrace thy consort as her loving husband (AV 18.1.3: 4241). Shall we do now what we never did before? Shall we righteously talk impurely now. Men are born of semen and so are women, such is our Kinship. Our mutual blood relation stands in the way of our wedlock (AV 18.1.4. 4242). When a doctor is desperate because the medicines have no effect on a patient then a doctor with a lot of experience injects the medicine by means of the umbilical point in the body. This method is the last chance to effect the syndrome. This indicates how important the umbilical point is. Here comes a link, made between the Maṇipūra cakra and the planet Venus (Śukra). The child here arises from fire, the main element in this cakra. In this cakra Candraghaṇṭā, the third Durgā, (the sound) and Lākinī live. From this cakra Parśurām (the God as defend or military power) and Śukra also operate. The consonant Ga the icon of fire is here under discussion.

The Nevli-kriyā or exercise with this cakra, is concentrated on this navel, the centre of the body, where the Ojas-energy (extract of sperm) lies. From the navel as centre of distribution, the breath has to push this energy upwards to the brains to serve as nutrition for meditation,[7] and the waste downwards with the air (force) called Apāna Vāyu. The Rīg Vedā mentions in this context 'Aśvins, who are rich in rain, ascend your golden chariot, a storehouse (of weapons); bring to us fattening food. (RV̇ 8.22.9-10). Food is regarded as medicine for purifying (koṣa or storehouse of quality, the Ānandamaya).

Emptying the lungs, maintaining the empty position and retracting the navel and pushing it out again physically

---

[7] Concentration and Meditation, Sri Swami Śivananda, The Divine Life Society, U.P., India, 1994.

activates the cakra. Then inhaling, holding the breath and again retracting the navel and pushing it out. Finally, inhaling, keeping the breath and subsequently retracting the abdomen.

It is mentally activated as it has been described in the discussion of the Mūlādhāracakra, but now with the primeval sound Oṃ Raṁ Oṃ. This sound is situated in a triangle and is produced by forming a triangle with the lips and pushing the tongue against the palate. When this sound is produced, the navel must be the main point of concentration.

Anāhata Cakra

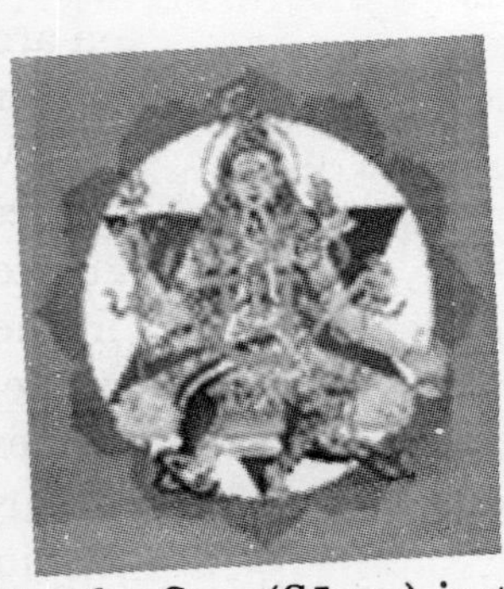

The Anāhata or heart chakra is located near the plexus cardiacus in the upper part of the back at the centre of the chest (breastbone) and opens towards the front. The name means 'unbeaten'. The brainpower, will power and guts, healing power, etc. are provided by this cakra in our body by the Sun (Sūrya) in the form of cosmic energy. The visible results in life are i.e. wealth, beauty, rest, peace, harmony etc. Here, the sense of touch is central, and it coordinates the heart, the chest and the chest cavity. This is the lowest part of the lungs, the blood, the blood circulatory system, the skin and the hands. It is connected with the thymus gland which is situated deep in the neck. Anāhata is the centre of the heart in which direct and conscious knowledge is central. The function of this cakra is to find a balance between the three cakras above the heart and the three below it. This is illustrated in a hexagram, which symbolises air and which is composed of two triangles, which overlap, and cut through one another.

The triangle directed upwards symbolises Śiva, the male principle. The other triangle which is directed downwards symbolises Śakti, the female principle (RV 10.90.12). When these two forces (Candramā and Sūrya) are united in harmony, a balance is reached. Male and female energy are balanced and the dissolving of the two energies which influence one another outside the body as well, is no longer a problem, as all relations become pure.[8] The level of sacredness within this cakra indicates the perception of the Divine mercy within all existence.

In the Subalopaniṣad, the heart of the gross body has been described thus: "In the middle of the heart there is a red lump of flesh in the midst of which there is the subtle Akāṣā. It is of white colour like the lotus, which blooms at night. It has developed in many ways. There are ten apertures of the heart in which prāṇa resides." (Ch. 4).

The shape of this lump of flesh is like a pear, tapering at the top and in which there are three main arteries which discharge blood. The lower part is large in which there are formations like the petals of lotus. In its midst, there is a small thumb like sheath. It has ten apertures like a large grape. In these apertures there is a flow of life through prāṇa. If it is struck there is a possibility of its failure. This is the lotus of the heart of the gross body.

Then, there is the heart of the subtle body, which is in the middle of the two breasts. In this heart, citta and soul are supposed to exist. This subtle body carries with it all the saṁskāras, good and bad, and is the cause of rebirth. This citta is related to the subtle and the causal bodies.The spiritually minded have given more importance to this heart. This is not a lump of flesh but it is subtler than the air and carries with it the subtle body. The spiritually minded have given excellence to this heart. The soul is supposed to reside in its citta.

Materialist doctors attach great importance only to the gross heart. It is considered to be the support of life. They try to keep it efficient in its functions and movement. This thinking of theirs is due to their materialistic attitude which accepts only what is seen directly or observed by instruments.

A birth of a child is a product of love. Love is born in the heart of people and is supervised and controlled by Śiva, the source of each Jīva (soul). In the Anāhata cakra, the child's own breathing of the child is started by placing it under the sun which is established in the Anāhata cakra (also called the

[8] Pure Yoga, Yogi Prāṇāvananda, Motilal Banarsidass Publishers Pvt. Ltd., New Delhi, India, 1997.

second button). The breath of people is Svara or vowel. The first vowel, which the child inhales, is the first vowel 'A' of AUM, and the lungs open up and start functioning. The child starts living with sounds in the heart. Heart and lungs are the vital bodies, which become active in the child. The conscience in embryo and in the growing embryo is stimulated here in the cakra. The mother radiates exclusive love in this stage of development and has a product of love in her uterus. Here we find the triad of love within the story of creation. The Big Bang is here presented in three characters, which have gone in advance, the AUM. Cosmic science arises, confessed in the growing embryo, in gestation, and is supervised by Ma Gāyatrī or Savitā (the Doctor of creation), the creating energy (also called Mā Kuśmāṇḍā). Savitā symbolises the twelve characteristics of the sun (the 12 petals of the lotus of this cakra) and this relates with one of the incarnation of Viṣṇu, Lord Śhri Rāma. Śiva and Kākinī are established in these cakras. The consonant Gha or air gets its important meaning in this cakra.

A person, who has realised consciousness of the fourth cakra, will find a subtle balance in body and mind.[9] He can master language, poetry and all other verbal skills, as well as the indryas or senses, desires and physical functions. His development has risen above the limitations of circumstances and the environment and radiates energy by itself. His life becomes a source of inspiration for others, because they experience composure and peace in his/her presence. Inhaling and exhaling deeply while alternately bending forward and sitting upright again physically activates it. This is done in the following manner: keep the head straight, together with the spine, stretch the hands above the head, inhale while thrusting out the chest, briskly lower the arms alongside the body, bend forward and then exhale deeply.

While activating this cakra mentally, you should concentrate as has been described at the Mūlādhāra cakra, but now with the primeval sound Oṃ Yaṁ Oṃ. When the Yaṁ sound is

[9] Hatha Yoga Pradipika, Swami Visnu-Devananda,Oṃlotus Publications, Motilal Banarsidass Publishers Pvt. Ltd., New Delhi, 1987.

formed, the tongue floats on air in the mouth. While doing this, you should concentrate on the centre of the chest.

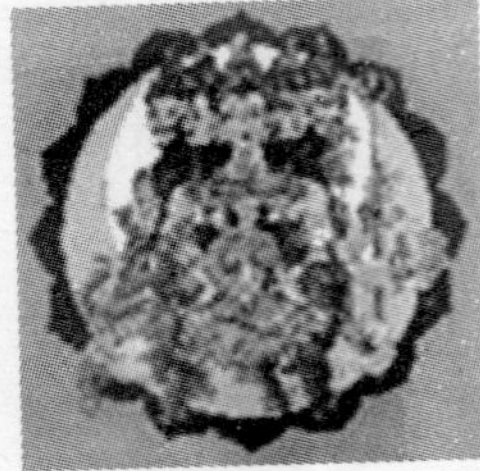

Viśuddha Cakra

The Viśuddha cakra is located near the plexus cervicalis (neck plexus) in the throat between the throat-holes and the larynx at the front and it opens to the front. Here the sense of hearing and Divine love are central. The brain power, will power and guts, healing power, etc. are provided by this cakra in our body by Mars (Maṅgala) in the form of cosmic energy. The visible results in life are i.e. wealth, beauty, rest, peace, harmony etc. In candid language we express these with Maṅgala or lucky. From its centre it coordinates the lungs, bronchi, gullet, speech organs (voice), throat, neck and jaws. It is connected with the thyroid gland and the parathyroid glands.

The name means Purity; the pure cosmic sound in the body. Elevation is an essential aspect of the Viśuddha cakra which must result in supersensory energy and speechless communication.[10] One understands non-verbal messages, as all energies become fine dusty matter because of the Ākāśa or ether, shining of its own. Ākāśa has the quality of anti-matter. In the cakra remain the five faces of Śiva. On the west (i.e. back) is Sadyojata; on the north (i.e. left) is Vāmadeva; on the south (right) is Aghora; and on the east (front) is Tatpuruṣa. Īśāna should be known as being in the middle.

Meditation on the cavity in the throat brings about tranquillity, serenity, purity, a melodious voice, control of speech and mantras and the ability to write poetry, interpret texts and understand hidden messages in dreams.

Besides that, the practitioner becomes youthful, radiant (Ojas) and a good teacher of spiritual sciences (Brahmavidyā). The Atharva Veda says 'The scholar is the ruler of the universe by his vigour' (AV 20.137.5). Here dwells the soul (Ātmā) of man, which is immortal and needs no addition, except for

---

[10] Meditation and Māntra's, Swami Visnu-Devananda, Om Lotus Publications, Motilal Banarsidass Publishers Pvt. Ltd., New Delhi, 1978.

being freed from dust only. The awareness in the fifth cakra is Soham, That I am, composed of Sa (that) and Aham (I am).[11] He comes to realise 'That I am, I am That' and because of that embodies sat-cit-ānanda, 'being, consciousness, bliss'. The voice of someone who lives from his fifth cakra penetrates as far as the heart of the listener. In this cakra all elements of the lower cakras-earth, water, fire and air-are distilled to their very essence and merge into Ākasa or ether. Earth merges into water and remains in the second cakra as the essence of smelling. Water evaporates in the fiery third cakra and just stays there as the essence of taste. Fire enters the fourth cakra and stays there as the essence of form and vision. The air of the fourth cakra enters Ākāśa and becomes pure sound. Ākāśa embodies the essence of the five elements, and has no colour, smell, taste, texture or form - it is free from all coarse elements.

In the fifth cakra space or ether are central. There a gestation of identity steps into the child. The Viśuddha cakra has been connected with the top planet, where a call centre (of sounds) takes place within the creation, because Lord Śiva blesses creatures as Īśāna (RV 10.90.2). The Atharva Veda proceeds with 'The Supreme Being is blissful. He is the lord of the animate and in-animate world' (AV 20.121.1). Here is Śiva a Dikpālaka, as the compass of eternal love. The section of compass is creating a platform for protection in a ritual sacrifice at the Pūjā ceremony. All creatures from this planet have granted their love (particularly of people) in the cosmos in their previous life. (RV 10.90.7;. In this hymn we find the mixture of the ingredients for the creation of man. Creation is a product of the sixteen faculties is signified in the sixteen steps of Pūjā (BhT. 2.6.13-16). Here the sixteen Svaras or vowels endow the child with latent knowledge of its own identity.[12] The alphabet is a photo of a typical identity or energy in the cosmos. Pronouncing the character is calling that particular energy. These sixteen energies are seated on each leaf of this cakra and rotating around the soul. The cakra

---

[11] The science of Prāṇayāma, Swami Śivananda, The Divine Life Society, U.P., India, 1997.

[12] Hatha Yoga, The hidden language, Symbols, Secrets, and Metaphor, Swami Śivananda Radha, Jaico publishing House, Bombay, 1998.

is a 'dynamo' which charges energy for circumstances on different levels. This is comparable with several kinds of energy that we need daily, i.e. lights, microwave, freezer, radio, TV, telephone, car etc. whom these cakra has on its leaves, and rotates around the soul like planets around its core.

This cakra is the second step where Svara or music affects the child. This cakra also produces blue light where the young man becomes disco minded. The cosmic thread (Gotra) here becomes visible within the process of creation. The Rīg Vedā indicates this with "The sons inherit the ancestral property" (RV 1.73.9). The soul in this cakra uses previous karma or credit balances, which are present within the cosmic line. And also among other things which of the sacrifices in the framework of the Śraddha or dead worship. It seems that the soul as the owner of the body is using a very small part. It stays here in the narrowest part of the body which is the connection (the neck where the Viśuddha cakra sits) between the divine (head) and the human (rest of the body). For this reason one concentrates on singing with Mālās(Chains) on the neck for maximum output. Through singing the Svaras arise love in the heart and these can be unconscious mumble sounds. A child in the womb reacts, slightly at this stage to these kinds of sounds. Devi Skandamātā, Kātyāyani and Sākinī have taken its place here. With Sākinī Sanātana Dharma arises for the first. This is a universal principle for every creature. In this cakra Siddhi and Nidhi start developing. The consonant Nga here is the icon for space.

In the exercises, the throat and vocal cords are central. The cakra is activated as follows: inhale, make a swallowing movement and bring the chin towards the chest. Then bring the chin back into its normal position, let go the breath, make a swallowing movement and bring the chin towards the chest again. Thereafter turn the neck clockwise and anti-clockwise. Then move the head up and down. Now, with the tailbone pulled up, inhale during ten counts and then bring the chin towards the chest. Hold this breath for 40 counts, and while in this position pull in the stomach as deep as possible and then slowly release the air in 20 counts. Now, quickly in a row, withdraw and release the Adam's apple.

The cakra is mentally activated as has been described with the Mūlādhāra cakra, but now with the primeval sound Oṃ Haṁ Oṃ. Forming an oval opening the lips and pushing the air from the throat outwards produces the sound Haṁ. When this sound is produced, the throat must be the main point of concentration.

Draft of life between the 5th and the 6th cakra the Lālana cakra is located. This cakra produces Māyā (illusory energy) in the human being as a prototype of the Māyā in cosmos. Both supernatural strengths and opulence are possible to obtain by means of yoga and pūjā (sacrifice). It is only when a person can resist by hard disciplines that the temptations of the Lālana cakra can grow up to the sixth cakra. This cakra serves as a misleading and materialistic area in the field of disciplines. They who become boasted by the Lālana cakra, become wizards, but they miss the capacity to release themselves. Supernatural strength is indispensable for achieving salvation. All these strengths remain both in the micro cosmos (people) and in the macro cosmos (universe).

In holy sacrifice or pūjā we symbolically use the extract of our body and that of the cosmos. The sacrifice of Pañcāmṛta is a mixure of five elements earth, water, fire, air and ether. Pañcāmṛta is an evaluation of a forth going process; a crosscheck of the mathematics or formula. These five elements are here symbolically visible in Dugdha (milk), Dahī (yoghourt), Ghī (churned butter), Madhu (honey) and Śarkarā (sugar). Milk is the first element that corresponds with the start of knowledge. A new baby is practising knowledge by the technique of breast-feeding. It proves that the newborn has knowledge and expertise of the process of feeding. This implies that this is not its first life. We find the link of these Pañcam in the science of language. This is the primary science of every creature. This corresponds in the alphabet with the first five consonants (Ka, Kha, Ga, Gha and Nga) which means the growth of the body (space, air, fire, water and earth). Knowledge is sound and sound is eternal (Sanātana), starting with the Big Bang, the primordial Sound. In this context, Ka indicates the sperm (milk), Kha for fertile (yoghourt), Ga for creation (butter), Gha for training (honey) and Nga for development or growth (sugar). The essence of creation and creatures is reflected in the colour of honey. After all, honey is equal to love. Love and God are similar. This colour expresses the maturity of wisdom and meditation for absorption and to merge in God (Sāyujya). Cosmic science expresses this as Srimad, the prefix at Bhagavad or Bhāgavatam; the preamble before salvation. In short, Śrī is spirit and Mad is maturity and both make spirituality. With Bhaga (fate) or Karma (ripeness) we have the access to penetrate and to sustain Godly-Bliss-Power.

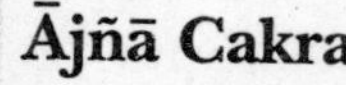

Ājñā Cakra

The Ājñā cakra resides in the plexus medulla, a spongy tissue in the internal bone at the nerve centre of the pineal gland, which is one finger above the base of the nose in the centre of the forehead and approximately two fingers inwards. It opens to the front and is the centre between the eyebrows. Brainpower, will power and guts, healing power, etc. are provided by this cakra in our body by the Jupiter (Bṛhaspati) in the form of cosmic energy. The visible results in life are i.e. wealth, beauty, rest, peace, harmony etc.

From this location it coordinates the little brain, ears, nose, paranasal sinuses, eyes, nervous system, forehead and the face. It corresponds with the pineal gland or hypophysis. The name means 'Authority'. Here the third eye of man is located, the Svanetra, the organ of clairvoyance. The aura of a clairvoyant manifests itself in such a way that everyone who finds himself in its presence comes to rest and becomes sensitive to the subtle frequencies of the AUM-sound that stays in him. All desires are in fact the acting of tattva or qualities. When one settles down on the location between the eyebrows one raises oneself above. All kinds of desires, which motivate man in life and make him move in a great number of directions. Some worship predominantly the masculine or right side of the conjoint male and female figure (Ardhanārīśvara).[13] Some, the Saktas, predominantly worship the left, and call Her Mother, for She is the Great Mother (Magna Mater), the Mahādevi who conceives, bears, and nourishes the universe sprung from Her womb (Yoni). This is so because She is the active aspect of Consciousness, imagining the world to be, according to the impressions derived from enjoyment and suffering in former worlds.

The whole process of evolution is due to the presence of the will to life and enjoyment, which is a result of Vāsanā, or world-desire, carried from life to life in the Saṁskāras, or impressions made on the subtle body by Karma, which is guided by Īśvara. In its reaching forth to the world, the Self is not only endowed with the faculties of the subtle body, but with the gross objects of enjoyment on which those faculties feed. There, therefore, comes into being, as a projection of the Power (Śakti) of Consciousness, the gross body of matter called Sthūla-Śarīra.

One now concentrates on one point and becomes Trikāladarśi, an expert of the past, the present and the future. The nerve flows, Iḍǎ and Piṅgala are limited by time. Up to the fifth cakra the yogi is also limited by time, but because Iḍa and Piṅgala end in the Ājña, the yogi proceeds to the Śuṣuṁṇā, the spinal cord, which is Kālātita, i.e. beyond the reach of time. He no longer risks a relapse. A spiritual turn is impossible because as long as he is in his physical body, he is in a constant situation of non-dualistic consciousness. He is now ready for understanding the inner meaning of cosmic science and to produce draw it. Someone who develops himself with the Ājñā cakra reveals the Divine in himself and reflects the Divinity in others.

A typical behaviour with the Ājñā cakra is that the pineal gland stretches out as far as the third ventricle and is surrounded by the cerebrospinal fluid Amṛta or the nectar of life. Amṛta is a clear, watery fluid that flows from the Soma cakra (the moon cakra), located above the Ājñā cakra. It moves through the empty spaces (ventricles) into the brains and along the spine. An experienced yogi leads this Amṛta to

---

[13] Yoga & Ayurveda, Self-Healing and Self-Realization, David Frawley, Motilal Banarsidass Publishers Pvt. Ltd., New Delhi, India, 2002.

the stomach and can fast for long. The pineal gland ensures that this flow passes evenly.

When someone enters de Ājñā cakra the astral light around his head will form an aura. As in this situation the yogi fully controls his breath and mind, he finds himself with all his acts in a continual state of Samādhī or contemplation. Contemplation is a situation of non-differentiated cosmic consciousness, because every duality must cease to exist.[14] Whatever he requires he realise, just like his ability to bring up images from the past, the present and the future. This is the result of merging the Iḍa(lunar flow), Piṅgala (solar flow) and (the neutral central flow) in the Ājñā cakra. In this cakra the syllables of Sohaṁ (from the fifth cakra) are transformed into Haṁsa. Now he is Haṁsa: those who fly, because he meditates on the Ātmā or the self in the Bindu.

We Can Fly

Bindu is a 'point' that symbolises eternity in the syllable AUM which is infinite. The word Haṁsa also means 'swan', a bird that flies to places unknown to common people. He who stays in this consciousness is called Paramhaṁsa.

Life means struggle and battle. This can bring victory or defeat, reward or death. This starts before birth; even before fertilisation. The victorious seed cell that won the race to reach the female egg was rewarded with the creation of a new life. During the race, millions of seed cells perished. May I also refer to the many caterpillars that perish before only a few of them can become butterflies? And to the flower buds that are not promoted to flowers or fruits? Life is ora et labora. Pray and work with an uncertain outcome.

By meditation is usually understood a devout reflection on Creation or the Creator. To prove how important meditation is to bring about an evolution in the human mind, followers often refer to the metamorphosis, which takes place in the cater pillar. In the first phase the embryo develops into a larva. Then the larva becomes a caterpillar. After having contributed

[14] Patanjali's Yoga Sustras, with the commentary of Vyasa and the gloss of Vachaspati Misra, Munshiram Manoharlal Publishers Pvt. Ltd., New Delhi, India, 1998.

its 'share' to the symbiosis it seeks out an unobtrusive spot and builds a pod in which it shuts itself to undergo the metamorphosis. In the pod only a small quantity of air is present which has to be consumed economically. When the time is ripe the caterpillar rips open the pod and draws in fresh oxygen (Prāṇa or life force) which enables it to spread its wings and to fly out as a butterfly. Behold the miracle: the caterpillar is no longer a caterpillar but a butterfly. Thanks to the metamorphosis a butterfly is able to cover greater distances with less effort than a caterpillar.

Thanks to the metamorphosis it becomes the subject of admiration, whereas caterpillars suffer aversion. Thanks to the metamorphosis its social value is so much greater than that of a caterpillar since it can through pollination contribute to growth and bloom of nature, whereas a caterpillar because of its burrowing activities exercises a negative influence on nature, which is the reason why it is being exterminated. Without the butterfly many plants would become extinct for lack of pollination in the required manner and neither would reproduction take place. Due to its evolution the butterfly has thus become a useful creature. Yoga, the withdrawing into oneself and losing oneself in meditation and systematic reflections of a positive nature, can therefore improve the quality of the practitioner and can have a positive impact on society. If the tiny caterpillar can realise its aim of life intuitively, how high then can man reach with his superior mind? In other words, man can become a super human being by making use of this technique. This, in its turn, can be of importance to attain Mokṣa faster or even to travel in the mind throughout the universe.

The metamorphose of a caterpillar is changing instinctually of conformation due to the quality of the second sheath or Prāṇāmaya koṣa. People on the other hand are born in the fifth sheath or Ānandamaya koṣa. People cannot be compared with a caterpillar. The performance of the caterpillar is a visible result of possibilities on the field of increasing the secret power in our body.

Turning the eyes to the left and to the right and keeping a straight back and sitting in the tailor position physically activates the cakra. And then making a circular motion with the eyes, clockwise and anti-clockwise. Thereafter looking up and down with the eyes while they are up and down. Then putting the little fingers in the ears and saying the word AUM three times whereby the M is held longer each time. Now bend the body to the front and make a circular motion with the upper part of the body, clockwise and anti-clockwise. Then activate the whole body through the Bhastrika (bellows) Prāṇāyāma. These are alternately quick, deep and forceful short breathings via the left and right nostrils (L-R-R-L) in which the pace is increased more and more, like a train building up its speed. Subsequently, through the Śuṣumṇā Svara (the dia-phragm), in and exhaling fast and deeply with both nostrils, like a steam engine. And finally inhaling fast and very deep, and exhaling en bloc with great force.

The cakra is mentally activated as described with the Mūlādhāra cakra, but now with the primeval sound Oṃ Kṣaṁ Oṃ. Closing the jaws and lips and concentrating on the forehead, between the eyebrows produces this sound OM. By focussing the eyes on the tip of the nose, the nerve flows and the Mūladhāra-cakra are stimulated and the Kuṇḍalini (cosmic energy) which is located here, is activated.[15] By applying this method to another cakra during concentration, one can make the Kunǎlini rise and make the relevant chakra, which has already been activated by concentration, even more effective. The technique of focussing the eyes on the tip of the nose is thus a powerful method via which the effect of concentration can be doubled. There are two reasons why stimulation of the perineum, the location of the Mūladhāra-cakra in the physical body, also arouses the Ājñā. In the first place the Kuṇḍalini which resides in the Mūladhāra is aroused by this exercise. No cakra can be aroused, unless it is activated by a Kuṇḍalinī that has been stirred up. In the second place the

---

[15] Kuṇḍalinī Yoga, Swami Śivananda Radha, Motilal Banarsidass Publishers Pvt. Ltd., New Delhi, 1992.

Ajña is in direct contact with the Mūlādhāra via the Iḍa-Piṅgala and Śuṣumṇā-nadi, which come together at these two points.[16]

Ājñā is the authorisation or admission by means of knowledge and wisdom to spirituality. Spirituality is the basis to achieve Mokṣa (salvation). This is comparable with a guaranteed money order. This cakra is also the third button. Pressing on the button is the start of the finishing touch. The child is the seed between human society and godly world (head). Godly principle is the third button that implements in this cakra, located in the forehead. The study starts with the concentration. The process of learning starts in the forehead through the hidden energy behind this button. In a long study the forehead becomes warm. We experience this in daily practice. Study means Self-sacrifice. In the Ājñā cakra the cosmos is present as a pinhead which is called Bindu (zero point) and stands under control of the energy called Vāmana, the microscopic cosmos. From this Bindu the entire creation or the Sindhu has arisen (see figure 38).

Figure 27 The Bindu
The electron is the Bindu

Figure 28 The Sindhu
From this Bindu the entire creation or the Sindhu has arisen

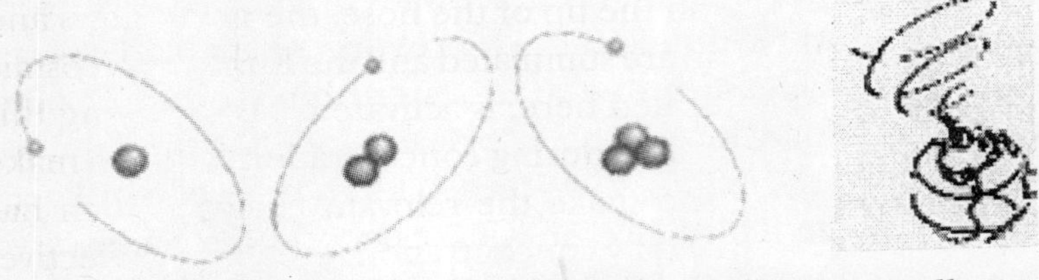

In figure 27 the electron is the Bindu. This is a small part of Śiva as Parambindu (Bhāvyam, Spirit), the smallest point. The multiplying effect starts from this point (RV 10.90.2). Parambindu is the cause of this entire (visible world). Proton and neutron are called the food of the creation. This figure shows the multiple effect on all branches of science (theory and practice). The most visible part of this formula we can find in each of our finger (phalanx) and in reference to the

[16] Kundalini Yoga, Swami Śivananda, The Devine Life Society, U.P., India, 1994.

three modes of our activities (good, bad and between). Modern science explains that the nuclear energy is the energy released (Gvam) during the splitting or fusing of atomic nuclei. The energy of any system (Bhūtam), whether physical, chemical, or nuclear, etc. is manifested by the system's ability to function or to release heat or radiation (Bhāvyam). The total energy (Tattva) in a system is always conserved, but it can be transferred (Amṛtam or ambrosia) to another system or changed in form (reincarnation). This is a confirmation of the process that happens in the Ājñā cakra. The lubricant in this process is also the binding agent, Love (Īśāna) as eternal ambrosia. The atom theory is linked with (re)incarnation. In physics we quote: creation is a process of expanding.

The AUM of the 4th cakra is here in extractible form present in the Bindu. Higher energy forms (deva's and devi's), here in micro form, develops the Citta or mind in the growing child in the womb. At this stage all agencies and senses are further developed in the growing process, so called the data bank of the mind. The baby child gets experience here with the Kāla-Śakti, the notion of time and the latent divine potentials to create. This quality is originated from Mā Gaurī, the white Goddess or energy that dwells in this cakra. Here is time linked to rhythm and the biorhythm of the 2nd cakra. With these capacities the child starts functioning. Beside interactions for activity, Śānti or peace is added to the volume of capacities (YV 36-17: 1889). The eleven sorts of Śānti are present in the Third Eye or Ājñā cakra. These Śāntis are cleaning the mind and purifying the soul. In meditation we go through this process to the Sahasrāra cakra for Samādhi or contemplation. jñānamudra is the connection of the forefinger with the thumb. This is the visible form of wisdom, which a yogi needs to merge with the Great Architect of the universe. Here is the forefinger the identity of the yogi and the thumb is God. The circle between these two is the visible wisdom as condition to become invisible and to merge (from Sākāra to Nirākāra). (RV 10.90.9). In the hymn the word Sādhya is the merging of the individual with the Almighty. The medium for this churning is knowledge, wisdom and devotion. The new identity of the individual here is Ṛsi or seer. After this ritual the slogan Śānti, Śānti, Śānti is the evaluation of the internal evolution and anticipation of new identity. These three Śānti at the end of each meditation session indicate the three states of Samādhī, i.e. Savikalpa (with an object in the mind), Nirvikalpa (without an object) and Nirvāṇa (without the seed of the mind). These processes of going into retreat are with an object in the mind, without an object in the mind and without mind in the object. Modern science announces this in the pedagogy the tabula rasa, blank sheet.

The above mentioned Śānti is available everywhere. Even in the womb of a woman a growing baby can take a rest in its movements. This is called the dancing in the womb in correlation with the Cosmic Dancing, the Naṭrāja, in the reincarnation cycle. With small brakes during work one can absorb much more than constantly in the move. In the educational science 5x3 is more than 3x5, which means that god üiva gives the child the third eye at this stage with five elements in all the three bodies. With this eye the child is able to see the gods, due to the capacity of absorbing astral knowledge. God mostly performs in astral posture. So, to the child it is not difficult to see the deva's and devi's in the womb, even strongly, it is in touch with them. Even after birth a baby smiles in its sleep and laughs with them. The baby is communicating by its third eye with God Śiva, the primordial Guru in the form of Bṛhaspati with the child. To survive and to pass life it needs a Guru.

The Gurucakra is located between the Ājñā-and the Somacakra. This cakra is the dwelling of Mother Gaurī.The child needs mother love. The first item in life after mother is the breast that the child finds after searching. This is the starting point of self-management of the thrashed little child. Milk is the first result of this effort. Bṛhaspati in this cakra is the male Guru for education and self-management. This energy must ensure that the child develops itself after birth as a strong personality. The blessing comes mostly from female energy. These supernatural capacities are the scarce items in life. The opulent Gaurī is the leading force of all demigods or energies (devis̃ and devta's). They are together in microform in the Ājñā cakra. The number of these energies or angels is 330 millions. We find this total by dividing the digit 1 with 3. One stands for God and three the qualities in the cosmos (1:3). The division is endless. This is the mathematics of creation within Trinity which is always present. This cakra is the dome of this triad. Also the eight supernatural capacities for self-realisation are found here. The Androgyne body consists of number 2 for the two kinds of bodies. Cosmic science multiplies this number (2) to the power of three instead of the 8 supernatural powers. On the scale from baby to salvation we become from 2 to 8, and are able to open the third eye.

A cross check of this chakra produces the following powers: Śiva, Kālarātrī, Gaurī, Hākinī, Vāmana, Bṛhaspati, Sarva Devi's and Deva's, Sarva Pitras and Pretas (ancestors). As mentioned before, are these forms and principles of the same God. The Rīg Vedā points out "May Sarasvatī, who has seven sisters, who is dearest amongst those dear to us, and is fully propitiated, be ever adorable. Seven Sisters - Saptasvasa: either the seven metres of the Vedas, or the seven rivers." (RV 6.61.1-10). Here we can also refer to the primarily sound or svara's (souls) as the first scale of music after the Big Bang, SA-RE-GA-MA-PA-DHA-NI, as the component and grade of creatures in the process of creation. If there is no music in life, life becomes a walking grave.

At this stage all mysteries of cosmos are revealed by means of the 16-steps of pūjā. People here become theoretically 'dressed' with the 16 Saṁskāras (sacraments) and 16 Śriṅgāras (vogue). These aspects must be applied after the birth in life to activate inner qualities. People become a jewel in the surroundings of birth. Depending on the karma (level of absorption) one is able to follow this education. Bṛhaspati is also the Guru of the first priests (guru) in the cosmos. He is Bṛha or Mahāguru. Bṛha means the increase in wisdom. In the Rīg Vedā we find him in this context as a Director "We have wandered, gods, into a desert where there is no track of cattle: the vast extant earth has become the protectress of murderers: direct us, Bṛhaspati, in our search for cattle: show the path, Indra, to your votary they being astray." (RV 6.47.20). Above mentioned is the implication between all creation and creatures. This applies both within positive and negative energies, called Suras and Asuras (also known as Diti and Aditi). Here it can be added that people get a property of Purohita. This property enables her to help others. Only with knowledge and wisdom is it possible to help others. Purah means place, surroundings and Hita means helpful or helping hand. The first mantra of the Rīg Vedā gets its blueprint here. Devi Hākini (the Visarga-the Ha-consonance and Rīg Vedā 10.90.2.) is the main ruler in this Cakra. In the Puruṣa Sūkta (RV 10.90.15) it is indicated that the double dots (Visargas) appear in the form of Vāmana, the multiplication-or cloning process. This small circle around a space is called Parikramā. The white colour of this cakra has to do with wisdom, which is compared to milk.

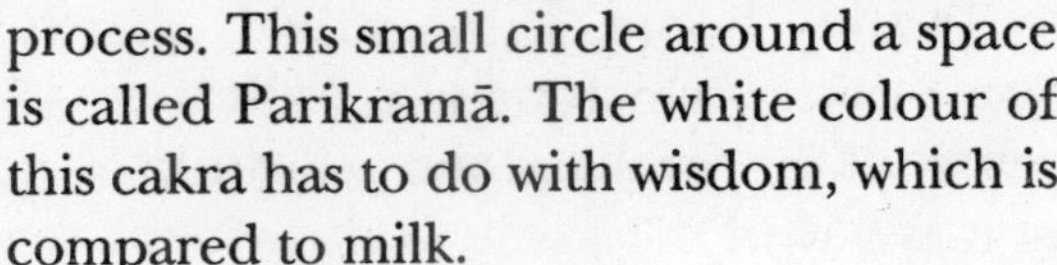

Sahasrāra Cakra

The Sahasrāra-cakra is situated in the region of the crown in the centre of the skull (plexus occipitalis), adjacent to the back part of the head, and opens upwards. This cakra regulates every aspect of the body and mind. The brain power, will power and guts, healing power, etc. are provided by this cakra in our body. With the link with Saturn (Śani) of this cakra we gain cosmic energy. The visible results in life are i.e. wealth, beauty, rest, peace, harmony etc.

When the "gate of Brahmā" is open in this cakra one can leave the physical body and enter the astral world of causality. As has been mentioned earlier, in Sanskrit this spot is denoted as Brahmdvāra or the entrance to Brahmā, the impersonal God. This is the crown of the skull under which the great brain is situated. It is connected with the pineal gland (epiphysis) that is in the brain. Sahasrā means "Thousand or Thousand-petalled." In the Rīg Vedā (10.90.1), it is explained with Sahasrā what God looks like: One with many noughts in every area. This cakra-space is also called Sūrya ('empty') or niralambapuri (abode without support: universe as roof). The Satyam-loka is situated here. This is the level of truth and reality. The inner Guru or Paramātmā is here in charge. The Guru is also denoted as the Mahāśakti, the Superpower. Swami Satyananda Saraswati specifies this cakra as Bindu Visarga and locates it at the back of the head where the Brahmanas tend to cultivate a tuft of hair (Kapārdinam, Curki or Tonsure). As a translation for the concepts Bindu and Visarga he respectively states 'point' and "pouring drop by drop." Another specification of this cakra is the term Somacakra. Soma is nectar for the gods and also means moon. The cakra is associated with the production of sperm.

In Cakra's, Energy Centres of transformation, published by Destiny Books, U.S.A., 1994, Harish Johari situates the Soma-cakra (which he also indicates as Amṛta-cakra) in the centre of the forehead above the third eye and makes mention of it as one of the smaller cakras in the seventh cakra. To him the seventh cakra is the Sahasrāra-cakra. There are more writers who denote the Sahasrāra as cakra, such as Swami Śivananda Radha in his book Kuṇḍǎlini yoga, published by Motilal Banarsidass in 1978, page 274. I further refer to the book by Helen Knopper: Lexicon of Yoga published at Bert Bakker, Amsterdam, 1976, page 101. Soma as well as Amṛta means nectar, elixir of life. By nature, nectar continuously seeps downwards from the nirjhara-or Brahmā guphā, the hollow between the cerebral hemispheres and when it reaches the Maṇipūra-cakra (number three), it is burnt by the solar energy of the solar plexus. Here the physical male semen (Bindu) unites with the lunar female energy because it is a combination of bhoga and yoga, of lust and disengagement. As we see the Bindu is a small cakra below the Sahasrāra. She is located in the region between the Ājñā and the Sahasrāra. This cakra is a channel with the nectar or Soma. Bindu and Curki are the front wheel (front cover) and the back cover of this channel. The Rīg Vedā mentioned in this context: 'We solicit riches of our friend, (Soma, Śiva as Īśāna), the chief of charioteers, the wearer of a braid (of hair), the lord of infinite wealth.' (RV 6.55.2). The yogi lengthened his tongue until it reaches the space between the eyebrows and is then introduced in a reversed position into the mouth searching for nectar in the Soma channel where the nectar for immortality flows (RV 6058; SV 1574; YV 33.97). This nectar replaces hunger and thirst and the yogi is then able to practise yoga for a long time.

Subsequently the author puts the Sahasrāra on the scene, which is supposed to be located on the crown of the head. 'It is not really a cakra but the abode of highest consciousness. In the Sahasrāra the mystic union of Śiva and Śakti would take place, the union of consciousness with matter and energy, the individual soul with the Supreme.[17] When Kuṇḍalini awakens, it ascends through the cakras to Sahasrāra and merges into the source from whence it originated. Matter and energy merge into pure consciousness in a state of intoxicating bliss, the goal of yoga. Having attained this, the yogi gains supreme knowledge and passes beyond birth and death.

Harish Johari situates the Soma-cakra (which he also indicates as Amṛtacakra) in the centre of the forehead above the third eye and makes mention of it as one of the smaller cakras in the seventh cakra.[18] To him the seventh cakra is the Sahasrāra cakra. Soma as well as Amṛta means nectar, elixir of life. By nature, the nectar continuously seeps downwards from the Nirjhara-or Brahmā Guphā, the hollow between the cerebral hemispheres and when it reaches the Maṇipūra cakra (number three), it is burnt by the solar energy of the solar plexus. The Vedas quotes this as "O Indu, bring us wealth in steeds brilliant and quickening all life; And make us better than we are." (SV 1056) and "From whom we have accepted thus thousands and three-time ten besides. Swift runs this giver of delight." (RV 9.62.22-24). Here the physical male semen (Bindu) unites with the lunar female energy because it is a combination of Bhoga (lust) and yoga (disengagement).

---

[17] Light on Prāṇāyāma, Prāṇāyāma Dipika, B.K.S. Iyengar, Harper Collins Publishers India Pvt Ltd, New Delhi, 1993.

[18] Chakra's, Energy Centers of Transformation, Harish Johari, Destiny Books, USA, 1987.

Energy One

Lord Śiva as Kameśvara gives the ability to retain semen. Therefore meditation on Kameśvara results in the subsiding of the ego and the yogi who finds himself in the Soma-cakra experiences Brahmānanda (the bliss of Brahm). Kameśvara or śakti has calmed down now that she has become one with her lord. She is no longer the spitting snake with the raging fire. He who meditates on this cakra and has stopped the downward flow of the nectar becomes immortal in this physical body. This process happens by doing the mime Khecari-Mudra (Khe is ether, Cari is moving). The yogi can now stop the process of aging and by doing so he stays young, full of vitality and stamina.

Hiroshi Motoyama has, in an exquisite manner, put into words what kind of things happen when this cakra is set to motion.[19] The inner sun is lighted in the body of the yogi and the aura of light that surrounds him becomes radiant. At this level the frequency of AUM which lasts infinitely manifests itself in the yogi; he is clad in and covered by vibrations and beams of light. The yogi receives complete control of the Prāṇa, which becomes so fine (sūkṣma) the total amount of Prāṇa in his body is said to have the size of a thumb. At his level several energies cooperate to help and to keep the 'metamorphose' in the yogi. There are energies as the Mīna (the fish or Matsya below the Mūladhāra for movement and on the Sahasrāra cakra the Vārāhī Devi is the protecting energy as a board. Between both ends the Gandharvas are music, sounds (consonances) and strengths with their important due to keep the balance resulting in the integration of the gross and subtle bodies. All these energies function for cohesion at the time of the flow of Energy One.

If someone would hold a piece of glass before the nose of the yogi, it would not steam up. The level of happiness (Sukha) rises when body and mind are internally balanced. When the state of Samādhī is reached and the physical body becomes completely motionless, immortality sets in. In this state there

---

[19] Theories of the Chakra's, Bridge to Higher Conciousness, Hiroshi Motoyama, Uitgeverij Ank-Hermes bv, Deventer, 1990.

is no activity of the mind, no person who knows, no knowledge, anything that can be known. Up to the sixth cakra the yogi can get into a trance in which activity and form still belong to consciousness, but in the Sahasrāra cakra Prāṇa moves upwards and reaches the top. The mind settles in the absolute emptiness of the Sūnyamaṇḍala as Mātrās for the soul, the space between the cerebral hemispheres. At that moment all feelings, emotions and desires merge into their very first root. The union is reached. The yogi is sat-cit-ananda (truth-bliss). Here citta (consciousness) is like a screen, upon which the reflection of the cosmic self is seen, through which the Divine is reflected. In the presence of the cosmic self everybody can experience the Divine and realise the Divinity in himself. Here the concentration is focussed on the fontanel and in meditation the sound changes into the image of AUM or GOD; the becomes visible invisible.

In general the technique follows these lines: a prescribed Āsana (posture) is assumed in combination with certain Mudrās; the eyes may be kept open or shut and focused on the roof of the head or between the eyebrows. For some minutes Prāṇāyama (breathing) exercises are performed with the object of "collecting and concentrating on upward and downward breaths." There is then a sudden ceasing of the breath, followed by the propulsion of the collected air down towards the Mūlādhāra. The pressure of the upward and downward breaths arouses the Kuṇḍalini.[20] Another method is described thus: fill the interior of the body with Prāṇa (air), and after a time apply Kumbhaka (retention of breath). Then contract the heart, move the air downwards, contract the anus and direct the Prāṇa through a semicircular motion, left to right, around the Pericarp of the basal lotus (cakra).[21] This will warm and stir the Kuṇḍalini, which should be assisted by slow intonation of a secret Bīja-or rootmantra.

---

[20] The Secret Serpent, Datta, M.R., Motilal Banarsidass Publishers Pvt. Ltd., New Delhi, India, 1994.

[21] The Primal Power of Man or Kundalini Sakti, Narayananda, Swami, Rishikesh, India, 1950.

The Final and Secret Power

Kuṇḍalini or 'coiled' is the name of a potent occult energy symbolized by a serpent having three and a half coils, and sleeping with its tail in its mouth. It is often referred to as a goddess and she has its home in the subtle body of man. She is occupying a point near the base of the spine at the Mūlādhāra plexus, "two fingers above the rectum and two fingers below the generative organs."

In most cases the Kuṇḍalini lies in deep sleep throughout one's lifetime, and even its existence remains unsuspected. This is just as well, for, according to the adepts, no one should experiment with it or try to rouse it without explicit instructions from a guru, as the dangers connected with its awakening are very real and terrible. When aroused and let loose without control and direction it rages like a vicious serpent so that it becomes impossible for a man to resist its force. Whatever supernatural powers he acquires through it will only bring him in contact with the lower orders of evolution and diabolical forces. Complete moral and spiritual degeneration will ensue, resulting in the disintegration of the gross and subtle bodies, and irreparable harm both in this world and the next.

The Burning Train

Controlled awakening of the Kuṇḍalini is one of the main objects of several branches of Hindu occultism, including yoga and Tantrism. By appropriate exercises the "serpent of life, fire and wisdom" can be aroused and properly directed to energise the body and soul. Long training and preparatory disciplines are required for the arousal of the Kuṇḍalini, but no fixed regime exists, and methods vary considerably. The experiences accompanying the awakening also differ; they are believed to be conditioned largely by the traditional background of the pupil and are therefore entirely subjective.

Once the Kuṇḍalini is aroused she becomes stiff like a rod, and can be directed by a special secret process to start its journey up the Śuṣumṇa (central column). As the Kuṇḍalini moves upward it strikes against the downward facing lotuses (cakras) in order, starting from the lowest, causing them to undergo involution and bloom upward. In other accounts the ascending Kuṇḍalini is said successively to pierce, heat up and burn the various cakras. The cakras are stations on the railroad of the Secret Power. Locomotion is now the act or power of moving from place to place. Śuṣumṇa is the locomotive and Iḍa and Piṅgala are now the rails. As each cakra is animated, different 'signs' make their appearance: body heat increases, the skin sweats profusely, a stinging sensation 'like a scorpion' is felt. Simultaneously the occult powers (Siddhis) are released.[22] Thus, by raising the Kuṇḍalini to the Manipūra cakra (near the navel) power may be acquired over fire. Only a few adepts succeed in working the Kuṇḍalini as far as the Sahasrāra, near the brain. The complete process is known as Saḍ-Cakra-Bheda, "he six Cakra piercing."

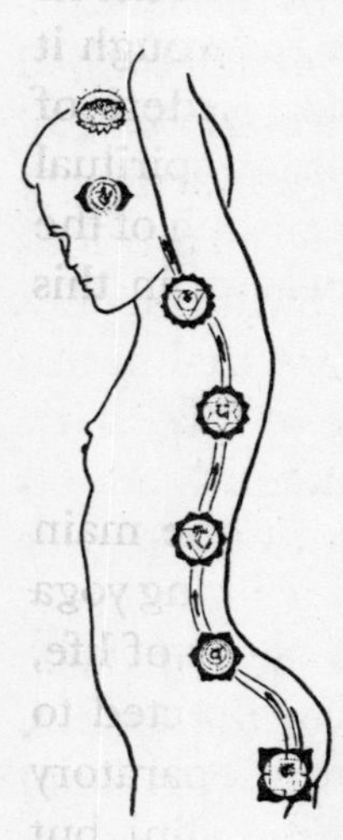

Some yogis hold that the Kuṇḍalini has only to break through three 'knots' (Granthi), namely, the Mūlādhāra or base (the knot of Brahmā), the Anāhata or heart (the knot of Viṣṇu), and the Ajñā or eyebrow (the knot of Śiva), to reach the Sahasrāra.[23] Contact between the Kuṇḍalini and Sahasrāra results in the flooding of the whole being with indescribable bliss.

Associated with the awakening of the Kuṇḍalini are various experiences on the occult planes. This are manifested, among other things, by different stages of awareness, as each Cakra is pierced (see figure of piercing).[24]

Figure 29 The Piercing of Kuṇḍalini Śakti through the cakras

[22] Kundalini, An Occult Experience, Arundale, G.S., Adyar, Madras, 1947.

[23] The Serpent Power; Sir John Woodroffe; Ganesh & Company; Madras; 1997.

[24] Figure: Wat is Yoga: Een inleiding tot universeel denken; Hans Wesseling; Uitgeverij Bert Bakker; Amsterdam, 1978.

When the yogi has pierced all six Cakras he listens for the inner sounds. At first many sounds are heard: the sound of a distant ocean; then a thundering; the sound of a waterfall; then a tinkling as of ornaments; then a drum, a bell, a flute, a bee. The head becomes giddy, the mouth fills with saliva, but the adept must carry on. The sounds become more internal and more and more subtle until, from the innermost core of his being he hears the Nā da, the voice of the inner silence, the 'unstruck' and unmanifested sound, the uncaused essence of Śabda, the Word.[25] Accompanying this is the experience of seeing dots of light, flames of fire, colored lines, dazzling geometrical shapes, and an 'effulgence', manifesting in progressive stages from the Marīcika, 'mirage', or illusive bright images, then smoke, then bright circles of light, then the Tāraka, 'star', a small intensely bright light seen between and in front of the eyebrows. This is followed by the Prakāśa, an inner illumination, which in turn is followed by the Samana-like experience of Jyoti, 'radiance', which has been described as 'the brightness of the Self which is like a universal flame of a lamp that no wind ever disturbed. Here is a new morning in life, according to the Vedas "The Morning knows all precious things, the Goddess knows her grace to man: Swift runs this giver of delight." (SV 1058). Rest and peace are vital in this stage and the Cosmic Śānti Pāṭha (exchange of rest) starts here. The innermost core of his being simultaneously adopts rust, peace and harmony working successively to the higher stage that carries on:

Dyauh-Śānti: if directed at the powers of Deva - or Svahaloka, the space of sounds above ancestors, specific for the Angles. Antarikṣagvaṁ-Śānti: if directed at the powers of Pitṛi - and Pretaloka also known as Bhuva-world where the ancestors reside. Pṛthivi-śānti: if directed at the powers of Bhūloka also known as Earth world. Āpah-Śānti: if directed at powers of water and waters of the oceans. Ośadhayah-Śānti: if directed at powers through homeopathic road. Vanaspatyah-Śānti:if

[25] Hindu World (volume 1-2); An encyclopaedic survey of Hinduism; Benjamin Walker; Harper Collins Publishers India; New Delhi, 1995.

directed at powers of oxygen. Viśvedevah-Śānti: if directed at the powers of Viśva, the universe. Brahmaśānti: if directed at powers of the Creator. Sarva-gvam-Śānti: if directed at powers surrounding the one performing the ceremony. Śantireva-Śānti: if directed at all powers known and unknown. Sāma Śāntiredhi: if directed at the powers in vibrations, sound, music and the cosmos in conformity with Sāma Veda. (YV 36-17: 1889). Oṃ Śānti, Śānti, Śānti.

APPENDIX

Table 4a Cakras with all characters

Name	Mūladhāra	Svādhiṣṭhana	Maṇipūra
Meaning	Root	Self-abode	City of Gems
Location	Base/Earth	Sex/Water	Navel/Fire
Petals	4	6	10
Bija Mantra	LAM	VAM	RAM
Character on the leafs	Vaṁ, Saṁ, Saṁ, Saṁ	Baṁ, Bhaṁ, Maṁ, Yaṁ, Raṁ, Laṁ	Daṁ, Dhaṁ, Naṁ,Taṁ, Thaṁ, Daṁ, Dhaṁ, Naṁ, Paṁ, Phaṁ
Element	Earth	Water	Fire
Tanmatra	Smell	Taste	Sight
Symbol	Yellow Square	White Crescent Moon	Red Triangle
Sense Organ	Nose	Tongue	Eye
Motor Organ	Excretory	Urino-Genital	Feet
Coordinate and control functions	the spinal column, the bones, the teeth, the nails, legs, anus, rectum, large intestine and prọstate	the pelvic region, eproductive organs, kidneys, bladder, all bodily fluids such as blood, lymph, digestive fluids and sperm	the ten Pranas or essential breathings
Consonant	Ka (Creation)	Kha (Knowledge)	Ga (Elan)
Rhythm-Scale	Sa (Creation)	Re (Knowledge)	Ga (Elan)
God	Brahmā	Brahmā	Viśnu
Animalrhythm	Peacock (üadja)	Bull (Śabha)	Goat (Gandhar)
Animal (Pancatattva)	Elephant	Crocodile	Raṁ
Color	Crimson Red	Vermilion	Dark Blue
Nadi	Alambusha	Kuhu	Viśvodhara
Tissue	Muscle	Fat	Blood
Dosha	Kapha	Kapha	Pitta
Prana	Apāna	Apāna	Samāna
Planets	Moon (Soma)	Mercurius (Budha)	Venus (Sukra)
Demigoddess or Kinis	Dākini	Rākini and Cākini	Lākini
Lokas, celestial planets	Bhur	Bhūvah	Svah
Bodies	Sthūla (physic)	Ātmabhava (psyche)	Sūkṣma (astral)

Table 4b Cakras with all characters

Anāhata	**Viśuddha**	**Ājña**	**Sahasrā Padma**
Unstruck Sound	Very Pure	Command	Thousand Petalled lotus
Heart/Air	Throat/Ether	Third Eye	Top of head
12	16	2	1000
YAM	HAM	KṢAM	OM
Tam Tham, Kam, Kham, Gam, Gham, Ngam, Cam, Cham, Jam, Jham, Njam	Ām, Ām, Im, Iem, Um, Oem, Rm, Rim, Lrm, Lrim, Em, Aim, Om, Aum, Am, Ah	Ham and Kṣham	a thousand petals
Air	Ether	Mind Space	Consciousness Space
Touch	Sound	Thought	Consciousness
Gray Six Pointed Star	Azure Dot		
Skin	Ears	Mind	Consciousness
Hands	Vocal Organ	Mind	Consciousness
the lowest part of the lungs, the blood, the blood circulatory system, the skin and the hands	the lungs, bronchi, gullet, speech organs(voice), throat, neck and jaws	the little brain, ears, nose, paranasal sinuses, eyes, nervous system, forehead and the face	all aspects of the body and the mind
Gha (Yam)	Nga (Body)	Visarga (Multiply)	Śūrya Bindu (Invisible)
Ma (Puruṣa)	Pa (Prakṛti)	Dha (Contact)	Ni (Invisble)
Śiva	Jīva	Ardhanāri	Brahmā (SadāŚiva)
Deer (Madhyama)	Cuckoo (Pamcham)	Donkey (Dhaivata)	Elephant (Niṣada)
Deer	Elephant		
Deep Red	Smoky Gray	Silver White	Colorless
Varūṇa	Sarasvatī	Iḍa and Piṅgāla	Śuṣuṁṇā
Plasma	Prāṇa (bhur)	Subtle Prāṇa (bhuva)	Causal Prāṇa (svaha)
Vata	Vata		
Vyana	Udāna		
Sun (Sūrya)	Mars (Maṇgala)	Jupiter (Bṛhaspati)	Saturn (Śani)
Kākini	Sākani	Hākini	Yākini
Maha	Jana	Tapa	Satyam
Kāraṇa (causal)	Manas (mind)	Buddha (intellect)	Nirvāṇa (eternity)

Chapter 6

The beauty of The Beauty

Beauty is a social necessity
Love built on Beauty,
As Beauty, soon dies.

Why women... are so much more interesting to men than men are to women? We quote the charm of a person to express the excellence. A German actor and singer said, "The average man is more interested in a woman who is interested in him than he is in a woman—any woman—with Beautiful legs."

Śṛṁgāra is 'Saṁskāra'

Love and beauty are elements for every poet, a writer, even for that matter a researcher. They all work with the triad, creator-creativity-creation. The creativity is known as art, in which materials are shaped or selected to convey an idea, emotion, or visually interesting form. We also use the word art in a more general sense to encompass other forms of creative activity, such as dance and music, or even to describe skill in almost any activity, such as "the art of bread making" or "the art of travel." In surveying major issues of life, one must begin by prevalence of the spirit of goodwill. The exchange of goodwill is connected with marriage prospectives. It is the art of life and represents trends (also called Saṁskāras or Śṛṁgāras) of parents unto the newly weds and vice versa.

Ceremonial rites and rituals occupy a place of utmost importance in the life of a devout Hindu. In fact, every vital action namely, birth, initiation, marriage, death etc. are performed with its appropriate rite or Saṁskāra. The number of Saṁskāras has been fixed at sixteen; Marriage is the most important and elaborate out of these sixteen Saṁskāras. Manu enjoins that rituals must be performed in the case of a virgin for legalising the marriage and legitimatising children. Saṁskāra is purification or upgrading of the brain (cf. HOY; C. Baidjnath Misier; Krips bv; Meppel; 2000). This is a dedicated operation for the spirit. The spirit is the principle of conscious life (inner nature); the vital principle in humans, animating the body or mediating between body and soul. In the chapter Yoga, we have already indicated that the number sixteen takes an important place in Hinduism. This number represents aspects in capacity, worship, development both mental and physical etc. It stands for facets which make the external decoration of the woman complete.

Developmental Psychology claims that growth up to adolescence is the age-period between puberty and adulthood, in which generic maturity is reached, but not, complete mental maturity. This happens globally between 16-20 years. In this matter we refer to the most valuable gem of this era, the diamond. The diamond is a stone found in a pure form. It is a transparent, flawless or almost flawless piece of this stone especially when cut and polished that it is valued as a precious gem. Diamond in the rough can be compared to a person of fine character but lacking refined manners or grace. Saṁskāra is refining the spirit and increasing finesse and density. Saṁskāra and Śṛṁghara together transform a young lady into a woman wherein she becomes a desirable partner for adult life. Now she is ready to become a mother. A mother is the most valued and regarded figure on earth. The woman or man is comparable with a Diamond bird or a Bastard honey-bird seeking a partner in life. Honey is in the celestial food to survive. The mantras "Aum Yanmadhuno", etc. in the sacred books are a tribute to the purity and sweetness of Madhuparka: "O celestial beings! The luscious sweetness which lights up the body despite all the strokes (of time and circumstance); which is the quintessence of the honeyed juice of flowers (makaranda); which is the material cause of all vital food grains, and which irradiates the beauty of honey itself is most suited to Madhuparka, the manifold qualities of which are all centred in the food I eat".

Beauty Means Nectar

The beauty of nature is the sweet honey of energy for every creature. If the cock doesn't shout out every morning, the farmer will not be able to start his day on time. The sound of the cock serves as a morning alarm for the farmer. The beauty and the dewdrops on the leaves and grass at dawn is the honey of nature (YV 1.16). This should stimulate the human being to be pure and beautiful in the morning and be sure, he can make the most of the rest of the day.

The grandeur of the ideal Hindu marriage is entering into the spirit and the thought of the mantras and other Sanskrit books, which embodies Saṁskṛti or way of life and life-rituals. Śṛṁgāra or decoration is a part of the ideal, means upgrading the body, the outer nature. The decoration in a wedding is an integral part of the way of life of a Hindu. Marriage has rather strong emotional, even sentimental, connotations, which suggested the accompanying festivities, whether elaborate or simple. A bride is, at the time of marriage exquisitely charming and auspicious. She is at that time a goddess on earth and must be made up as a divine. The Kanyā or virgin (also called Gauri, white woman, pure) will now be promoted to being a woman. And everyone should look at this newly wed, be well disposed towards her and bestow on her prosperity as well as respectability and good luck. Hereafter, she is also able to obtain the position of a mother as soon as she bears children. Motherhood is the breakthrough for a girl or lady as an everlasting dream in life. Once this happens, life changes. At this particular occasion a lot of money and time are spent for preparation. We select appropriate clothing, jewels and other necessaries. Lipstick is also one of the attributes of Śṛṁgāra, that's why it always stays in a woman's purse. Lipstick illustrates the oneness between the woman and nature—the end product being the combination of Saṁskāra and Śṛṁgāra.

Every God and Goddess in Hinduism has been adorned with ornaments and colourful attire. The first Puruṣa's name is Hiraṇyagarbha. Hiraṇya means gold and Garbha means womb or development of life. Gold in this matter is a symbol of beauty (Śrī) and fortune (Lakṣmī), and development of life is associated with faith and rites (YV 31.22: 1679). These four elements are connected with the phenomenon Śṛṁgāra (YV 31.22: 1679). From the creation of the world, the aspects of beauty and fortune, also called honey and money, are important for every state of development of a human being. In this process of development, ceremonial observances are made and in propitiating the duties not only for attaining happiness and prosperity in the world (two sides of a golden coin) but also for final beatitude thereafter. Every duty has been defined in the Saṁskāras. Hindu Saṁskāras, a mirror of the faith and rites of the common people is more than those of the highly specialised religion of the priest. In this sense, the influence of the Vedas on the Hindu mind continues to be deep and ineffaceable. There is a general feeling that the continuance of the age-old Saṁskāras is a blaring reflection of the Hindu world-view.

Puruṣārtha

The affirmative attitude of Hinduism toward life has been emphasised by its recognition of four legitimate and basic desires: Dharma or virtue, Artha or wealth, Kāma or desire (sensual pleasure) and Mokṣa or salvation through communion with God or the Infinite. These four attainments of life are collectively known as Puruṣārtha. Of these, the first three belong to the realm of worldly values; the fourth is called the supreme value.

A person without wealth cannot gratify any desire; similarly, there can be no wealth in one that is destitute of virtue. He, therefore, who is outside the pale of both virtue and wealth, is an object of fear unto the world. For this reason, one should seek the acquisition of wealth with a devoted mind, without disregarding the requirements of virtue. They who believe in the wisdom of this saying succeed in acquiring whatever they desire. One should first practise virtue and then seek gratification of desire, for this should be the last act of one who has been successful in acquiring wealth. Even that householder, who observes the duties of his mode of life and who abandons sensual pleasure and attachment to action, does not find it difficult to obtain heaven.

Sensual pleasure is lust, which the seeker of salvation tries to avoid or conquer. If a person doesn't understand the meaning of lust, and how to use this in life, it will lead to destruction. The English poet and playwright, William Shakespeare, quotes the result in Sonnet 129:

"Th' expense of spirit in a waste of shame
Is lust in action; and till action, lust
Is perjur'd, murd'rous, bloody, full of blame,
Savage, extreme, rude, cruel, not to trust;
Enjoy'd no sooner but despised straight".

In a marriage ceremony the father of the bride requests a promise from the groom for assisting his daughter in realising these three: Dharma, Artha, and Kāma. The groom makes the promise by repeating three times that he will not fail the bride in realising these elements of life. These three goals in life make responsibilities bigger for the bride when she enters the new family. The last aspect, liberation becomes the responsibility of the groom.

The Hindu Marriage

Marriage is viewed as a sacrament and not a contract. A Hindu marriage is a life-long commitment between a wife and a husband, and is the strongest social bond that takes place between a man and a woman. Gṛhastha Āśrama (the householder stage), the second of the four stages in life begins with marriage and starting a household. For a Hindu, marriage is the only way to continue the family and thereby repay his debt to his/her ancestors. This stage of life a householder commences through Agni. "You, Agni, are the homestead's Lord, our Hotā priest at sacrifice." (RV 1.1; RV 7.16.5).

Hinduism views, marriage is not a concession to human weakness, but a means for spiritual growth. The British writer Stephen Leacock said: "Many a man in love with a dimple makes the mistake of marrying the whole girl". Man and woman are soul mates who, through the institution of marriage, can direct the energy associated with their individual instincts and passion into the progress of their souls. The Hindu marriage, Lagna Vivāha is the bonding of two souls in a matrimonial ceremony, performed according to Hindu rites. However, the marriage, as explained in Hinduism, is an institution not only of two souls (man and woman), but essentially bonding of two families, which after this ceremony holds a special relationship. Marriage according to Hinduism is a perfect union of man and woman spiritually, mentally and physically, essential for procreation and continuation of mankind.

Marriage is a social institution under which a man and woman establish their decision to live as husband and wife by legal commitments, with religious ceremonies etc., that is the legal or religious ceremony that formalises them to live as husband and wife, including the accompanying social festivities to officiate in a marriage. It is also possible without any legal sanctions. The holy books mention that the gods also get married and we learn about the marriage from words and music. These gods have an astral body. Our eyes are not able to see immaterial things. That is only possible when we open our spiritual eye, viz., the third eye.

Wearing a nice dress is not enough for a marriage and be married is not enough for liberation. Seeking to understand the dynamic interplay between loving relationships and the path of spirituality urges one to study Hinduism. In clear, candid language, God Rāma presents His vision of the potential that marriage and family life have to help us open our heart, expand our personality, and contribute to our governed and spiritual enfoldment. Marriage, according to Indian way of life, is a sacred relationship whereby man aspires to transcend life and its compulsions. An ideal Hindu marriage focuses on man truly loving his wife and the woman having Śraddhā or respect for her husband. Marriage is creating a new life for giving new birth. Marriage is thus a mantra, a marketing mix of the female and male love.

Parents and Their Sacrifice

Parents are proud of the performance of their children and would want them to participate in the activities of adults when they come of age. Parents help in finding the marriage partner, but at the end of the day the individual has the choice. There is no pressure or force, in fact in a way it eases undue worries for the individuals. This also does not mean that boys and girls cannot meet and choose their own partners. In fact more often than not it is they who may have met each other during their education or social groups and then on their request the parents arrange the marriage. This request is usually fulfilled, however if there is a reason for the parents to disagree, it is normally discussed and possibly resolved to a mutual solution.

The Holy Fire as Witness

Fire, produced by the priest, is omnipotent and it is He that adopts the sacrifice. This divine sacrifice is a visible dedication of the parties through this marriage. The wish and promises which one makes unto each other at this fire, are visible and audible to everyone. Following are the events for the search of the marriage partner, through to engagement, registration, and wedding, explained (endeavoured to) in brief. For this special purpose she must be dressed appropriately and shown to persons concerned, the gods, the honoured guests etc. The gods pay attention to this process of obligation and enter the place from the heavens where the parties from the sky are absent, they are represented by an 'agent' helping to link the couple. The bride and the bridegroom face each other, and the priest ties their garments (the bride's Sārī to the groom's shirt) in a knot, symbolising the sacred union. The bride and the groom garland each other and exchange rings. The sacrificial fire symbolises the divine witness, and as the sanctifier of the sacrament, is installed and worshipped. The Sāma Veda denotes that fire or Agni is the messenger of the worshipper when they sacrifice their oblations. The Rīg Vedā describes Agni as the oblation bearer, the Lord of wealth, the immortal and the best at sacrifice (RV I.12.6). The fire into which the oblation is poured is kindled by the application of fire produced by attrition. Bearer means that each time the fire is produced, new things are created. All riches are at Agni's disposal, and he is the most bountiful rewarded, both directly and indirectly, of the pious worshippers whose oblations he carries to the Gods (RV I.12.1). The Sāmagrī, consisting of crushed sandalwood, herbs, sugar, rice, ghee (clarified butter), and twigs is offered into the sacred fire to seek God's blessings for the married couple.

Another form of oblation is when the bride and the groom grasp their hands and pray to God for His blessings. Therefore we know that the blessings of Agni will result in the birth of sons. Valiant sons are necessary for rituals in life and also in ceremonies after the death of their parents. Due to the menstruation of the woman, Agni takes a great part in birth and growth. With Agni's blessings marriage will continue with all religious processes in the family and keep the devotion energy line unbroken. The elaborate marriage ceremonies provide a good example of the Hindu world-view. Especially for this occasion we build a marriage temple or Maṇḍapa in a hall or at home. The Maṇḍapa should be decorated with all kinds of jewels, ivory flowers showing birds of varied plumage buzzing and whistling in the rustling breeze. Of course, this decoration is also meant for worshipping Agni.

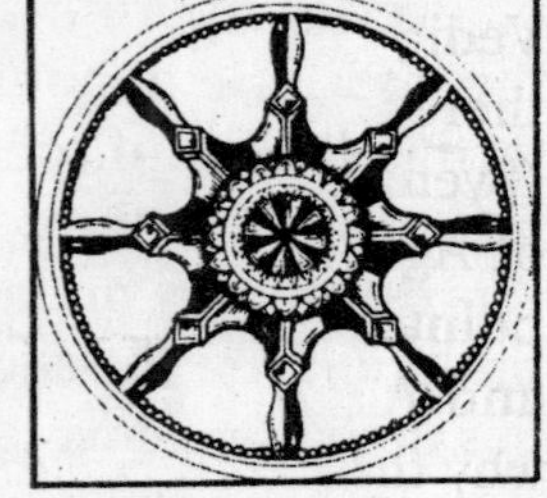

The Circle of Life

The mind and energy in the human body flow in circles viz. cakras. In the wedding ceremony the bride and groom also make seven rounds around the fire-pit to unite spiritually. The ceremony that is performed by circling round the small square shaped fire-place or Havan Kuṇḍa (firepit) is called Maṅgala Pherā. This happens in the centre of the marriage temple or Lagna Maṇḍapa. This 'wheeling' refers to the circles of the planets and the cakra's in the human body, called Agni-parikramā and Sāt-bhāwara. Seven times both by the bride and the groom, solidifies their marriage and declares them as husband and wife. Agnī-parikrama is circling around the fire, where mantras from the Rīg and the Atharva Veda are cited. She is divided in two groups, viz., three walk-rounds where the bride and groom go around the Agni-parikramā untied.

These three rounds, is the celestial part of the wedding referring to the first marriage in the cosmos of Lord Śiva as Soma. The second round is for god Gandharva who keeps every creation together. Gandharva is the energy i.e., which holds, sustains and enlivens our relation or body, and on which growth and decay of everything are dependent in our physical form. The gods Soma, Gandharva and Agni are involved with the physical development of a girl. This Gandharva region in the cosmos is the most important because it forms the embodied universe. It is the nervous system in our body. It has its heaven, atmosphere and earth. The third walk-round is for the presenting god Agni who merges both souls together. In the fourth walk-round the couple is tied to each other and Agni solidifies their marriage. God Agni (fire) transfers the celestial relationship into a materialistic or visible one for (re)production by means of sex.

The small square of the marriage temple is noticed as a Vedic alter for the bride and groom. In the Vedic culture there is another modification of alter in the form of a falcon (Syena). The falcon or Syena has been described as the form of Agni or electricity. This modification into falcon shape, points to the fact that the physical creation is run by Apah and Agni (water and fire) represented by falcon. This is why the Paurāṇic mythology has identified the falcon as the vehicle of Viṣṇu (created world). Alters were also modified to the shape of Ratha cakra or the wheel of a chariot with its navel and spokes. The wheel shaped modification represented the phenomenon of earth's revolution round the sun. Here the sun as being the navel and elliptic path of the earth being the circle of the wheel and spokes being the twelve zodiac signs or months of the year. In other words it may be stated that the wheel shaped modification symbolised the Kāla cakra or the wheel of time. This Kāla cakra has been described in the Rīg Vedā (1.164.2) as follows:

"The wheel (of time) having twelve spokes (months) revolves round the heavens, but it doesn't wear out".

In addition to terrestrial and astronomical representations as shown above; fire-alters also had equivalences in Adhyātma, particularly in physiology. The striking example of this is the Dārśic vedī i.e., the alter for Darśa-pūrṇamasa sacrifice. In fact, Darśa and Pūrṇamāsa are associated with the moon. Pūrṇamāsa means full moon and Darśa means new moon. Darśa-pūrṇamāsa sacrifice has two fold significances, one Devayajitva, i.e., astronomical another Ātmayajitva, i.e. physiological. In astronomical sense it refers to the phenomenon of origin or rising of moon. In physiological sense it symbolises the birth of a child. Darśa represents the old decaying man and Pūrṇamāsa is the full-blown young man.

Gandharva, The Rhythm of Life

Yoga is making a compromise with nature. If a person comes into contact with rain or a river, then it is better not to have a conflict with water and when outdoors no conflict with air. Natural elements greet people every moment of the day. This means that the external characteristics of nature must become coordinated with the inner nature of people. The well-known proverb says "if you get out off bed with your left leg", it means that that person is in a bad mood. To avoid this, it is better to coordinate the inner nature of sound with the sound of music. The essence is that the astral coordination itself is in the form of sound. Listen simply to your favorite music when getting out of bed. This improves the emotional condition of people and you are able to classify your day with improvement. The process of harmonisation to a better mental condition is called Gandharva (Go=sensual perception, Dhay=drink, in the form of consonance, melody and song). Fragrances too help in the harmonisation of people. In this sense one is able to define Gandhah as a fragrance (Iva=such as, just like).

The sound Gam is also the consonance of Brahmā, which multiplies himself, scattered in several forms or in number. Consonance Dha is the increase of capacity. This process is the same with people who have been classified on the eighth scale (read more in chapter 2 Understanding the Spiritual World). People are also placed on a scale. "Erect, to heaven has the Gandharva mounted, pointing at us his many-coloured weapons. Clad in sweet raiment beautiful to look on, for he, as light, produces forms that please us" (SV 1847). Gandharva (Vena) is also said to be the rising Sun. It means that if we wake up in the morning and see the light of the sun, our life should be colorful, harmonised with music tunes. This will make us feel better.

According to the reincarnation study human birth comes after a cow. A cow (Go) is an animal in which all devas stay and accompany. These devas ensure that grass is converted into milk, as a result of which they can complete their sacrifices. The conversion takes place with wisdom, which is white. The end product is milk. These sacrifices ensure that the soul of a cow adopts a human conformation in the next life. This milk is the consequence of a fourfold process (the four stomachs of the cow): first food, then energy, after that spirit development and finally knowledge. These four elements are described in the Veda such as the four koṣas, in our triple body, viz., Ka is fortune in materialistic body, Ūśa is fire in the astral; Ūśa is the morning light in our causal body. This process is called Ka or Earth, in the meaning of the well-being theory it indicates luck. The four Koṣas are: Annamaya or food; Prāṇāmaya is energy; Manomaya is spirit and Vijñānamaya is knowledge. The condition for this is that a combustion process must take place firstly to be able to raise itself to a higher consciousness, more strongly, from a physical towards a spiritual development of the person.

In the combustion process the body is associated with the Kuṇḍa and burning is fire. The four elements are the ingredients that are sacrificed in the firepit (burned). In the fire sacrifice, during a ritual, milk is for this reason the most important product. With this milk a mixture is made, which is called Pañcāmṛta (quintuple nectar). This mixture keeps also a link with the aforesaid four elements. Water (Jala) is food, sugar (śarkarā) is energy, honey (Madhu) is spirit and churned butter (Ghī) is knowledge. These four elements mixed with milk (Dugdha) ensure that the spiritual development comes in action: the ānandamaya or nectar of happiness. This is also the result of the combustion process in the body, the aim of a fire sacrifice and the blessing of all devas, which is present in milk.

The word Gandharva also has three characters. Ga, Dha and Va who is inferred of as the origin terms Gṛ (to want), Dhṛ (to bear, Dharma) and Vṛ(to be). Ga has to do with the Will (fire), Dha with the Virtue (earth) and Wealth (Dha also means Kubera) and Va has to do with the aspect of Self (Varuṇa, Vāyu, Viṣṇu). In a psychological way first people have to feel a tingle of the mind (will) to do things, then proceed to perform the action, then desires to move to a prosperous position, and at the end stage of life the final question will come: what's life? Gandharva gives the next answer: Gṛ(dhya): will (and desire) is life, Dhanad: wealth is life, Varuṇa: water is life, Vāyu: air is life, Viṣṇu: space is life.

Such as mentioned above that the sound Ga has to do with fire. As soon as the element fire moves in an active form, it is called desire or wanting. This character one finds during and after the marriage. The God, which is charged with the conductance of wants and wishes, is Gaṇeṣa. His appearance is in the form of an elephant. He is the god symbolised by the cosmic wisdom, the destroyer of obstacles and the bearer of all divine consonances. The last one translates itself in the large ears of the elephants. In the cosmos one speaks of elephants power (EP), and on the earth one speaks of horsepower (HP). The cosmic elephant is the bearer of the universe, named Airāvata. This elephant is the vehicle of the king of the sky, called Indra. He moves himself in astral form in the cosmos, and this translates itself in people in characters as tolerance and non-violence. The cow on the other hand is the physical form of these characters. The development of people occurs at scale level between these two appearances.

The sound Dha has to do with the element earth. The physical form of earth is prosperity and the astral form is Lakṣmī, the Divine Mother. She is frequently represented with elephants, which blow golden coins from their trunk; this also means, in relation with the aforesaid characters, that prosperity cannot be abused. By abuse of prosperity, pride and violence arise. At that moment in the cosmos, Lakṣmī will take a decision and these elephants will crush these imposters. Prosperity (Riddhi) is intended for healthy and long life. This is called the blessing of nature: divine nectar. This nectar is in the form of artistic qualities in nature. All nature that we behold is the mother aspect of God, because in nature we find beauty, gentleness, and kindness, flowers, birds, and the beauties of nature, all speak of the Mother aspect of God-the creative motherly instinct of God. When we look at all the good things in nature, we feel a tenderness rise within us; we can see and feel God in nature. The Divine Mother is so beautiful! But remember, in Her higher manifestation even that beauty is formless. She is in everything. Her divine, compassionate love is expressed in the raindrops. Her beauty is reflected in the colours of the rainbow. She offers fresh hope to mankind with the rose-tinted clouds at dawn. Above all, be ever conscious of Her presence in your heart.

Varuṇa represents the element water, also called Soma in the Rīg Vedā (RV 7.85.3: 5819). Varuṇa is one of the most interesting creations, of the Hindu mind, because, though we can still perceive the physical background from which he rises, the vast, starry, brilliant expanse above, his features more than those of any other Vedic god have been completely transfigured, and he stands before us as a god who watches over the world, punishes the evil-doer, and even forgives the sins of those who implore his pardon. In the Rīg Vedā an exceedingly high position is ascribed to Varuṇa. He is chief of the Ādityas, "inviolable, imperishable, eternal being," sons of Aditi, an abstract, mysterious creation representing Infinity, who may best be regarded as a personification of universal, all embracing Nature or Being. The name Varuṇa is derived from the Sanskrit Var 'to cover.' He is, therefore, the god of the heavens covering all things. Birds flying in the air, the rivers in their sleepless flow cannot attain knowledge of his power and wrath. But he knows the flight of the birds in the sky, the course of the far travelling wind, the paths of ships on the ocean, and beholds all the secret things that have been, or shall be, done. Suffering people look up to the sky and when they see the clouds, laden with life-giving waters, floating in from the ocean, they become happy.[1]

The Rīg Vedā gives a description of people who are seduced by other things in life. "It was not our own will, Varuṇa, but some seduction which led us astray—an intoxicating draught, passion, dice, and thoughtlessness. The stronger perverts the weaker; even sleep brings unrighteousness." (RV 7.86.6: 5827) Gandharva is the chorister of Indra's heaven. Indra there is attended by troops of Apsarās (dancing girls) and Gandharvas (heavenly musicians). Vac (the goddess of speech) once said when she wanted to bring the Soma to the Gods: "The Gandharvas are fond of women". Beauty and the rhythm of life are always fond of each other.

Vāyu is the element of air. A history in the Rīg Vedā teaches us, the importance of Vāyu. "When Soma was first brought to the notice of the gods, a dispute arose as to who should have the first draught. At length, it was agreed to come to a decision by having a race. Vāyu (the wind) first reached the goal, Indra being second. Indra tried hard to win, and when near the winning post proposed that they should reach it together, Vāyu taking two-thirds of the drink.

---

[1] Gods of India; E.O. Martin; Low Price Publications; Delhi; 1999

Not so," said Vāyu, "I will be the sole winner." Then Indra said, "Let us come in together, and give me one fourth of the draught divine." Vāyu consented to this, and so the juice was shared between them" (RV 2.113-7).

Nowadays the Hindus are a temperate race and Soma, in his Vedic character, has ceased to be worshipped. The name, however, is still given to the Moon, together with that of Chandra. In the later Vedas the word Soma is used interchangeably either as the god of the intoxicating liquor or as the ruling of the moon over the night. The subtly beguiling character of the Queen of the Night may account for this. The Gandharva takes us on a fascinating journey in order to explore the future of human relationships. He guides us through songs and melodies the history of thought to arrive at a deep understanding of our evolutionary moment-the expansion of human consciousness. Like a good storyteller, the Gandharva makes sure that we can hear breathlessly more, and how we can put ourselves on this path to a better world.

Viṣṇu is symbolised as space, also called Sound (Nāda) or Brahmā. There are two states of this Brahmā-one with and the other without shape; one perishable, other imperishable. These are inherent in all beings. The imperishable is the Supreme Being; the perishable is in all the world. The blaze of fire burning in one spot diffuses light and heat around; so the world is nothing more than the manifested energy of the Supreme Brahmā; and inasmuch as light and heat are stronger or feebler as we are near the fire or far off from it, so the energy of the Supreme is more or less intense in the beings that are more or less remote from it. Brahmā, Śiva, and Viṣṇu are the most powerful energies of God. Vaikuṇṭha is Viṣṇu's abode situated on Mount Meru and is made entirely of gold. It contains pools of water on which float blue, red, and white lotuses. Viṣṇu sits on a throne glorious as the mid-day sun; on his right is Lakṣmī like a blaze of lightning. He is called the holy being.

Essentials in Marriage

Below we describe some essentials of the Hindu marriage.

The first is touching the heart or Hṛdayasparśa. The bridegroom comes over the bride's right shoulder touches her heart saying: "I hold your heart in serving fellowship; your mind follows my mind. In my word you rejoice with all your heart. You are joined to me by the Lord of all creatures." The second is wearing the Maṅgala Sūtra, the marriage chain. The groom performs this by tying the thread containing the marks of the Soma (Śiva) around the neck of the bride. After tying, she becomes a Suhāgina or married woman. This is vitalised by the Sindūradāna, the sacred holy red powder, the visible sign of a married bride. The groom places Sindūra (vermilion, a red powder) on the bride's hair. This is the last decoration of women in beauty. With this act beauty becomes undying and marriage becomes alive.

After these two performances the couple is ready for blessings. The groom's parents and guests bless the couple and offer clothes or flowers to the bride (now their daughter-in-law), symbolising her joining the groom's family. The congratulation ceremony follows, where the close relatives and friends would throw rice around the couple's foreheads and give presents.

Modern science confirms the unity of two souls as the goal of life. The Pythagoreans taught and practised a way of life based on the belief that the soul is a prisoner of the body. The merging of two souls in a marriage is the freedom from that prison. A person can also achieve freedom at death, and reincarnate in a higher or lower form of life, depending on the degree of virtue achieved. Virtues should be practised in the stage of marriage. The last stage or the highest purpose of humans is to purify their souls by cultivating intellectual virtues, refraining from sensual pleasures, and practising various religious rituals. The Pythagoreans, having discovered the mathematical laws of musical pitch, inferred that planetary motions produce a "music of the spheres", and developed a "therapy through music" to bring humanity in harmony with the celestial spheres. The above mentioned marriage ceremony in a "small temple" is a celestial sphere and the music is comparable with the mantras and blessings.

The guests and the couple are part of the witnesses of the marriage ceremony. The parents, priest, officials, gods and angels, all sign this marriage with their blessings and wishing that this ceremony culminates into a happy marriage. Yearns for love for each other is also sensed and supported in the heavens. There is nothing so lovely as to be a beautiful united and blessed soul. This Beauty is a gift of God and we should cherish it as such.

The Last Greeting of the Bride

The last performance is when the bride says farewell to her parents, relatives and friends. The ceremony is very emotional and almost all members of the bride's party will have tearful eyes (joy in hearts). The musicians will play the emotional Bidāyee song "Babul ki Duvanye Leti Ja..." to symbolise the severing of her ties with her parental home, and to start a new life at her husband's home. A British librettist and playwright W.S. Gilbert wrote a poem about this part of life as follows:

Take a pair of sparkling eyes,
Hidden, ever and anon,
In a merciful eclipse.

Beauty with Intelligence

The most beautiful dress was worn by Miss D in a ball-room in New York. She was a very beautiful Indian woman. She was not called the belle of the evening, but belle of the season. She was beautiful and graceful, winning and attractive in her manners, so amiable and lovely, that the belle pickers, who picked all to pieces, could not find anything to say against her.

Every poet or writer knows that every city has a belle and this time it is Miss G. Ever since her girlhood until now you will never see any change in her. Not only is she beautiful, but always mild, gentle, amiable and lovely, and remarkable for her talents and superiority of education. Beauty with intelligence is required in a person, and certainly for a lady. Philosophy also asks if there is a difference between the beautiful and the sublime. To admire or desire a lady in her aspects and qualities is more important in this society. The world famous English poet and playwright William Shakespeare (1564-1616) points out in the play Antony and Cleopatra (Act 4, Scene 14) the following sentence:

ANTONY I will be
A bridegroom in my death, and run into't
As to a lover's bed.

The Irish poet and playwright, W. B. Yeats (1865-1939), supports this in The Wind Among the Reeds, "He Wishes for the Clothes of Heaven" as follow:

But I, being poor, have only my dreams;
I have spread my dreams under your feet;
Tread softly because you tread on my dreams.

Bridal Dress

The bride's wedding dress in India is glamorous with a superb glow and shine. It has a magical touch to it. It is a gorgeous silk Sārī from Benares or the South with intricate golden brocade and tinsel work. It is either cream or red in colour. These days, special bridal Sārīs are obtained from India. In the ancient Vedic period, the bridegroom's womenfolk made the bridal dress by hands. A few decades ago, the brides had special ties and dyes Sārīs known as Cunaris. In fact, it is the tradition in Bhojapuri culture for women to wear these ties and dyes Sārīs on marriage occasions. Some years back, plain georgette or chiffon materials were bought and embroidered with silk threads, Jari work, Badla (tinsels) and synthetic pearls. The ensemble had a matching Coli and beautifully made matching undergarments stitched elaborately in lace works. The U.S. author James Hillman said: "If God-given and man-made are unnecessary, even false, opposition, then the city made by human hands is also natural in its own right...Cities belong to human nature; nature does not begin outside the city walls."

Beauty Designs

Since time immemorial man has tried to enhance his human form by the use of adornments and the application of pastes, colours and marks. Both men and women have sought to increase their Beauty in the above manner in various civilisations and countries. Tattooing the skin on various exposed parts of the body with indelible marks, designs or figures as a mark of beauty is known in many cultures. Many contemporary tribal men in Africa, Asia and Latin America still wear their ethnic jewellery. Today, with the pop culture emerging, it has become fashionable for youths to have one ear lobe pricked and wear a stud or a pendant. But nowhere else have jewels had a greater place in religious life and been associated with divinity, blessings and protection, power and glory, success and prosperity as in India. Gods and goddesses, celestial beings, men and women and children alike, wear jewellery in the Indian society. But it is during the Vivāha Saṁskāra that both the bride and the bridegroom assume their most magnificent bloom. Their elegance, charm, glamour and glitter captivate the gaze of one and all. And since the dawn of history, women in particular have tried to make themselves more alluring and attractive. Beautiful or plain, each woman may spend hours each day indulging in Beauty rituals and treatments guaranteed to enhance her inherent charms and sensuousness. No other day is as bright, glamorous, sensational and more appropriate for this ritual than the marriage day. On the occasion of marriage the bride embellishes herself. This embellishment rite is known as the Solah Śṛṁgāras among the Bhojapuri Hindus.

Solah Śṛṁgāras

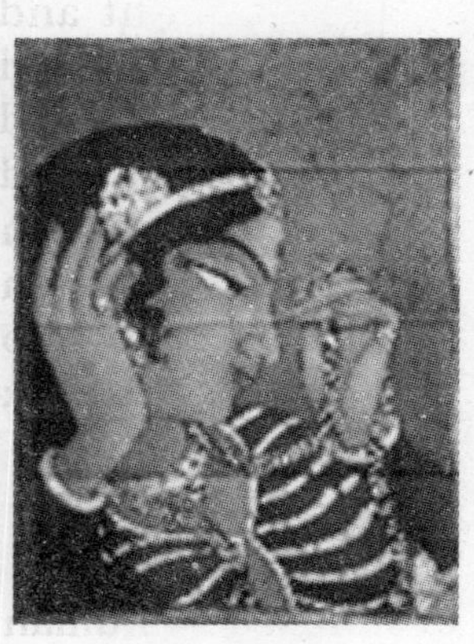

The Solah Śṛṁgāras symbolise the culmination of the basic feminine urge for Beautification. Painting and decorating of the body to enhance it has been an elaborate art of Hindu society. It was not a mere cosmetic process but had an under-current of deeper significance—a philosophy.

And the roots go deep into Indian traditions. The smooth running of life was regulated by a number of disciplines and rituals in the ancient Vedic society. These rituals encompassed even the aesthetics. The artist creates a world in which Beauty, as much as truth, is an end, foreshadowing that absolute freedom which is the goal of human will. Art is individual, not social, but it fulfils a great human purpose. The basis for one's response to Beauty exists in the structure of one's mind. The Solah Śṛṁgāras rituals were evolved for the requirements of health, hygiene as well as for divine and aesthetic sense. C.G. Jung once said that man's most vital need is to discover his own inner reality through the cultivation of a symbolic life. To discover this inner reality, he has to discover inner beauty and the way to inner beauty is through outer beauty. Did not Keats say "A thing of Beauty is a joy forever?" Beautiful conveys closeness to perfection, which gives intellectual and/or spiritual satisfaction as well as sensual pleasure. The body is an expression of one's psyche and the house of the inner self-manifestation of the greater Self-the All Pervading-God. Beautifying the body is preparing it as an abode of God for the act of welcoming divine qualities as a first step in worship.

All bodily preparations: bath, perfuming, libations, decorations are but outward preparations of the body as they are the chief instrument of worship. It is then that the Śakti, female energy, the creative power of Śiva in man, is awakened. The ritual marks are regarded as cosmic cross-points. By being adorned for the nuptials, the bride is being prepared as a representation of Lakṣmī, the goddess of wealth (prosperity). Beautifying the body today is a mere mechanical and physical process, to emphasise the sensual rather than the divine.

Hindus (Indians) have expended limitless energy and creativity in the invention of ornaments that celebrate the human body. Adorning the visible, material body, they feel, satisfy a universal longing for ornament but are incapable of touching the counterpart, namely the human spirit. Indeed rarely is a traditional Indian ornament simply decorative and devoid of inherent meaning or symbolic value. Symbols found in Indian jewellery act as a metaphorical language communicated from the wearer to the viewer. Such jewellery is created from an infinite reserve of symbolically significant forms and images, some obvious, some subtle, and some whose meaning is forgotten.

Complementary to such thought is the conventional view where the graceful form of a woman is said to epitomise ideal Beauty and mystery inherent in nature. Thus befittingly each and every part of the feminine physique including the head, torso, limbs, and between the appended parts-have consistently been used to support ornaments, often in ingenious ways. The Indian idea being that only things covered with ornaments are Beautiful. Poetry must overflow with rhetorical ornaments (Alaṁkāra), metaphors, alliterations, and other musical effects. The verb Alaṁkāra, "to adorn, to decorate," means literally "to make enough": for simple appearance without ornament is "not enough"; it is poor, disgraceful, shocking, except in the case of an ascetic. Hence is the stress on adornment of the women, who are but the poetry of nature.

Ornamentation not only serves to please the eyes of the beholder but also fulfils an auspicious purpose. The impulse to adorn stems from a deep rooted sensibility to mark every occasion of life with auspicious symbols, designs and figures in order to obtain good fortune and protection from evil. Thus a fully bedecked woman evokes in the viewer a deep and ingratiating feeling of tranquil contentment, springing from an intuitive realisation that evolving before him is an image of perfect beauty, symbolically conveying the richness and completeness which is but natural to nature.

The ancients who translated the abstract nuances of Indian philosophy into images of everyday reality went even further and canonised the adornment of the female form into sixteen different ornaments covering her entire being from head to toe. The choice of the number sixteen too is not without significance. It is a significant number among the Hindus, and corresponds to the sixteen phases of the life of the moon, which in turn is connected with a woman's menstrual cycle. This is another pointer to the feminine physiognomy being a microcosm of the rhythms of natural processes. Further a woman of sixteen is considered at the peak of physical perfection in her life. At this stage of her life the aspect of delight is most pronounced. Her nature is to play, seek new experiences, and to charm others to her. Her innocence attracts to her all that is true and good. Indeed it is common for deities to be described as eternally sixteen years old, which is considered the most beautiful and vigorous human age. In fact an important goddess is named after the Sanskrit name for sixteen (Ṣoḍaśī), and is visualised as having all the above mentioned qualities. This number is also related on the process of the creation of our universe.

The Śrīmad Bhāgavatam explains the sixteen elements of creation. "May the Lord, who enlivens the materially created bodies of the elements by lying down within the universe, and who in His Puruṣa incarnation causes the living being to be subjected to the sixteen divisions of material modes which are His generator, be pleased to decorate my statements. The elementary creation of sixteen items of matter are namely the five gross elements (earth, water, fire, air and ether), the five subtle elements (sound, form, taste, smell, touch) and the eyes, ears, nose, tongue, skin and mind is known as Sargās, whereas the subsequent resultant interaction of the modes of material nature is called Visargā (Bh.T. 2. 4.23 and 2.10.3).

The Ornaments

The sixteen ornaments have been said to make up the standard repertoire of feminine adornment. We enumerate a few as follows:

Bindi

The Bindi is a small ornamental dot placed at the centre of the forehead, between the eyes. The word itself is derived from the Sanskrit Bindu, meaning dot. Metaphysically speaking, it is the dimensionless point of infinite potential from which has originated all manifested existence. It is further said to signify the mystical third eye, an invisible organ of spiritual perception and second sight, traditionally said to be situated at a point little above the place where the eyebrows meet. It is regarded as the channel of supreme wisdom and sublime intuition, and is said to confer divine knowledge. Here it is relevant to note that the two eyes are often likened to the sun and moon. The third symbolic eye is then said to represent fire. The two eyes are capable of seeing only the past and the present, but the third eye gives potency to the perceptive powers making them see the future also.

Interestingly at some places men too adorn their foreheads with this 'third eye', but predominantly it remains a feminine trait.

Sindūra

Sindūra (vermilion) is a deep, rich blood-red powder applied in the parting between the hair. Exclusively used by married women it represents their marital status. Significantly this same powder is an essential ingredient in Hindu rituals (pūjā). In relation to women the notable characteristic is the colour of this powder. A vital red it is symbolic of fertility and the regenerative power inherent in women. At a practical level (especially in India where marriages are said to be made in heaven), it proclaims in loud terms the status of a woman committed irrevocably, and as passionately as the colour of her Sindūra, to a single individual, and thus being out of bounds for any other.

Tikā

The Tikā is a composite ornament composed of a chain with a hook at one end and a pendant at the other. It too like the Sindūra is worn in the parting of the hair. The hook holds the Tikā at the hair end, while the pendant falls on the exact centre of the forehead. This place is believed as the house of the 'ājñā' cakra. This cakra stands for preservation. Thus by adorning herself with this mark, a woman reiterates her status as the preservator of the order of the human race. Significantly this cakra is visualised as having two petals, and its presiding deity is Ardhanārīśvara, the half-male, half-female androgyne. This represents the ultimate union where no dualities exist. In Tantric terms this signifies the union of the male and female elements in nature, at all levels, including the physical. Hence this ornament is specifically associated with women about to undertake the vows of matrimony, uniting with her mate, and holding within her the potential to perpetuate the genealogy of the new clan she is thus becoming a part of.

Añjana (kohl)

"The eyes could never have beheld the Beautiful had it not been made Beautiful first". Ordinarily the eyes are a comparatively neutral and receptive organ, but when intent is added to the look it can charge the glance with irresistible power. Every feeling of the heart is transmitted through the eyes. The eyes can communicate feelings of reverence and sympathy, or love and lust.

The Indian poet usually longed to sink "in the depths below depths of the eyes of his beloved." Most poetic similes about eyes in Indian poetry are drawn from nature. Eyes are like the narcissus, the almond, the lily, or "like fishes with their long, flashing glide."

Kājala

A morning bath is a popular habit in India, and sprinkling the eyes with cold water is a necessity on account of the tropical climate. There is an existence of a popular powder (technically the sulphide of antimony), also known as Kājala, which has been used from time immemorial both to brighten and strengthen the eyes, and to darken the eyelashes.

A silver or ivory pencil or a fine camel's hair brush is dipped in the kohl and passed along the borders of the lids with a light and gentle hand, taking care to carry the line of shading a trifle beyond the angle of the eyes. This will cleanse the eyes and give them a large, almond shape, delightful to look at.

"A fair maiden's transformation into lovely womanhood, when she comes of age, is indicated by the transfer of restlessness of her feet to her eyes, the orbs whereof keep always on the move," says an Indian sage. "When the slow music of time begins to sing a sad song into a woman's ears towards her prime, the flashing of the eyes is then a very good exercise, winking an excellent one."

Thus the highlighting of the eye is an acknowledgement of the maturing of a young girl in all her aspects, though the symbolism remains primarily physical. Often a poet would address a heroine's eyes "as deep as the sea". Outlining with Kājala establishes two discernible banks to these fathomless oceanic streams. The erotic sentiment dominates the adorning of the eyes. Large eyelashes, it is believed, make large eyes. Therefore the Indian artist drew long spears of hair for the eyelashes he painted.

Also kohl, freely applied, will make each lash not only dark and bright but also so long that it is seen in full even when the face is turned aside. The eyes size is increased by drawing a short, fine pencil mark outwards from the corner of the lids where they join. Thus is created that sharpness in the glance that can let an Indian poetess say with pride to her lover: "My eyes are not eyes, beloved, but arrows of light; My eyebrows are not eyebrows, but swords for your Destruction."

The easiest way of preparing kohl at home is by burning a cotton wick soaked in mustard oil and then collecting the smoke that arises in a silver spoon. A silver pencil is then dipped into it and passed along the eyelids. This is said to blacken the eyes and preserve them against the sun and air. The eyes change to moonstones, brilliant, glinting and flashing fire, as, in the words of Kalidasa, "they are weighted over by the eyelids and half closed under the deeps of their palaces."

Natha or Nose Ring

The nose was once believed to be exclusively concerned with smell, but is connected with emotional responsivity also. In fact occultists go further, believing it to be the 'seat' of the sixth sense. Further there is known to be a close connection between the nose and the sexual reflexes. It is a medically established fact that swelling of the nasal spongy tissues and congestion of the nose occur during sexual excitement in human beings. The nasal passages of women swell, and occasionally bleed, during menstruation. Indeed Wilhelm Fliess (d. 1928), friend and associate of Sigmund Freud, found a relationship between the nose and the female sexual apparatus, and held that certain gynaecological complaints could be cured by cauterizing the appropriate parts of the nose.

In males there is believed to be an affinity between the nose and the virile member, and from ancient times it was thought that a large nose was a sign of a large male sexual organ. Similarly, a woman with a little nose is believed to have a small sexual apparatus. In a parallel custom, in a number of north European countries, and in England under the law of Canute (d. 1035), the punishment for adultery for both men and women was amputation of the nose, not only to cause disfigurement and loss of physical attractiveness, but also to symbolise punishment for the offending genitals. In India, the deflowering of a virgin is symbolically referred to as the removal of the 'natha' or nose ornament.

Thus the Indian aesthetic befittingly adorns the female nose with an inspired ornament, which highlights its amorous connotations. Indeed amongst the many jewels with which the Indian woman adorns herself, the nose ornament is perhaps the most seductive. Ornaments for the nose take on a variety of shapes ranging from tiny jewelled studs resting on the curve of the nostril, to large gold hoops that encircle the cheek with graceful pendant pearls dangling provocatively just above the upper lip.

One can imagine the ornament making a very soft, sighing sound, like breeze moving over Pīpala leaves, as the head moves. The length and position of nose ornaments often came in the way of comfortable eating, prompting the Abbe Dubois, a Christian missionary who lived in south India in the 19th century, to observe in amasement: "The right nostril and the division between the two nostrils are sometimes weighted with an ornament that hangs down as far as the under lip. When the wearers are at meals, they are obliged to hold up this pendant with one hand, while feeding themselves with the other. At first this strange ornament, which varies with different castes, has a hideous effect in the eyes of Europeans, but after a time, when one becomes accustomed to it, gradually seem less unbecoming, and at last one ends up thinking it quite an ornament to the face."

An integral part of traditional bridal jewellery, many aristocratic families have a special natha brought out at weddings to be worn by the bride. This is now perhaps the only occasion on which today's urban woman wears the natha, evoking its powerful seductive charm.

Hāra or Necklace

The neck is an important occult centre. Because necklaces are often worn near the heart, they can be used to work on emotions, or to attract or strengthen love.

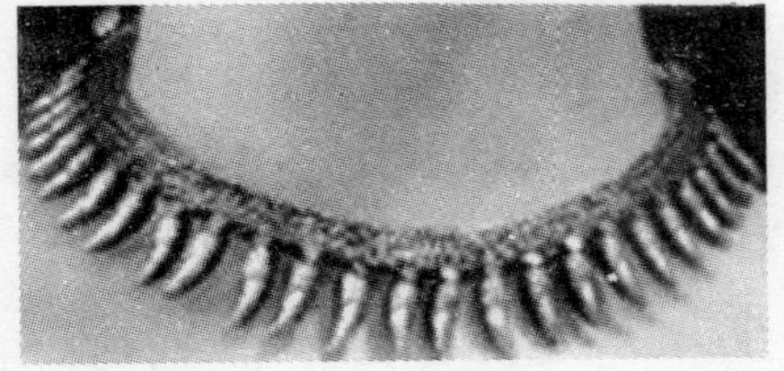

Figure 30: Necklace

By wearing a necklace of stones for example, it is believed that we are binding ourselves with their powers. From earliest times protective pendants, necklaces and strings of beads, as well as elaborate ornamental collars, were worn around the neck to bring good luck and avert the evil eye.

Indeed among all the kinds of jewellery, necklaces have had the maximum number of magical properties assigned to them. In some cases, they were designed as amulets or charms to insure good health or wealth to the wearer. Such necklaces could be very simple, with a gem or carving carrying the burden of the charm, or they could be very elaborate, glittering with gold and gems.

In all probability the form of the necklace was visualised with the explicit purpose of distracting the eyes of the viewer from the wearer's face and eyes-and thus protecting the wearer from the dangers of the mysterious Wicked Eyes. The necklace hence also served as a protection against any attempt at hypnotizing, since such an effort would have had to start with a concentrated gaze at the wearer's face, an attempt which the necklace effectively undermined. A necklace in this manner acted as a powerful restraint against undesirable gentlemen trying out their charms on virtuous maidens.

Most likely, the predecessor of the necklace in India was a fresh flower garland, to which there are a number of references in literature. One of the more important designs of the necklace is known as Campākalī, i.e. 'buds of the Cāmpā (Michelia champaca) flower'. Many others derive inspiration from the jasmine flower, the fragrance of which has strong erotic connotations. Even today, despite the emergence of paper and plastic flower garlands, the custom of offering fresh flower garlands has retained its charm.

Karṇa Phūla

The Karṇa Phūla is the ear flower. From earliest times long ear lobes have been regarded as a sign of spiritual development and superior status. Among the distinguishing marks of the Buddha, and a sign of his greatness, were his large ear lobes. Homer (d.c. 800 BC) and Aristotle (d. 322 BC) reputedly also had the same characteristic. There is believed to be a close connection between the ears and the sexual reflexes. The fleshy ear lobes, absent in all other primates, are not, as they appear to be, useless appendages, but erogenous zones which in sexual excitement become swollen and hypersensitive. In ancient times severed ears were offered to the Mother Goddess as a substitute for the male organs. In Egypt, devotees offered their ears to the goddess Isis, and till the early decades of the Christian era, sculpted ears were offered at the Shrine of the Great Mother in other parts of the Middle East.

The boring of ear lobes has been widely practised in all parts of the world from early times. The purpose of this operation is not only to facilitate the wearing of earrings for Beauty, but also to protect the wearer from evil influences, the adornments serving as talismans. The practice was also thought to have some therapeutic value. In certain places, ear piercing was believed to be good for the eyes; it also sharpened the mind and drew off 'bad humors'. One historian attributes the piercing to the desire to punish the ears for overhearing what they should not hear. The earrings, in turn, were the consolation for the pain and suffering. It was believed that the more decorative and expensive the earrings, the greater the consolation.

Early sculptures demonstrate that ear ornaments were an important constituent of Indian female attire. To the married woman, the ear ornament was (and is) auspicious. Additionally a woman's wealth was conspicuously visible and the ear ornament became a statement of her status and power; elongated ear lobes were considered a sign of Beauty and wealth-the longer the lobe, the greater the woman's wealth. By appending ornaments to almost every part of the ear, the woman also ensured a continuous state of mental and physical well being. Indeed recent studies have identified the ear as a microcosm of the entire body-"the point of vision in acupuncture is situated in the centre of the lobe."

The Indian woman's bejewelled ear offers a sight that prompted the exclamation: "European ladies are content with one appendage to each ear, while the females of Hindustan think it impossible to have too many."

Ancient Prākrit and Sanskrit literature describe girls wearing fresh flowers in their ears. A range of floral earrings of gold, silver or precious stones that have been popular over the centuries in India suggest that the forms of flowers were, almost literally, translated into precious jewellery. Most ear-ornaments are virtually bunches (Jhumkā) of fruits and flowers. A particular type, known as the Karṇaphūla, i.e. 'ear-flowers' is considered particularly auspicious. These are an important, universal, large, round metal flower-form earring, with a central stud at the back being the equivalent of a flower stem.

The choice of the flower as the inspiring shape behind this conception is of certain significance. Flowers in addition to being natural erotic stimulants, by virtue of their association with Kāma, the god of love, are also essentially a concise symbol of nature, condensing into a brief span of time the cycle of birth, life, death and rebirth. In addition, it also reflects gentleness, youth, spiritual perfection and artless innocence, qualities which are but the fundamental attributes of feminine character.

Often they are so heavy that the ear lobe dilates to the extent that the long-hanging earrings worn in the widened orifices touch the shoulder. Foreign travellers were fascinated by the sight of elongated ear lobes and have recorded their astonishment.

Bangles

Bangles are one of the oldest art objects in India, the bronze statuette of a dancing girl excavated at Mohenjo Daro epitomises the antiquity and the universality of wrist ornaments in India. She stands in the nude with one arm at her hip, the other arm completely weighed down with a collection of bangles. From then on the variety and shape of wrist ornaments spanned the gamut of nature's materials and human creativity.

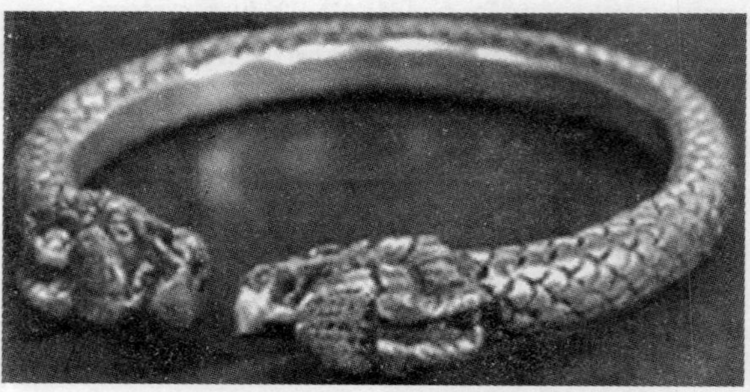

Figure 31 Bangle (Kuṇḍala)

Indeed more than any other single jewellery form in India, the bangle has been crafted from the widest veriety of materials. Ancient fragments testify that bangles were made from terracotta, stone, shell, copper, bronze, gold, silver and almost any material that lent itself to craftsmanship. Bangles, made from Lāc and glass in a plethora of colours, are a common sight in India even today. For simple plain circlets of metal, to ones decorated with etched and repousse designs, to fabulous examples with bird and animal-head terminals and studded with gems, these circlets symbolise the potent energy of the suṇ The German philosopher Johann Gottlieb Fichte considered Beauty a moral virtue.

The artist creates a world in which Beauty, as much as truth, is an end, foreshadowing that absolute freedom which is the goal of human will For Fichte, art is individual, not social, but it fulfils a great human purpose.

Mehndī

"When she puts henna on her hands and dives in the river, one would think, one saw fire twisting and Running in the water." Unlike a real tattoo, which is permanent, some decorative patterns created on the skin with stain or dye are not immediately removable but, depending on the dye strength, can last for three or four weeks. Mehndī, the Hindi term for "henna," is one such temporary tattoo.

Men agree that Mehndī patterns on a woman evoke thrilling, erotic sensations, perhaps because they associate Mehndi with a maiden's initiation into mature womanhood.

The custom of applying elaborate Mehndī patterns to the hands and feet is a symbol of satisfaction and happiness in marriage among the Hindus. This belief derives partly from the dye's red colour, universally considered to be auspicious; and which is also the colour of a bride's dress. Mehndī is commonly applied to propitiate Gaṇeśa, the elephant-headed god, son of Śiva, who overcomes obstacles and is always invoked to attend a Hindu marriage ceremony. It is also considered very dear to Lakṣmī, goddess of wealth and fortune. Indeed if ever there was a plant associated with luck and prosperity, it is the henna bush.

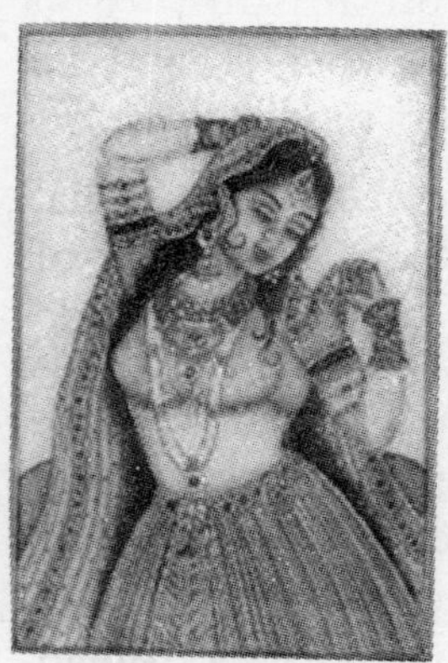

Figure 32 Dressing

Mehndī has a great significance in all Eastern wedding traditions, and no wedding is complete without the decoration of the bride's hands and feet- in many cultures on both the front and back of the hands right up to the elbow, and on the bottom half of the legs.

Mehndī is carried out on a bride's hands and feet the night before the marriage celebrations begin, often known as the 'Mehndī Ki Rāt' or night of henna (Rāt meaning night). A party of the bride's women relatives spend several hours at this joyful task, during which they sing appropriate songs, teasing her about her future:

"Oh, how sleep is hard to come by, once her hands have been adorned with the Mehndī of her beloved." "Oh, friends, come and decorate my hands with Mehndī, write my beloved's name. Just see, how auspicious this occasion is." "Everyone's fate is held within the lines on our palms, it is on these palms that Mehndī paints such Beautiful pictures." The Mehndī night is something like a hen night in the West, with all the bride's female friends and relatives getting together to celebrate. For the bride, the process is therapeutic in calming and preparing her for the event.

Mehndī signifies the strength of love in a marriage. The darker the Mehndī, the stronger the love. The colour of henna specifically has symbolic significance because red is the colour of power and fertility. Many brides believe that the deeper the colour of the Mehndi, the more passionate the marriage. The design itself is important, too. Sometimes the groom's name is incorporated into the bride's complex Mehndī tattoos, and it is a delightful task to try finding it-often taking up hours to accomplish. After marriage, Mehndī may be applied to a woman on any auspicious occasion, such as the birth or naming of a child.

Mehndī designs are an aspect of folk art requiring a well-developed decorative sense. Though the community perpetuates old patterns, innovative designs may also be introduced, which gradually enter the communal design repertoire. But an interesting aspect is that whatever be the innovation or tradition, only vegetative motifs are used. Thus henna is an attempt to symbolically link women with the vegetative and organic nature of Nature, along with its associated concepts of birth, nourishment, growth, regeneration etc.

Additionally, the purpose of tattooing is mainly apotropaic: to it is credited an evil-averting, magical function. Especially in animist societies, the tattoo serves to repel the forces of evil believed to be constantly active and attempting to gain advantage over the unwary, unprotected individual, causing misfortune, illness, or even death. In India, it is believed that an auspicious occasion like a marriage, requires an extra protection against evil forces. This is because such occasions are celebrated with much pomp and show, amidst a high profile, making the probability of their being noticed by negative forces very high. The application of henna is thus an attempt to safeguard against any such dark influences.

Besides being a lavishly colourful cosmetic, Mehndī is also supposed to have many healing qualities; many herbal doctors still recommend the use of Mehndī for some ailments, such as dry skin and to hasten the healing of cuts and scratches. It also acts as a hair conditioner when applied on the head and is also said to stop hair loss by strengthening the roots of the hair.

According to Loretta Roome, a henna expert, in societies where Mehndī is traditionally practiced, marriages are often scheduled to coincide with ovulation. "That's part of the intention, "she said. "It's a fertility rite. Henna is the colour of blood, representing the breaking of the hymen. In fact, Muslims call Mehndī 'love juice."

The remaining elements are part of the wedding attire which do not have a significant scientific connotation namely, finger ring, pāyal (anklets), tagari (belt), hansuli in the shape of Omega etc. therefore do not need elaborate explaination.

Gṛha Lakṣmī and Mahā Lakṣmī

The Gṛha-Lakṣmī or the wife in the family is the wealth and health of the family on earth. Whereas Mahā-Lakṣmī maintains wealth and health of the Viṣṇu family in the heaven. Gṛha-Lakṣmī focuses on the policies of the Mahā-Lakṣmī to improve quality of life of the family on earth. All supernatural powers are gained from the Mahā-Lakṣmī. This is called the Nidhi (behaviours), Riddhi (wealthy), Siddhi (cosmic power). The Gṛha-Lakṣmī co-ordinates financial and all other activities in the home. We can say that Gṛha is the wife or mother and Mahā is the Super Mother. This also refers to the soul and the Super Soul.

The Lakṣmī has been described in Śrī Sūkta and a hymn in the Rīg Vedā. "The supreme appears in the form of Viṣṇu to uphold and protect the world. The operation is done through the power of Viṣṇu for which the terminology is Lakṣmī. She is the Brahman revealed in its mother aspect as creator and nourisher of the three worlds. Her description appears in the Śrī Sūkta, where she has been lauded in golden words and in glorious terms (...). Just as there is no difference between Power-Holder (Viṣṇu) and Power (Lakṣmī) (...). She is the presiding deity of all divine manifestation.

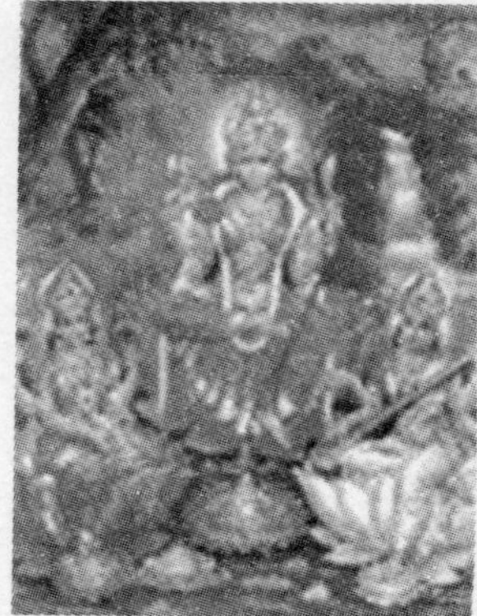

The characters, syllables and words in the fifteen verses of Śrī Sūkta, collectively form the sound body of Lakṣmī, the presiding deity of this hymn. As it has come to us from the state of consciousness of the Ṛṣi (seer), the substance is Cit, the creative energy in Vaikhari or gross form of sound. The universe is conceived and born of sound. Light is nothing but a sound of a particular frequency. All that we see in these worlds in solid, liquid, or gaseous state has emanated from sound. Even our mind is the crystal of sound. Nāma (name) is sound from which Rupa (form) has come. In short, Śrī Sūkta is a Siddha Mantra and is a radiant mass of energy. By proper Sādhana, the Jīva or soul can raise itself to a divine status. We mention below the translated version of the presiding deity of this hymn.

"Invoke for you O Agni, the Goddess Lakṣmī, who shines like gold, yellow in hue, wearing gold and silver garlands, blooming like the moon, the embodiment of wealth. O Agni! Invoke for me that unfailing Lakṣmī, blessed by whom, I shall win wealth, cattle, horses and men. I invoke Śrī (Lakṣmī), who has a line of horses in her front, a series of chariots in the middle, who is being awakened by the trumpeting of elephants, who is divinely resplendent. May that divine Lakṣmī grace me. I hereby invoke that Śrī

(Lakṣmī) who is the embodiment of absolute bliss; who has a pleasant smile on her face; whose lustre is that of burnished gold; who is wet as it were, (just from the milky ocean) who is blazing with splendour, and is the embodiment of the fulfilment of all wishes; who satisfies the desire of her votaries; who is seated on the lotus and is Beautiful like the lotus. I resort to that Lakṣmī for shelter in this world, who is Beautiful like the moon, who shines bright, who is blazing with renown, which is adored (even) by the gods, which is highly magnanimous, and grand like the lotus. May my misfortunes perish. I surrender myself to Thee, O Thou resplendent like the Sun! By Thy power and glory, plants like the Basel tree have grown. May the fruits thereof destroy through the grace of all inauspiciousness rising from the inner organs and ignorance from the outer senses. O Lakṣmī! I am born in this country with the heritage of wealth. May the friends of Lord Śiva (Kubera, Lord of wealth and Kīrti, Lord of Fame), come to me. May these (having taken their abode with me), bestow on me, fame and prosperity. I shall destroy the elder sister to Lakṣmī, the embodiment of inauspiciousness and such evil as hunger, thirst and the like. O Lakṣmī! Drive out from my abode all misfortunes and poverty. I hereby invoke Lakṣmī (Śrī), whose (main) avenue of perception is the odoriferous sense (i.e., one who abides mainly in cows); who is incapable of defeat or threat from anyone; who is ever healthy (with such virtuous qualities as truth); whose grace is seen abundantly in the refuse of cows (the cows being sacred); and who is supreme over all created beings. O Lakṣmī! May we obtain and enjoy the fulfilment of our desires and our volitions, the veracity of our speech, the wealth of cattle, the abundance of varieties of food to eat! May prosperity and fame reside in me (thy devotee)!"

The Rīg Vedā (4.8.7) remarks the enjoyment to fulfil our desires in the following hymn: "May riches, envied by many, devolve upon us day by day, and (abundant) food awaits us." The underneath hymn in the Śrī Sūkta in the Rīg Vedā, refers to our dynasty in heaven.

"Lakṣmī! You have progeny in Kardama. (Hence) O Kardama, may you reside in me. Make Mother Śrī with garlands of lotuses to have Her abode in my (ancestral) line. May the (holy) waters create friendship (they being of adhesive nature). O Ciklita (progeny of Śrī)! Reside at my home; and arrange to make Divine Mother Śrī stay in my lineage!

Invoke for me, O Agni, Lakṣmī who shines like gold, is brilliant like the sun, who is powerfully fragrant, who wields the rod of suzerainty, who is the form of supreme rulership, who is radiant with ornaments and is the goddess of wealth. Invoke for me O Agni, the Goddess Lakṣmī who shines like gold, blooms like the moon, who is fresh with anointment (of fragrant scent), who is adorned with the lotuses (lifted up by celestial elephants in the act of worship), who is the presiding deity of nourishment, who is yellow in colour, and who wears garlands of lotuses.

Invoke for me O Agni, that Goddess Lakṣmī, who is ever unfailing, being blessed by whom I shall win wealth in plenty, cattle, servants, horses and men."

The underneath hymn refers to Lakṣmī as the Cosmic Power.
Om Mahā-Lakṣmī Ca Vidmahe Viṣṇupatnai Ca Dhīmahi
Tanno Lakṣmī Pracodayāt ˇOm Śānti, Śānti, Śānti.

"We commune ourselves with the Great Goddess, and meditate on the consort of Viṣṇu; may that Lakṣmī direct us (to the Great Goal). Om May there be Peace, Peace, Peace.

A fantastic and perfect life is there.

Chapter 7

Youth and Health

Physical and Mental Health

Youth in a sense has nothing to do with political history. It is a metaphysical endowment, an essential factor, a structure, a conditioning. Youth is in itself so amiable, that were the soul as perfect as the body, we could not forbear adoring it. In the time of youth both mental and physical effort is required because effort contributes to health. Some psychologists regard mental health as the ability to maintain a balance between positive and negative emotions, such as elation and sadness. The Russian novelist and playwright Nikolay Gogol (1809 - 1852) said "As you pass from the tender years of youth into harsh and embittered manhood, make sure, you take with you on your journey all the human emotions! Don't leave them on the road, for you will not pick them up afterwards!" In this view, a person who displays emotional extremes in either direction is less well adjusted. Other psychologists emphasize the role of one's environment in influencing well being. This perspective sees mental health reflected in a person's overall happiness in various domains of life, such as social relationships, work, and community life.

With the exception of yoga and meditation the effort of a person needs a lot of energy from our energy stock. The practitioners of yoga and meditations have identified a number of distinct dimensions of mental health..These include self-acceptance, or self-esteem, characterised by a positive evaluation of oneself and one's past experiences. Personal growth reflected in one's sense of continued psychological growth and development. This means that one's life has purpose and meaning; positive relations with others; environmental mastery, the capacity to manage effectively in the surrounding world. Autonomy, a sense of self-determination and the ability to control one's own life is necessary. Self-acceptance, relations with others, environmental mastery, and autonomy usually improve as a person ages and gains life experience. However, many people find that their personal growth and sense of purpose in life begin to decline in midlife. A wise man in his midlife period would say 'No wise man ever wished to be younger'.

The wise yogīs harmonise their mind and intellect to visualise the Supreme Being through their meditation (RV. 5.81.1: 1244). The yogi knows that at the beginning of this universe only the seed was created. It is a disputable fact that auditory and visual cognitions cannot take place in the absence of contact with the mind. Moreover when a person becomes deeply immersed in sleep, he cannot see, hear, smell, touch and taste any thing. Furthermore in this stage he becomes deprived of the power of feeling pleasure, pain, fear, longing or loathing. Not only this, he cannot even think or articulate sound.[1] Now as the mind performs all the functions of the body, then, what can be the ground for postulating the existence of the soul? It is only the soul, which remains immanent in the body of all beings that actually accomplishes bodily movements and activities. It is this eternal soul who feels the sensations of colour, smell, touch, sound and taste. It is he, who feels pleasure and pain.

If a human being is mentally okay then his physical health improves day by day. The practice of sport is one of the means to stay healthy. A human needs sport or physical fitness, that's the ability of the human body to function with vigour and alertness, without undue fatigue, and with ample energy to engage in leisure activities, and to meet physical stress. Muscular strength and endurance, cardio-respiratory integrity, and general alertness are the overt signs of physical fitness. It

---

[1] The Naradiya Purana; Dr. S.S. Upadhyaya; Srimati Kumud Kumari Upadhyaya; Muzaffarpur, Bihar; 1983.

is usually measured in relation to functional expectations, that is, typically, by periodic tests measuring strength, endurance, agility, coordination, and flexibility. In addition, stress tests ascertain the body's accommodation to powerful, sustained physical stimuli, which in turn is used to analyse fitness. If individuals accommodate to the stressors, they are said to be fit.

The level of physical fitness can be influenced by regular, systematic exercise. Moderate activity will maintain the individual at a level that is usually adequate to handle ordinary stress. If the fitness level is to be improved, however, it is necessary to participate in more intensive exercise that overloads the physiological systems and thus promotes change. Exercises that demand total body involvement improve and maintain fitness most effectively, for example, jogging, running, swimming, vigorous dancing, cycling, and brisk walking. Organised games and sports, which have long rest periods within the play design, have only minimal influence on fitness. We always say "eat healthily to a certain limit". Sports are also an activity, which one does with a limit. An excess of sport activity means injury, fracture and blackouts. We need the energy-reserve to live and to survive. In development of the youth nowadays, they need assistance in the areas of drug and alcohol prevention, delinquency prevention, health and fitness, career exploration, and education enhancement. These factors are also destructive of our energy stocks. A British poet and critic, Matthew Arnold (1822-1888) remarks the following about youth's agitations:

> "And sigh that one thing only has been lent
> To youth and age in common-discontent."

The nature of youthful experience is greatly affected by cultural and economic norms. The passage from youth to adulthood is frequently acknowledged by ritual formalities. Idealised youth is embodied in enduring themes of art, literature and mythology. In Greek mythology, the goddesses Aphrodite and Persephone were beloved because of their beautiful youth appearances. Aphrodite is the goddess of love and beauty and the counterpart of the Roman goddess Venus. Persephone is the personification of the revival of nature in

Spring. Both goddesses were seen as the fertility of the earth or the youth in heaven. The youth in heaven has been described in the Sāma Veda as beauty, full of courage, truthful, flowery wealth (SV 14.3.2).

As mentioned above about the capacity to manage effectively in the surrounding world and the ability to control one's own life, the youth also needs rules of scriptures. The Veda replies that youth is pure, a richly shining period of a human being, and a period of intelligence to be honoured in the future (RV 6.48.7). In every civilized human society there is some set of scriptural rules and regulations, which is followed from the beginning of creation. Youth without knowledge of the scriptures will be called demoniacs. The Bhagavad Gītā (16.7) says "Those who are demoniac do not know what is to be done and what is not. Neither cleanliness nor proper behaviour nor truth is found in them. The demons are not clean, either externally or internally. One should always be careful to keep his body clean by bathing, brushing teeth, shaving, changing clothes, etc. To assist youth not to become demoniac persons in this civilised world, organisations should undertake three tasks:

1. consider the needs of youth and appraise the facilities and resources for serving these needs;
2. recommend procedures and programs which seem to be most effective in solving the problems of youth;
3. popularise and promote desirable plans of action through conferences, publications, and demonstrations.

Nowadays mostly people think very economically about the use of electricity, gas and water because we know that these resources will not available for a long time. Similarly, we should also think of our own energy stock. Our energy sources too are limited. The number of breathings that people has are 700 millions. Compare this with a bank balance; we don't use up the money in one day. You can be young without money but you can't be old without it. The essay of the English philosopher Francis Bacon (1561-1626) responds of Youth and Age "A man that is young in years may be old in hours, if he has lost no time." However, a good ratio of income (energy stock) and expenditure (breathings) makes a good balance between body and spirit. This bank assessment we don't spend all in one year, but in daily proportions to regulate health and our cycles of life. If you don't do this, then the so-called process-servers will enter your accommodation as sickness phenomena: you become bankrupt. A daily slogan 'buy now before it's too late' refers to the right time of spending energy. In the entertainment world we also say 'buy your tickets on time'. Another popular expression nowadays is 'God is a DJ'. Each musical tone is determinative of movement and breathing. This breathing is regulated by the Prāṇas, life energy, in the body. In the Atharva Veda the Prāṇa is compared to a gentle or erotic whip (Pasha, Madhua) which keeps the senses (the horses) busy, or ensures that the horses continue to trot (AV 8.1.2, 3: 2032, 2033). The horses must be controlled to trot to the correct destination. This destination which is reached by the Prāṇa is called Prāṇāyāma (Prāṇa: life energy; Ayama: destination, aim). With Prāṇāyāma it is possible to extend life (Diṛgh-āyu), to slow down old age and ensure that death (Yama) stays away (stay healthy) (AV 8.2.11: 2062).

The Inner Guide

It is obvious that we have an inner guidance system, a connection to our Higher Self or Inner Being, or whatever name we choose to give this Higher Intelligence. This inner guidance system functions through what we call our intuition or instinct. It speaks a very simple language. Either it feels good, or it doesn't. All the rest is just politics. We are told that we should move with feelings that are good, and not with that doesn't feel good to us. We are told to trust this inner voice. When we don't follow this inner voice we feel tension. This tension moves the inner intuitions, which effects the fire flow in the body. The body becomes weak and a strong hyperventilation can be the result. The Yajur Veda advices to control the fire system in our body, becoming a guard of our breath (breath is life), stay healthy in voice and action, and keep your body and style in good shape (YV 3.17: 82).

The Inner Clock

Biorhythm or Biological Clocks (inner clock) are internal physiological systems that enable organisms to live in harmony with the rhythms of nature, such as the cycles of day and night and of the seasons. A lot of people have a big problem waking up early in the morning. It seems sometimes that there exists an inner bell, which does not run right with the alarm clock, which forces us to get out of bed. Others, on the other hand have problems, going to bed at night. It proves that a lot of effort has to be put in the system of 24 hours, without the aid of pills or tablets. Generally we split our day of 24 hours in three parts. One part to work, one part to relax and one part to sleep. From this one is able to conclude that our biorhythm is programmed on a 24 hours system. Such biological 'timers' exist for almost every kind of periodicity throughout the plant and animal world, but most of what is known about them comes from the study of rhythmic biological cycles recurring at approximately 24 hours intervals (circadian). Circadian rhythms cue typical daily behavior patterns even in the absence of external cues such as sunrise, demonstrating that such patterns depend on internal timers for their periodicity.

We know that no clock is perfect. When organisms are deprived of the external cues, which the world normally provides, such as light, they display a characteristic 'free-running' period of not quite 24 hours. As a result, free-running animals drift slowly out of phase with the natural world. In experiments in which people are isolated for long periods of time, they continue to eat and sleep on regular, but increasingly out-of-phase, schedules. Such drift does not take place under normal circumstances, because external cues reset the clocks each day. Our biorhythmic system is also dependent on light, particularly bright light. Light is the most powerful synchroniser of circadian rhythms. The Veda called this light the inviolable means to reach the beloved station. The brightness of light is an instrument to reset the conditions of our body. This resetting process ends up in a healthy feeling with a bright mind. (YV 1.31: 31). Some philosophers say that the mind has only a form which is commensurate (similar) with the body with which it may, for the time, be connected; it contracts or expands like light placed in a jar or a house as the case might be. And thus they say that non-interruption and repeated are proper. It is the manifestation alone of the self-existing mind that expands or contracts, and that it is this, which has the necessity of the operation of the exciting causes of virtue. These exciting causes are two-fold, external and internal. The external are those that staid in need of body as an instrument, such as praising, giving of charity, and the performance of obeisance. The internal are those that strand in need of the mind alone, such as faith.

The Effect of Light

Recent studies on humans have shown that the amount of artificial indoor light to which people are exposed per day can resynchronise the body's cycle of sleep and wakefulness. People can inadvertently reset their body clocks to an undesired cycle by such activities as shielding morning light with shades and heavy curtains or by reading in bed at night by bright lamplight.

These two kinds of light, respectively shielding and brightness have been described in the Veda as the Aśvinas, the twin Light-Gods. The impulse of light makes sure that a person becomes vivid in his activities. Their impeller and vivifier is the Great Sun who distributes in respective portions to every creature. This portion functions in the biorhythm of every organism (YV 1.10: 10).

Many organisms also make use of rhythmic variations in temperature or other sensory inputs to readjust their internal timers. When an internal clock's time is very different from the external time, complete resetting sometimes requires days. The inner body is also in confusion. This phenomenon is well known to long-distance air travelers as getting a jet lag. The pressure of the air, the light shield in the aircraft and the irregular breathing are the cause that the conditions in the body change very quickly. To regulate the pressure we should acclimatise in the second layer of mid-air, the earth. The next is controlling the ranges of light and practice the right positions in order to firm our breath (in-, out- and up-breath) and strength (YV 4.14: 702). Humans can acclimate to extreme conditions through changes in normal physiological processes. Persons who move from a temperate to a hot, dry climate undergo changes in heart rate and body temperature such that in time they perspire less, and their perspiration contains less salt. Although at an altitude of 7600 m (25,000 ft) most persons need to breathe high-pressure oxygen for survival, through gradual acclimatization they may become able to breathe unaided.

Acclimatisation may also refer to psychological changes occasioned by a change in environments, as from a rural to an urban setting. The inner clock recovers after a long flight one hour per day of the time difference between the past and the present location. If the environmental difference is extreme, changes take place in the structure and physiology of the organism. Each organism, however, has certain limits of temperature and other conditions within which it can survive.

Apparently, biological clocks can exist in every cell and even in different parts of a cell. Hence, an isolated piece of tissue removed from an organism for example, the eye of a sea slug will maintain its own daily rhythm but will quickly adopt that of the whole organism when restored to it. Environmental factors are important for any organism in this world. Also the development in growth depends on these factors. Daily rhythm means that we are able to unite the air inside the body with the air outside. It incites us to greater efforts in life and gives us more self-confidence to stand firmly on any area. With a good biorhythm it is possible to strengthen your vital power. This power can be shown in society, viz. searching solutions in achieving wealth, in helping people and functioning better in politics (YV 5.27: 192).

The Inner Voice

Ignoring the inner voice could be the cause of bad feelings. The voice must get louder. This is the next level of communication: emotions. As we move further in the direction that feels not-good, we experience more and more emotions that feel not-good, and at a certain point we could say "I should have listened to myself when I thought of going in the other direction". That means that we heard the inner voice. Otherwise, we could not have said, "I should have listened". Listening to the inner voice means that we are able to stop ourselves going the wrong way. The inner voice is a powerful weapon, which we can use to destroy demonic impulses of the heart. That voice is the director, the wise adviser and the right sound in our heart. The inner sacrificial sound sends a message straight upward to the brain. After that, we should try to understand the signal, which can be godlike, lengthened life, future pointed, joyful and peaceful (YV 5.17: 182). And that sounds good! Yes, indeed music has a high value and expression. Especially for the youth, they have an enormous range of tastes and skills. The speed of modern communications made it possible for the youth to evaluate innovations in their style more quickly. The result of these features is that, today originality is more valued than in any previous era, and that diversity and rapid change have become the most prominent general features of music. Today music seems to encompass a bewildering variety of procedures and approaches. This was the emphasis on sounds, their qualities, textures, densities, and durations. This element began to take precedence over all others, including melody, which might not be present at all, and harmony, which might be treated merely as one component in a series of sound complexes. This harmony effect is good for the youth and certainly for their health.

If we still move on into the direction that doesn't feel good, the inner communication reaches the physical level. First the inner voice will be stronger, then it will stimulate the breath and further it will have affect on our vision. The result from that level is that the emotion creates a symptom that reflects an idea of creating an identity or our own reality. The Veda underlines the cleaning of the voice, the breath and the eyes (YV 6.14: 222). This is the beginning of understanding the message from the inner sound or movement. Receiving and believing the message means that the symptom doesn't remain for long. Symptoms that are created by decisions are easier to remove, because the symptom is based on consciousness and awareness.

The symptom of creating an illusionary vision can also have effect on the other organs of the body. The word 'cleaning' in the Veda means the disinfectional treatment of the following symptoms viz. not listening with attention, being nervous or having stomach problems, sexual limitations and pain in the back. The solution is to be conscious about the inner voice in the mind and be aware of the fact that this sound should be heard inside the heart. Taking a deep breath before getting emotional or as the Veda says "increase the fullness of breath, the fullness of the eyes, and let the ears become stronger. Be filled, cleansed and united" (YV 6.15: 223).

Consciousness Energy

The Ancient Hindu traditions that have been studying consciousness for thousands of years have left a map behind. The map contains the consciousness that the body represents and uses the language of the cakras. Cakra means 'wheel or vortex', because that's what it looks like. Each cakra is like a solid ball of energy interpenetrating the physical body, in the same way that a magnetic field can interpenetrate the physical body. The cakras are not physical. They are aspects of consciousness in the same way that the auras are aspects of consciousness, and more dense than the auras, but not as dense as the physical body. Consciousness travels in the body in the form of Prāṇa (inhalation) and Apāna (exhalation). It has illumined the physical body of living-beings (SV 631). They interact with the physical body through two major vehicles: the endocrine system and the nervous system. We have seven main cakras in out body. And each of the seven cakras is associated with one of the seven endocrine glands, and also with a particular group of nerves called a plexus. Thus, each cakra can be associated with particular parts of the body and particular functions within the body controlled by that plexus or that endocrine gland, associated with that cakra.

Your consciousness, your experience of being, represents everything that is possible for you to experience. All of your senses, all of your perceptions, all of your possible states of awareness, can be divided into seven categories, and each of these categories can be associated with a particular cakra. Thus, the cakras represent not only particular parts of your physical body, but also particular parts of your consciousness.

When you feel tension in your consciousness, you feel it in the cakra associated with the part of your consciousness experiencing the stress, and in the parts of the physical body associated with that cakra. Where you feel the stress depends therefore on why you feel the stress. When someone is hurt in a relationship, they feel it in their heart. When someone is nervous, their legs tremble and their bladder becomes weak. When there is tension in a particular part of your consciousness, and therefore in the cakra, associated with that part of your consciousness, the tension is detected by the nerves of the plexus, associated with that cakra, and communicated to the parts of the body, controlled by that plexus. When the tension continues over a period of time, or reaches a particular degree of intensity, the person creates a symptom on the physical level. Again, the symptom served to communicate to the person through their body, what they had been doing to themselves in their consciousness. When the person changes something about their way of being, they are able to release the stress that had been creating the symptom, and they are then able to return to their natural state of balance and health.

Secret Map

How to read the map which the old traditions left behind? Let's find someone who is feeling stressed about something that was happening in his or her life at that time. Let us examine the map of consciousness that the cakras provide, in order to understand the language of the symptoms that are associated with each cakra.

In order to complete this map, however, we also need to look at ourselves, as each is a polarity of yin and yang, feminine and masculine characteristics. For most people, their right side is their yang side, their will side, their acting or active side, and the left side is their yin side, their female side, their feeling or adaptive side. These parts are similar to that of the Ardhanārīśvara (Śiva-Śakti) as mentioned before.

Polarities

For people who were born left-handed, this polarity is reversed. Thus, for a right-handed person, their right leg can be described as their will leg, or their male leg. This is the foundation of their will, but for a left-handed person, their left leg would be their male leg or will leg, and so on. Thus, we can talk about the will arm, or the will eye, or the will nostril, etc., and which side it is on will depend upon whether the person is right-handed or left-handed at birth. The inner two parts of our body are linked with the cakras in our body. Each of the cakras is energy vibrating at a certain frequency, in a logical and orderly sequence of seven vibrations. As we move up the scale, the elements become more and more subtle, moving through the five physical elements of earth, water, fire, air, and ether, to the spiritual elements of inner sound and Inner Light.

The heaviest element is on the bottom, the lightest on the top. It is a logical and orderly sequence. Everything is liable to gravity. We find this sequence in color, sounds and other non-physically things. The colors of the spectrum also represent a series of seven vibrations in a logical and orderly sequence, as do the notes of the musical scale. Thus, we can put the heaviest vibrations or the longest wavelength on the bottom and the lightest on the top, and a particular color can be used to represent a chakra in its clear state, as can a particular musical note. Music played in a certain key vibrates a particular cakra, and we feel a particular way when we hear that music. Our relationship with a certain color says something about our relationship with the part of our consciousness that the color represents. In the same way we merge the relations between another people. Inner and outer contacts are dependent on sound or vibration.

Youth Fix

Those who have a desire to prolong their youth should

frequently change the flow of the 'vital' breath from one channel to the other. Besides this, they may attempt, under a yogi's guidance, the inverted gesture (Viparita Kāri Mudrā) every morning and evening.[2]

There are three basic ways of breathing:

1. Breathing in and out through the nostrils;
2. Inhaling through the mouth and exhaling through the open nostril;
3. Breathing in through the open nostril and out through the mouth. If each of these three ways of breathing is done for about 4 minutes every morning there will be few illnesses and a healthy, long and trouble-free life.

The vital' energy that lives in the region of the heart is called Prāṇa. Prāṇa flows in and out with the physical breath. During normal breathing, the inhaled 'vital' breath is 10 angulas or inch long, while the exhaled breath is 12 angulas long. Thus we lose a lot of 'vital' energy during daily respiration. This can shorten our life considerably. Now, each exhalation/inhalation takes about 4 seconds to complete. The rate of respiration and the length of the 'vital' breath is increased by physical action, viz., eating increases the length of the 'vital' breath to 18 angulas, walking to 20 angulas, running to 24 angulas, sexual intercourse to 60 angulas, and so on. If the rate of exhalation/inhalation is reduced, and the flow of 'vital' energy checked, we can easily increase our life span and gain control over our environment. The other name for life is age. Life should be protected against affliction such as poverty, disease and crises as these too are the cause of confusion and distress and can decrease longevity (YV 5.9.174).

To perform the above-mentioned Mudrā, first lie supine on a flat, hard surface and a woolen cloth. Stretch the arms right above your head. Now gently raise the legs together making an angle of 45^{0} to the ground. The knees must be kept straight. After achieving this, raise the legs further to make a 90^{0} angle to the ground. Now raise the buttocks and trunk by supporting the body with the palms held at the waist. In the final position,

---

[2] Secret Power of Tantrik Breathing; Swami Sivapriyananda; Abhinav Publications; New Delhi; 1996.

the body should be at an angle of 45^0 to the ground, with the legs held vertical. Accompany this gesture with quick, forceful exhalations from the lungs. This Mudrā can be performed for about 10 to 20 seconds at a time. Many yogīs can do this Mudrā for as long as 3 hours, but this is achieved only after long practice under a Yogi-Guru's instructions.

Inner Guideline

One's health and character are reflected in its breathing pattern. In general, people who breath short are weak, nervous and very unreliable, whereas those, who breathe long and deep, are reliable and happy. If someone gets excited his breathing pattern changes rapidly, because he will breath shorter. If someone rises to higher ideas, his breath becomes slower. This means that we are able to analyse our own strong and weak potentials. It is comparable with the SWOT (Strengths, Weaknesses, Opportunities, and Threats) analysis, which is used for industrial analyses. The process of utilising the SWOT approach requires an internal survey of strengths and weaknesses and an external survey of threats and opportunities. Structured internal and external examinations are necessary for a good and qualified practice and for good breath control.

Above all a practitioner (Sādhaka) must have a controlled life free from vices. Do good and reap good for your success, happiness, prosperity and good health. If a man attains the Siddhi of any Deva and has His blessings then he doesn't need to use any Yantra. One will obtain the answers of all his questions; will be bestowed with health, wealth and happiness. In addition all his desires will be fulfilled. But these methods are very difficult. One has to perform them with complete faith and confidence. We provide a few guidelines for the Sādhaka which are common for all.

1. The Sādhaka should either do idol Pūjā or Mānsic pūjā which means that a figure of a Deva be kept in mind.
2. The practice should be started after taking a bath, wearing new or clean clothes, using a good scent on the body.

3. The place should be clean and noiseless, free from any bad smell. The best places are: river, canal, pond etc., where you can sit in seclusion.
4. Your diet should be free from meat, wine and other intoxicants. Sexual relations be avoided.
5. Always think of your Deva, where ever you are and whatever work you are doing. Keep your mind clear from all bad or unwanted thoughts.
6. While doing the Mānsic Pūjā, keep the figure of your Deva in your mind, bathe him in the mind.
7. Recite the mantras with a rosary.

Śrī Yantra and Health

Yantra means an instrument, apparatus, talisman or mystical diagram but definitely not a magic or Jādu Tonā as is commonly believed.[3] During Kali Yuga, when the majority of the people had a materialistic mind, people according to instructions could not do Sādhanā or meditation of Mantra. The short cut is Yantra and Tantra to fulfil desires and attain success. Some of these Yantras are dealing with specific aspects of life, like possession, birth of child, good business, lawsuits, love, friendships and enemies. Yantras are also used for prevention of fear and bad influences, to prevent abortion, to return a missing person, for good health, wealth and happiness.

Yantra is usually translated as a machine, but in the special sense of the Tāntric tradition refers to the Devi in her linear or geometrical form. Every aspect of Devi has her own mantra and Yantra. The divinity of the Yantra always occupies the centre or apex. The different parts or petals and lines of the Yantra are usually arranged in concentric circles (Maṇḍalas) and contain rays or sub-limbs of the Devi. The Śrī Yantra has nine of these Maṇḍalas, each filled with various aspects of the Devi. The Yantra of Devi Lalitā is Śrī Yantra. This Śrī Yantra is said to be a geometric form of the human body, which implies that goddess as macrocosm, is one with human being as microcosm. Lalitā means 'She who plays'. All creation,

[3] Practicals of Yantras; L.R. Chawdhri; Sagar Publications; New Delhi; 1990.

manifestation and dissolution is considered to be a play of Devi or the goddess. Mahā-Tripura-Sundarī is her name as transcendent beauty of the three cities, a description of the goddess as conqueror of the three cities of the demons, or as the triple city (Tripura), but really a metaphor for a human being.

Lalitā or Tripurāsundarī is the 16th day or full moon, with her 15 digits. Each of the 15 Nityās has a certain number of arms, the totality of arms (= rays) of the whole circle being 108. Because any unit of time is taken as a microcosm or parallel of any other valid unit, each of the 15 Nityās has 1440 breaths.

One lunar fortnight is 21600 breaths - which is the number of a whole cycle or process. The breaths of a human being during one day and night are 21600 - 10800 of which are solar, the other 10800 being lunar. This device shows the unity of the 15 Nityas, time, space and a human being.

Lalitā loves pūjā or worship. Her mantra is called Vidyā or knowledge, specifically female knowledge, or the goddess, and in this context it relates to the magical diagram. She is a red flower, so her diagram is a flower too. The Tāntric tradition views its symbols as having a gross aspect, a subtle aspect, and a supreme aspect. In terms of Lalitā, the gross form is the image of the goddess with her four arms and so forth, the subtle form is as Yantra, and the supreme form is her mantra, all three being the goddess in different aspects. Behind the sometimes-colorful symbolism is deep wisdom coupled with practical methods for realising oneself.

The creation of the Śrī Yantra is described in the Yogini Hṛdaya (Heart of the Yogini Tantra (I.6-16).

"From the fivefold Śakti comes creation and from the fourfold Fire dissolution. The sexual union of five Śaktis and four Fires causes the cakra to evolve. O Sinless One! I speak to you of the origin of the cakra.

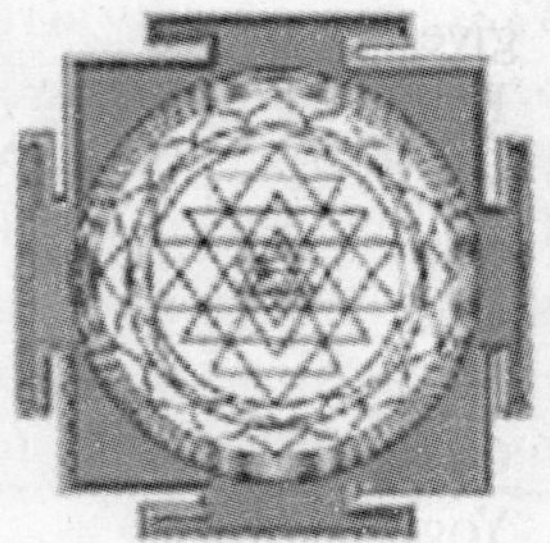

"When she, the ultimate Śakti, of her own will (svecchā) assumed the form of the universe, then the creation of the cakra revealed itself as a pulsating essence. From the void-like vowels with the Visarga (:) emerged the Bindu, quivering and fully conscious. From this pulsating stream of supreme light emanated the ocean of the cosmos, the very self of the three mothers.

"The Baindava of the cakra has a triple form, Dharma, Adharma and Ātmā, and Mātri, Meya and Prāṇa. The cakra of nine Yonis is the great mass of consciousness bliss and is the nine fold cakra and the nine divisions of the mantra.

"The Baindava is placed on a dense flowery mass and is the Citkāla. Similarly, the Ambikā form of eight lines is the circle of the vowels. The nine triangles quiver forth the effulgent form of 10 lines. Śakti, together with her surrounding nine blossomed forth the 10 Trikonas. The second quivering form of 10 lines has Krodhiṣa as first of the 10. These four cakras, of the nature of light, create the 14 - fold form, the essence of perception." At the very heart of the Bindu or centre of the Śrī Yantra is that which caused it to emanate. This is Kāmakālā, consisting of the three Bindus or potentials. One is red, one is white, and one is mixed. The red Bindu is ova, the white Bindu semen, and the mixed Bindu the union of Śhiva-Śakti, the individual as potential Śrī Cakra.

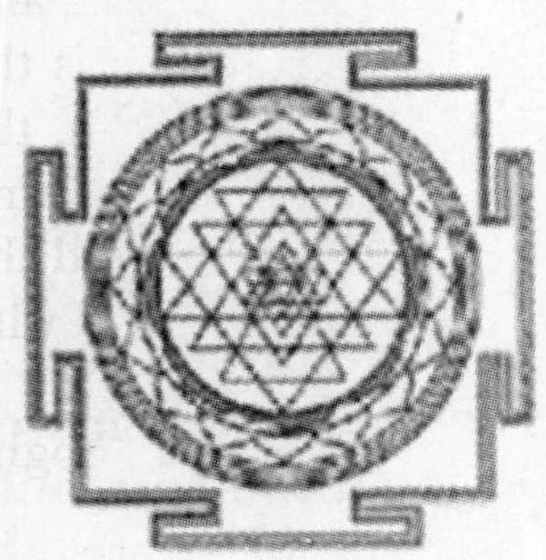

Father and Mother are represented in Śrī Vidyā by two limbs or aspects of Lalitā known as Vārāhi and Kurukullā. The semen of Vārāhi, the father-form, gives four alchemical Dhātus to the child. The ova of Kurukullā, the mother-form, gives five Dhātus to the child. Consciousness enters via orgasm. The three Bindus, collectively known as Kāmakāla (digit of sexual desire), are the root potential of sun, moon and fire. It is like sun and moon coming together in an eclipse, or the seed from which the plant-the human being grows.

The whole circle of eight petals is called the 'All Exciting Cakra'. The Śaktis in the mandala are called the Very Secret Yogini. Presiding here is Tripurā Sundarī. Her Vidyā is *Hriṁ Kliṁ Sauḥ*. She is described as swaying because of her love intoxicated state, with her eyes full of bliss. She smiles with passion. She shows the Mudrās dispelling fears and granting boons. The eight Śaktis in each of the eight petals of the Maṇḍala are described as Śaktis of Speech, Holding, Walking, Excreting, Pleasure, Abandoning, Concentration and Detachment. They are described as sapphire blue, holding noose, goad, dispelling fear, and holding blue lotus. Their names (like Ananga Madana) all convey terms of loving sexuality. The gem is cat's eye. The time is day and night (21600 breaths).

The whole Maṇḍala of 16 petals is called 'Fulfiller of Desire'. The Śaktis in the circle are known as the Hidden Ones. The presiding form of the Lalitā is Tripureṇi. Her Vidyā (mantra) is Aiṁ Kliṁ Sauḥ. She is described as ornamented with all gems, carrying a book and a rosary. The 16 Yoginis in this Maṇḍala are associated with the attainment of desires by the cultivation or strengthening of power over mind, ego, sound, touch, sight, taste, smell, intellect, steadiness, memory, name, growth, etheric body, revivification, and physical body. They are described as the Nitya Kalās. Each holds a noose, a goad, pot full of nectar, and makes the sign of giving. They are very red.

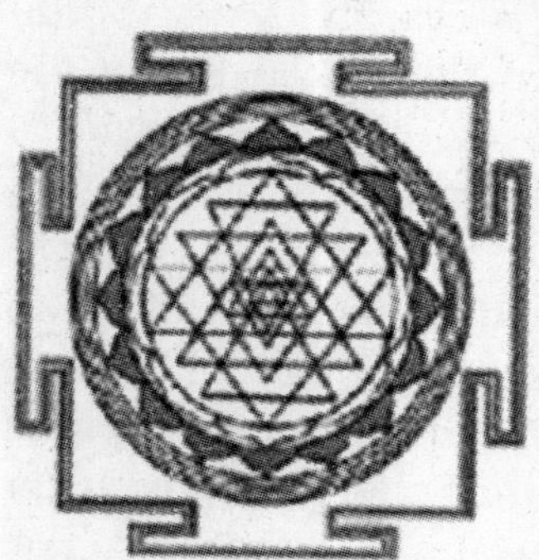

Her redness surpasses the redness of the China Rose, vermilion, or the pomegranate flower. She is clothed in red garments, holding an effulgent noose and a goad. She sits on a red lotus, and is adorned with red gems. She has four arms and three eyes, and She holds five arrows and a bow. Her mouth is filled with various pieces of betel mixed with camphor. Her beautiful gazelle like body, smeared with red powder, is the vanquisher of the God of Love. She wears the most beautiful kind of clothes, and is adorned with every kind of precious gem. She is the Mother Who gladdens creation, the cause of happiness in the world, causing all love in the world, creating the world, the Devī made of Mantra, great good fortune Sundarī, consisting of

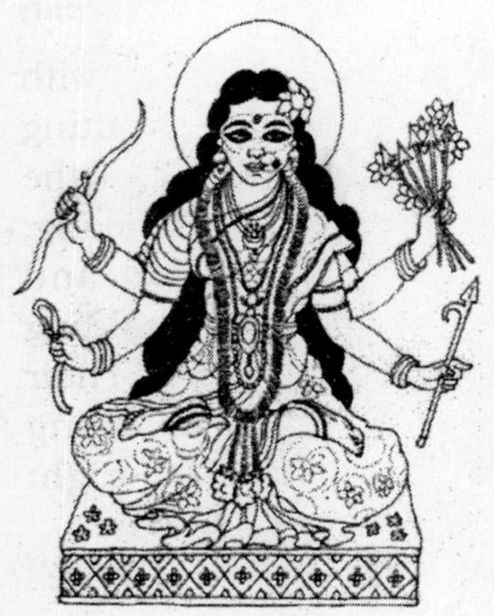

all wealth, eternal, supremely blissful and joyful.

A Yantra should be worn in any finger or in the neck as directed by the Guru with mantras. Before wearing the next method must be followed for proper use. Before wearing, the Yantra should be purified with gaṅgā water. After that, put a Tilaka of red vermillion (Sindūra) and put in the smoke of incense while sitting in a comfortable Āsana. Final the Yantra be dipped in scent or sprinkle scent over it. Then the person should recite the mantras, which have been recited by the Guru. The Śrī Yantra with Bīja should be inscribed on a gold plate, and be worn as a talisman. The Bīja-mantra must be recited 1,000 times daily for 45 days. Honey, Trimadhura, curds, milk and spiced rice of various kinds are food specific for offering. It is used for the attainment of all worldly desires, health and happiness.

Chapter 8

Pūjā

Survival of the Fittest

Human needs food to survive. For this reason we do a lot of actions, good and bad. The cosmic norm is that people should not think nagative, because bad thoughts are mainly the obstacles of mind development. Anyway, food creates mind and mind regulates growth. Food and growth correlated, academies found that the rule in the biotope is that one kilo growth of a meat-eater needs 10 kilo meat of another animal. The herbivore eats ten kilo plants to grow 1 kilo. In the sense of proportion the carnivore needs 100 kilo plants to grow one kilo. In the same scale we can put 'time'. Each 24 hours in heaven is one year on earth. We experience this in one of the death ceremonies according to the pitṛyajña that takes place every 6 months. After some one's death, the sixth month ceremony happens due to the dinner for the dead person and after one year for the breakfast. As soon the dead person arrives in heaven the soul has to visit the Dharma Rāja, the Judge in heaven. Death is a door opening from one aspect of life to another. If we want to survive every negative thoughts of life, to develop our mind and to grow spiritually, we ought to learn the concept of death. In addittion, death is placed on a high level in Pūjā performances.

What is death? Death is cessation of bodily or physical activity, of physical and organic function, of physical consciousness. Death is a transition from one state of being to another, a change of the form of consciousness to another plane, astral or mental. Ice becomes water, and water becomes steam, vapour, and invisible gas, according to the degree of vibration. So is life in the physical, astral, and mental planes. Death does not end your personality and self-consciousness. It merely opens the door to a higher or lower form of life. Death is only the gateway to a fuller life. Death is not extinction of personality. It is merely the cessation of an important individuality. It is only a change of form. Life flows on to achieve its conquest of the universe, till it merges in the Eternal. It is not the end of life. It is an aspect in the chain of lives. Death is a natural incident in the course of life, in the cycle of birth and death. It is necessary for your evolution. A new life starts after death. The process for the physical body is taking up the coffin for conveyance to the cemetery reciting the following Mantra. "O man! Death has separated the soul from this which becomes lifeless; take the corpse to the cemetery, situated at the southern outskirt to perform his burial, or crematoria" (AV 18.2.27).

Death means back to physically nothing or zero (ash). The new beginning is a restructure of this ash; of the five gross elements to a new body, type of life. The Jīva reincarnates constantly in bodies to achieve the bodiless. In reality, God needs a body to create (Brahmāṇḍa), and human needs a body to liberate himself. Vedic Science expresses this body relation as the Āṇda (Soul) and Piṇḍa (body). The upāniṣads named this relation as Bindu (Soul) and Sindhu (Supreme) or the Jīva (creative) and Śiva (Lord).

The human (Soul with body) is in Hinduism known as Nara or Nārī (man or woman). Nara indicates growth and progress of knowledge, analyse and syntheses.

Therefore the soul, carried by the astral and the carnal body, needs vitamins. After death the physical body is left behind on the earth. The triple form of our human body total is a product of 27 aspects and equal to that of the materials of the macrocosm. The logarithm of the aspect of the cosmos is three to the power of three (3^3), for more details we refer to chapter 2 Understanding the Spiritual World. We have equal body parts of god that present the material world for creation. In this sense, we are god. The physical body is a product of five aspects, the five gross elements, ether (space), air, fire, water and earth. Also compared with our left hand with five fingers. The right hand too has five fingers. They stand for the five main prāṇas or the vital energies. The veda named the vital energies as follows:"O Lord of knowledge, get up and awaken the deities by means of sacrifice. Increase the age, vitality, generation, animal wealth and fame. Make the sacrificer prosperous" (AV 19.63.1). These energies are 'parts of breaths' to control and regulate several sections in our body. The Vital breaths dwell in the following parts:

* Heart, Prāṇa
* Arms, Apāna
* Stomach, Samāna
* Throat, Udāna
* Total Body, Vyāna

The left hand joint with the right makes life possible.As soon the gross elements are not able to take breath into the body, death penetrates instead of in this life if want to continue with building on existence, we all need to join our qualites also in order to grow according to the rituals, death awareness, and controlling the Vital breath. The Veda adds that we are able to "attain the following qualities by means of sacrifice: Longevity, vitality, power of seeing and listening" (YV 9.21).

Ātmā Pūjā

Pūjā teaches people how to use and control the incredible force of the subconscious. Anyone can learn the powerful technique to change life, i.e. of the combining spiritual wisdom within the influences subconscious mind.

At every ritual ceremony Bṛhaspati is honoured as the first one in the section Svastivācana (introduction or invocation). This goes as follows: 'May the Master of vast knowledge, May Mighty God prosper us. May the Nourisher of all, the Author of all the Vedas prosper us. May He, the Giver of all comforts like the horse, prosper us. May God, the Lord of all the elements of Nature, vouchsafe us prosperity. May God, the Lord of all the elements of Nature, safeguard our prosperity.

Sixteen Steps

The number 16 can be traced in human bodies. For instance, the Viśuddha cakra where the soul, as part of God, resides has 16 lotus leaves. Both the upper and the lower jaw of human beings have 16 teeth. Food (sacrifice) must be milled by teeth before it can be consumed. Cheeks are moved both by the powers of Viśuddha and Ājñā (third eye) cakras to mill it. This process is called Svāhā just as in a Homa ceremony. In this connection we see the correlation between the Yajña and the Ājñā. First the food passes the Viśuddha where man is central, the so called Ātmapūjā. Then it goes in Ojas form (essence of food) to the brains where godly energies of Daivic-Śaktis originate. Finally I point out that a normal Pūjā consists of sixteen steps. Every form of worship, sacrificial ceremony and yoga in its original form goes back to God or Purūṣa, as described in the Purūṣa Sūkta or the hymn of God.

Pūjā, a Societal Map

Pūjā consist sixteen steps of holy sacrifice. We can classify the sixteen steps into four divisions. Each division has an essential core that is related with society, human and nature. In each division there is a question of life that is possible to answer with the pūjā system. Our question is: Who am I? Pūjā answers: you are a Ātmā or Soul. Where am I? You are a micro cosmos on earth within the macro cosmos. What is my destiny? Your destiny is to be enlightened. How to reach the goal? You can reach the goal by the path of spirituality. The devotee solicits to become enlightened, a Member of the Cosmic Parliament, a firmament of Super light. Becoming a member means that he or she is getting an Immaterial Master Card. In the business world you also have to go through four stages to get a Master Card, viz. application, screening, solvability and gratifying. This last stage is called in spirituality the Sāyujya (Mukti) or salvation, end of births. We can also divide the four components in life stages (Aśramas). Brahmcārya (celibacy) is the stage full with desires to obtain knowledge and practices. Gṛhastha (marriage, household) is the stage of sharing those desires, knowledge and know-how (diversion). Vānaprastha is reaching the mental state to go back to the source (conversion). The last stage is Sanyāsī, the end of desires and reaching the Zero-point.

Table 5: The First Division

Pūjā steps	Performance	Meaning	Societal Values	Life needs
Āvāhanam	invocation with flowers	to call, invitation	opening and definition of the objectives (SWOT)	appreciation
Āsanam	welcome with rice and flower	to place, to give a seat	location, logistics, definition of the objectives	social status
Pādyam	foot washing	to (show) respect	basics, laws and fundamentals	basic norms
Arghyam	water offer, washing hands	to honour with water	choices of definitions	respect

The first division is comparable with the four stages of an interview, viz., invitation, seat, respectful conversation and a drink. In work, business and organisations, these management values take a main part of the acts, viz. the objectives, logistics and positions, fundamentals and decisions. In the examination of staff qualities and processes of the organisations, every personnel should be aware of the SWOT-analyse: Strengths, Weaknesses, Opportunities and Threats. This analyses makes it is possible to measure the needs in the organisations.

Every human has life needs. The first one is desire for approval and recognition. This desire is a healthy motive, but the desire to be acknowledged is better, stronger or more intelligent. It means when you eat a fruit, think of the man who planted the tree; when you drink water, remember the spring. This is called appreciation of life, nature and human being.

Social status is a part of the social stratification, which is division of a society into a hierarchy of wealth, power, and status. This status is the main first step of civilisation with a cultural unity. This cultural unity is based on norms and values, and principles of family traditions. The fourth principle is respect. In another way of speaking: one should not insult the river god while crossing the river. Respect for humanity, nature and all creatures are very important in this pūjā performance. This is the drive-in of life.

Table 6: The Second Division

Pūjā steps	Performance	Meaning	Societal Values	Life needs
Acamanam	sprinkling water (three times)	threefold purification	development of mind, speech and action	parenthood, master, wisdom
Snānam	ceremonial bathing	cleaning the outer and inner body	life without illness	health and youthful
Vastram	Dressing	colourful life, social expression	cultural, and aimed to the climatic changes	beauty and protection
Yajñopavitam	sacred three threads (Gāyatri)	study, training and progress	science, growth and power distribution	body, mind and spiritual steadiness

These four steps are compared with the first stage of life, celibacy (Brahmcārya), within the four life needs. In the Yogic Science, this stage is called the Yama, the virtues aimed to be a qualified person whose thoughts are non-violent, and Niyama, the standards and norms aimed to be a respectful individual. These four steps of pūjā ought to give a good place in society, in ceremonies, and in managerial fields. This place is called the Sālokya, the place of the demigods; the destiny of the beginning (Sa). Characteristics of this division are to be involved in general society meetings and to participate in decisions.

The second division of pūjā concerns the advancement of the above mentioned stage and growing to a new identity (Sārūpya). The most stable and therefore most healthy pride is based on deserved respect from others, rather than on external forms or celebrity and unjustified praises. When people are making decisions on issues of ethics and rights, it calls for respect for all cultural differences and opposes any kind of cultural change imposed on one society by another. We should know that people derive their individual identity and sense of dignity from their own cultures. People are born to and die in a culture. This ethical stance (or Āsana) reflects the cultural practices as basic human rights. These threefold, viz., identity, dignity and rights are called in the pūjā, Āchamanam or achievement. In the early level of development, children strive to maximise pleasure and avoid punishment, the cleaning process or ceremonial bathing (Snānam). Children at this level consider the needs of others only to the extent that meeting those needs will help the child fulfil his or her own needs. During the next period, which is characterised by conformity to social rules (so called the climatic changes), the child demonstrates respect for and duty to authority. In other words: a human owes respect to the living; to the dead, he only owes truth. The child also seeks to avoid disapproval from that authority. As the child matures, his or her moral judgment is motivated by respect for legally determined rules and an understanding that these rules exist to benefit all (Vastram or social expression). Beginning in adolescence, the child develops the ability to think logically about the future and to understand theoretical concepts. These stages are from cognitive development to stages of moral development.

Table 7: The Third Division

Pūjā steps	Performance	Meaning	Societal Values	Life needs
Gandham	sandal paste, vermilion powder, perfume	cleaning the air, the senses	nobility	cleaning of the environment, good neighbourhood
Puṣpam	flowers, grass (Dūba or sex), raw material mix (seeds)	sacrifice from the heart	fertilization (micro cosmos)	reproduction, descendants
Dhūpam	incense (static fire), wisdom	fragrance	dispelling heavy emotions and evil thoughts	morals, peaceful area
Dīpam	lamp shining (dynamic fire; emotion)	inner purity and peace	tolerance, non-violence	world peace

Futuristical thoughts and these developments are the three threads of pūjā, the Yajñopavitam or the secret threads ceremony expresses the relation between the child and the cosmic Mother Gāyatrī: This is a hyperlink between the micro and macrocosmos, a Śiva-Jīva meditation. We are part of and in a cosmos. This is also the stage of development of mind, speech and action, which is very important in the second stage of life, the Gṛhastha. This stage is also a start of parenting, to develop skills, taking responsibilities of nurturing and teaching a child. The head of the family becomes a leader and is the decision-maker.

In the third division I would say God must be glad, one loves His world so much. In this stage we are talking about cleaning the air and environment (Gandham), fertilisation (Puṣpam), dispelling evil thoughts and a peaceful area (Dhūpam) and world peace (Dīpam): a truly God's world, in which we want a solid relationship with Him (Sāmīpya), based on His desire (Mīp). Virtue begins when a human dedicates himself actively to the job of gratitude. In the philosophy we call this morals or ethics. This is concerned with norms of human conduct, as distinguished from the formal sciences, such as mathematics and logic, and the empirical sciences, such as chemistry and physics. The empirical social sciences, however, including psychology, impinge to some extent on the concerns of ethics in that they study social behaviour. For example, the social sciences frequently attempt to determine the relation of particular ethical principles to social behaviour and to investigate the cultural conditions that contribute to the formation of such principles.

The development of the family moral goes to say that the members in the family are well trained to take decisions. The leader is remoted and the power is distributed in the first echelon. The growth and progress in the field of leading power and management is handed over to other people or members (of the family). This is the beginning of nobility, and well being, characterised by continuing personal growth, a sense of purpose in life, self-acceptance, and positive relations with others (a good neighbourhood). The third stage of a human life is the recluse of domestic life. This is the beginning of the stage of ascetic life. The woman in this stage is clean from menstruation and ready to fully participate in sacred processes. In the study of yoga, man's activities concern moral conduct, learning, tranquillity, self-discipline, breath and mind control on a higher stage. Our biorhythm system is also dependent on light (Dīpam), particularly bright light. Light is the most powerful synchroniser of circadian rhythms (read more in chapter Youth and health). The Veda called this light the inviolable means to reach the beloved station. The brightness of light is an instrument to reset the conditions of our body. This resetting process ends up in a healthy feeling with a bright mind. (YV 1.31: 31). A main part of biorhythm is reproduction. Reproduction is a process whereby all living organisms produce offspring. It is one of the essential functions of plants, animals, and single celled organisms, as necessary for preservation of species as eating is for preservation of the individual.

The Kaṭhopaniṣad (6.18) gives an impression of the Light as follows: "Always dwelling within all beings is the Ātmā, the Purūṣa, the Self, a little flame in the heart. Let one with steadiness withdraw himself from the body even as an inner stem is withdrawn from its sheath. Know this pure immortal light; know in truth this pure immortal light."

Table 8: The fourth division

Pūjā steps	Performance	Meaning	Societal Values	Life needs
Naivedyam	food, fruits	challenge hunger in the world	social care, healthy food supply	nourishment
Tāmbūlam	betel leaf	cleaning of the mouth (Kunda or fire pit)	be fluent in speech and in a language	communication
(Pra)dakṣinām	coin, micro-cosmic circulation, salutation	a godsend, present	charity, donation	wealth
Prārthanā	glory to god, human and all creatures	purifying errors in life, body, mind and brain	greatly honour, forgiveness, One in All, All in One	harmony, humanity

The fourth division is mainly based on the liberation of material objects. We come on the earth as children of God and go back as a manager for the company of the Supreme. As long as we are not completely grown in spirituality, we will wander around within the creation, and will never find the way to God (Sāyujya). Yuja is the pipeline or light tunnel. Capable management and action in the process of dissolving (body) and resolving of the soul in the Super Soul can lead to liberation where you're stable in the God's world. The process has been described in yoga as Samyama.

In the hierarchy structure the leader in the past becomes an icon in this stage. Symbolically, he takes decisions, which means that these pass through the organisations or the family, and are accepted in society. It happens in the name of the 'lord'.

In this fourth division, food (Naivedyam) and communication (mouth cleaning or Tambūlam) are very important. Human beings require food to grow, reproduce, and maintain good health. Without food, our bodies could not stay warm, build or repair tissue, or maintain a heartbeat. Eating the right foods can help us avoid certain diseases or recover faster when illness occurs. The second, communication is the process of sharing ideas, information, and messages with others in a particular time and place. Communication includes writing and talking, as well as nonverbal communication (such as facial expressions, body language, or gestures), visual communication (the use of images or pictures, such as painting, photography, video, or film), and electronic communication (telephone calls, electronic mail, cable television, or satellite broadcasts). Communication is a vital part of personal life and is also important in business, education, and any other situation where people encounter each other. In short, food and communications are growth and understanding the Spiritual Being.

The two other needs in life are wealth and harmony. Wealth has an economic value, which has several characteristics. First, an object must have utility. It must have, or be suspected of having, the capacity to satisfy some human desire. Discovering uses for things previously not regarded as useful can increase wealth. Second, economic goods must be in scarce supply. Finally, an object must have measurable economic value.

Because the only common unit of value today is money, the worth of goods must be expressible in monetary terms. Some economists also regard a definite skill in performing a job as human wealth; as such skill has a determinable market value. Wealth in the shape of coins circulates everywhere. This teaches us to donate because money doesn't stay forever with someone. A gift should be seen as a godsend or greatly honoured. Harmony is the right and desirable relationship of parts to a whole, whether in nature, society, or an individual. Just like music that produces a kind of pleasure which human nature cannot do without. Harmony can be compared with the origin of the leisure society, which is dreaming of living like a master. One of those masters is the Dalai Lama, who has developed his philosophy of peace from a great reverence for all things living and upon the concept of universal responsibility embracing all mankind as well as nature. The Hindu quotes the growth, understanding, wealth and harmony as All in One and One in All.

A Normal or High Society

The quotient of qualities is growth and knowledge (skills) that we need to survive primarily. The next table shows the Qualities Quotients (QQ). Once we are educated, we have to join the society to contribute and change the quality. The more we learn to manage the more responsibilities we are given. Thereafter we become a captain in the world society. We can find the mirror of our world in the world of the gods and goddesses. They too have managers who provide daily services. Clever people and learned have changed to continue their business in the metaphysical world. This world is open for new blood and ideas, captains of industry.

In every phase of life we deal with a lot of mental threats which a human has to conquer by training and disciplines, non-attachment and purification. These four components are also the chariots to reach liberation. Without training and discipline true freedom cannot survive. There are people who strictly deprive themselves of all things eatable, drinkable, and smokable, which have in any way acquired a shady reputation. They pay this price for health. And health is all they get for it.

Learning is good in and of itself. It is just like pouring honey on a book, so people would know that learning is sweet. So they can go forth into society with well-developed bodies, fairly developed minds, and beloved hearts. We know that smooth seas don't make a skilful sailor that's why we strive to train them to be useful for society and for the glory of our humankind. God helps those who train themselves. The best way to really train people is with an experienced mentor. Mentoring requires special skills, but it does not require hierarchical position. An uncontrolled person is a danger in society, for his own and other people's life. In this situation, future life ends up in crises and the person becomes an obstacle in society. The proper function of man is to live, not to exist. You should not waste your days in trying to prolong them but use your time better. The table below is like a united exertion weave: societal mosaic.

Table 9: Qualities Quotient (QQ)

Life phase (4) (Aśrama)	**Stages of life (4)**	**Strengths of life (4)Puruṣārthas)**	**Kinds of duty in life (4)**
Brahmcārya	celibacy	duty, work (Dharma)	employer, professional cleaners, servants
Gṛhastha	household	wealth, money (Artha)	businessman, cultivator, farmer, inventor, artist
Vānaprastha	recluse-life	attraction, sex (Kāma)	ruler, construction-workers, army
Sanyāsa	renunciation	liberation, freedom (Mokṣa)	teacher, priest, academic, policy makers
Levels of training (5) (Abhyāsa)	**Disciplines (5) (Yoga Sādhana)**	**Steps of management (5)**	**Measurements quality (5)**
Yama	good virtues of life	planning	shared values
Niyama	standards, norms	expertise	skills
Āsana	physical postures	staff training	staff
Prāṇāyāma	breath control	control	strategy
Pratyāhara	withdraw of the senses	responsibilities	structure

Stages of non-attachment (3) (Vairāgya)	Degrees of disciplines (3) (Samyama)	Technical disciplines (3)	Measurements grades (3)
Dhāraṇā	concentration	technology	systems
Dhyāna	meditation	direction	style (steadiness)
Samādhi	contemplation	efficiency	science
Steps in purification (4) (Mokṣa)	**Liberations (4)**	**Economic principles (4)**	**Stages of womanhood (4)**
Sālokya	holy region	place	Hastini (elephant)
Sārūpya	physic equality	Price	Śankhini (conch shell)
Sāmīpya	desire resemble	product	Kṣatrini (sword-release)
Sāyujya	cosmic united	promotion	Padmini (lotus-flower)

The table above gives an idea of the structure of our society and our future. We refer to the below mentioned hymns which explain the essentials, correlated with the elements in the table.

"We worship you for pleasant fields, for good roads, and for riches: may our sin be repented off" (RV 1.97.2). In this hymn, there is a matter of working areas in society (the fields), duties and responsibilities (repentance), management tasks and disciplines (good roads).

"Wide fields, vast treasure, (spacious) pastures has the much-knowing (Indra) bestowed upon his friends: the radiant Indra with the leaders (of rites, the Maruts) generated the sun, the dawn, the earth, and fire" (RV 3.31.15). This hymn sums up all the aspects of the phases of life and methods of training and exercise. Expressed as wide fields (duties in life), vast treasure (strengths of life), spacious pastures (degrees), radiant (technical), leaders (managers), sun (measurement), dawn (womanhood), earth (economics) and fire (liberation). If we are to live our lives in peace and harmony, and if we are to achieve our ambitions of improving the conditions under which we live, we must have both freedom and discipline. For freedom without discipline is anarchy; discipline without freedom is tyranny.

"The greatness of the strength of the many-worshipped Puṣaṇa is universally lauded; no one detracts (from his praise); his praise displeases no one. Desirous of happiness, I adore him, whose protection is ever nearly; who is the source of felicity; who, when devoutly worshipped, blends with the thoughts of all (his worshippers): who, (thought) a deity, is united with the sacrifice" (RV 1.138.1). We find here an impression of the strength of life, the Puruṣarthas. There is no detraction in work and duty (Dharma), desires and happiness are adored (Artha), the source of felicity is passionate (Kāma) and unification (Mokṣa), is a fact. Moral, like physical, cleanliness is not acquired once and for all: it can only be kept and renewed by a habit of constant watchfulness and discipline.

"Aśvins, causing the barley to be sown (in the fields that had been prepared) by the plough; milking (the clouds) for the sake of Manu; destroying the Dasyu with the thunderbolt; you have bestowed brilliant light upon the Ārya" (RV 1.117.21). The twins Aśvins in societal meaning is reward and punishment, and production and profit. In all four duties of life we experience this. The hymn qualifies the employer (to be sown), the businessman (milked clouds), the farmer (plough), the soldier (destroyer) and the policy (law) maker (Ārya), the managers. All of them must continuously discipline themselves to remember how it felt the first moment.

"Through fear of you, Indra, all the regions of the firmament cause the unfallen (rain) to descend: the heavens, the earth, the mountains, the forests, all the solid (universe) is alarmed at your approach" (RV 6.31.2). The manager is a full-time professional (Indra) whose decision is of overriding importance for the whole organisation and branches (regions). Descending the rain means that all the employers are doing their jobs with the fear or precaution that of making mistakes. Management concerns all the three principles of the technical development (heavens), the astral or internet technology, the five steps of management (earth), the three grades of measurements (mountains), and the five qualities of measurement (forests). The only safeguard of order and discipline in the modern world is a standardised worker with interchangeable parts. That would solve the entire problem of management.

"Those provident and intelligent sisters, (the rays of light), conceived of the same womb, (ever) united (with each other), and dwelling in the same abode, metre out (all things): knowing (their functions), and bright shining, they spread in ever new (directions) throughout the radiant firmament" (RV 1.159.4). This hymn denotes the sisterhood in the behaviour of women. There are four very important elements in the development of a woman, viz., beauty, battle, beat, and body (the four B's). Padmini (beauty) means bright sight and intelligence, Kṣatrini (battle) is calculated (metrics) in all sectors, Śankhini (beat or rhythm) means spread in new directions like sound waves from a conch shell, Hastini (body) means knowing the functions in which she is operating. These are skills for the present life and the knowing of things in advance for lives in the future. Though, motherhood is the most important of all the professions, requiring more knowledge than any other department in human affairs.

Pūjā, A Micro Yajña (Seven Days Happening)

The principle in the whole creation is eating and to let eat. Academics say: "the survival of the fittest." The whole life and beyond is a big ritual of eating, born; eating, let eating and born again; a cycle of birth and rebirth with different names and places. In cosmic science creation and dissolution are day and night of the Creator, in which the digit ten is the key. In daily life and in education we express ten, as associated with the highest. We find this in the Rīg Vedā as "Purūṣa who has a thousand heads, a thousand eyes, a thousand feet, investing the earth in all directions, exceeds it by a space measuring ten fingers." This hymn is decoding the cosmic secret. Number 1 stands for the bearer and the 0 is the womb. Born as a zero and become a hero. We find this number in the Śrīmad Bhagavatam too. He is transcendental, eternally existing in a form not exceeding nine inches. The sun illuminates both internally and externally by expanding its radiation; similarly, the Lord by expanding His universal form, maintains everything in creation both internally and externally.' In the physic science neither the sun nor the moon, are planets. Continuing about the theory of the digits we find the image of number 1 in Sanskrit as the position of the delivery. In the pose of perfection, number 9, we find this nature again. Modern science mentions that at the time of delivery the dilation has to be 10 cm. As mentioned before every new life needs ten aspects only for a new body (five gross elements and five pranas). The ancestor ceremony (Pitra pūjā) is a part of holy sacrifice in our life and continued by the family after death. We find the importance of the ancestor ceremony, in a number of the hymns of the Vedas. Learned people denote that 75percent of the Vedas consist hymns for the period after death. After death the soul remains between the moon and the sun, benefits depend on the results of the karma. This is the Bhuva area in the cosmos, an astral world. This area is the sojourn of the Pitris and pretas (deceased ancestors). The preta-loka is a separate part in the ancestor world without surplus of annual ancestor ceremony. The closer you get to the sun the higher is the karma. This shows that our soul is related with the planets in the cosmos. Before starting a pūjā or yajña ceremony we establish a holy area for the ceremony. Therefore we call energy from those who are protecting the creation and the creatures. This is also known as the Dikpālakas or the secret compass.

We pay respect to the eight guarding or deities. These are Indra (Lord of the Heaven) guardians of the east, Agni, the fire god of the southeast, Yama of the south, Nirati of the southwest, Varuṇa of the west, Vāyu of the northwest, Kubera of the north and Śiva of the northeast. In the midst is the finite centre of consciousness, the Jīva or the Individual Soul.

Mirror-Image of Heaven

The Rīg Vedā, edited by Dr. Ravi Prakash Arya, discloses the journey of life as follow: "Three are the spheres; two are in the proximity of Savitar, one leads men to the dwelling of Yama. The immortal (luminaries) or Amṛta (water) depend upon Savitar as a car upon the pin of the axle; let him who knows (the greatness of Savitar) declare it. The spheres or lokas which lie in the immediate path of the sun are said to be heaven and earth; the intermediate loka, Antarikṣa, or firmament, is described as the road to the realm of Yama, the ruler of the dead, by which the pretah, or ghosts, travel. Why this should not be considered equally the course of the sun, is not very obvious" (RV 1.35.6). In the air and light of the sun remains the Soma and is called Savitar, the male form of the Sun. The Soma also obtained from the Sindhu, the ocean (RV 4.54.6). Air, light and water are the most important elements of life. Without these there is no existence, that's why it is said to drink this Soma thrice a day. These threefold existencials are bonded with our health and well being (RV 4.55.3). In ecological meaning we should protect our nature and make this earth the abode of happiness (SV 1216).

Another part of happiness is the existence of delighted sounds or a self-contained composition. The term Arka, one of the names of the Sun, means song of praise, hymn, singer and splendour. All are related to different kinds of waves, tunes, sounds and voices of nature (SV 1205, 1206). Without air there is no movement of vibrations. This also means the conversion of thought into action, ideas into events, and meditation into movement. These waves or tunes change into sounds, which go forth like a sharpened arrow (RV 10.50.1-5). The tunes and waves are also related with Savitar (he who inspires), generator deity of the gods. He works in close conjunction with the other Vedic gods, such as the god of water, Varuṇa, and the god of thunder, Indra, as the source of all movement. Savitar grants immortality and worshipers pray to him for the forgiveness of sins. As an arrow has to strike its goal, in the same way a wise person uses his voice or wisdom (SV 1224) at the right time and place. Light travels like an arrow and time like a shuttle, and there is no water without waves. Nathaniel Hawthorne (1804-1864) writes in his play The Scarlet Letter, The Custom House "Human nature will not flourish, any more than a potato, if it be planted and replanted, for too long a series of generations, in the same worn-out soil. What he meant, is that human being should use his knowledge better, with strategy, and to enjoy his own growth in this life. The Greek philosopher, Aristotle (384 BC - 322 BC) adds this growth in life by saying "the soul is characterised by these capacities: self-nutrition, sensation, thinkings, and movement."

Standards of the Leader

Does capital punishment tend to the security of people? By no means. It hardens the hearts of men, and makes the loss of life appear light to them; and it renders life insecure, inasmuch as the law holds out that property is of greater value than life. A life is not important except in the impact it has on other lives. That's why people need principles or standards (qualities) considered worthwhile and desirable. Ideas and theories must be tested in practice, by assessing whether acting upon the idea or theory produces desirable or undesirable results. According to that, all must be tested with correlations to truth, knowledge, and morality.

The death ceremony is the sixteenth or last sacrament in human life (death). In this ceremony there is a water ritual, Amrita, for the travel of the immortal soul. According to the qualities in relation between God and man, and as mentioned before, we have several items in life with sixteen faculties on the way to perfection. Therefore it is important to perform simple daily sacrifices for the benefit of life after life. Each delivery is a New World for a soul. In the fontanel chakra ten is the leader. We must follow the Leader or Energy. In the process of liberation we have to increase the ten into one thousand, the merge that sounds as the meeting point in mahā samādhī, the platform for Śiva-Śakti at the top of the Sahasrāra Cakra. The hymn of the Rīg Vedā announces this as "Purūṣa, who has a thousand heads, a thousand eyes, a thousand feet, investing the earth in all directions, exceeds (it by a space) measuring ten fingers".

According to this principle this digit is the symbol for the beginning and for the end of life or creation. As soon as we increase our inner quality of energy to enter the zero (0-point) we change our density and are able to leave the body.

The soul or energy is as constant as sound, varying in density. The secret for liberation is to achieve zero-violence in the mind and in our actions, the zero-point. This whole world is bound by actions, except for those actions, which are performed for the sake of sacrifice unto the Lord. Since one has to work even for the simple maintenance of the body, the prescribed duties for a particular social position and quality are so made that that purpose can be fulfilled. Other kind of work done in this material world will be a cause of bondage. For both, good and evil work has their reactions, and any reaction binds the performer (BhG. 3.9, Nothing should be performed for sense gratification. Perform duties and actions without attachment for the purpose of sacrifice. This is the great art of doing work, and in the beginning this process requires expert guidance. This practice will not only save one from the reaction of work, but also gradually elevate one to transcendental loving service of God. This sacrificial performance is called Yajña.

Pūjā and Yajña

Customs and rituals are a part of all cultures. All cultures and religions teach that rituals are very important in devotion to God. The Hindu pūjā ceremony is unique in its form and difficult for a lot of people to discover the secret benefits of this process of evolution in man and society. Yoga is transparent to any person, as a physically formula for heath and youth, as well as for the development for spirituality. Even the fire God, Agni, has his customs or descendants in several forms. Yajur Veda formulates the birth of Agni: "Sovereign of men, Agni, you are born for the days (of sacrifice), pure and all irradiating, from the waters, from the stones, from trees, and from plants" (YV 11.27). The term Susuksani in Sanskrit signifies drying up, causing the evaporation of the earths moisture, or it may also mean destruction or consumption. Agni is produced from the waters, either as the lightning that accompanies rain or submarine fire; from stones by striking them together; or from trees or wood by attrition; from plants, such as bamboo, by mutual friction, causing the conflagration of a forest. These enumerations show to be for the most part personification of light, of luminous bodies, of divisions of time, of celestial phenomena, and fires adapted to peculiar occasions, as the full and changing moon, or to particular rites, or sacrifices with food, funeral fires, expiatory fires, and so forth. The Rīg Vedā (1.1) determines that Yajña makes an essential part of our life. The first mantra starts with the glory to Agni or fire (Agnimīle), the high priest (Purohitam) of sacrifice (Yajña), the divine (Devam), the ministering priest (Ritvija), who presents the oblation (to the gods) (Hotāram), and is the possessor of great wealth (Ratnadhātamam).

P̃ūjā and Science

In this scientific day and age when one doesn't take anything for granted, customs and rituals come under special research. Our ancestors have given us the gift of the rules of community worship in a temple for the welfare of people of the community as a whole and prosperity of the world. They were indeed wise and that these once seemingly meaningless and insignificant customs and rituals are full of meaning and help give us our very identity. They have given us the rules of prayers at home as essential for the welfare of the individuals and their family. The Rīg Vedā mentions the ancestors as follows "the people adore you, Agni, the protector of the people in their dwellings: they propitiate you as a benevolent sovereign: leader of a radiant host, you are lord over all offerings: you are the distributor of tens, and hundreds, and thousands (of good things) (RV 2.1.8). The basic and essential principle behind the prayer is the total surrender to God who fills the universe by His glory and is present everywhere and that without His command even an atom will not move.

Pūjā has anthropological and social significances too. Tracing back the history of the development of the techniques of Pūjā, we see a period, when the two powerful images in the whole poetic structure evolve: the images of the Sādhaka and the Sādhya. Sādhya, the Brāhmaṇa is represented as a royal guest and Sādhaka as a respectful host. The deity is welcomed with kingly respect, while coming with pomp and glory and with royal decorations on him and with a trail of attendants. He is entertained as a royal guest with feast, song and dance. While treating the Brāhmaṇa as a king, society was considering king as somewhat equal to Brahmā, which was then a social necessity. He was a guest, could be invited, and intimate relations with him could be built. The king was lovable; he was one who would protect the subjects. The kingship was, in short, not cut away from the people.

The technique of Pūjā evolved and was perfected through the centuries as part of the Tantra, Yoga and Vedānta philosophy. According to Vedānta, man is charged with a spark of the universal soul, Brahmā, which is omniscient, omnipresent and omnipotent. The ultimate purpose of human life is to realise the identity of his Self or Ātmā with the universal soul (macro-soul) from where Ātmā comes and get absorbed into it.

Fertilisation

The basic symbols of Pūjā go still farther back in human history. Carefully looking at the whole system, one could find a series of fertility symbols in it. The concept of deity as the union of Yoni (vagina) and Liṅgam (phallus), which probably goes back to the Indus Valley Civilisation, is a typical fertility symbol. Again, the pedestal is conceived as a lotus flower (the flower is surely to fertilize). To further this concept, there is Abhiṣekam, pouring consecrated water on the idol in the beginning. This is nothing but bringing about the symbolic Amrīta Varṇam, showers of nectar on to the pedestal, the earth or Prakṛti. The materials of Pūjā-Jalam (sacred water), Gandham (sandal paste), Puśpam (flowers), Dhūpam (fragrant fumes) and Dīpam (the lighted lamp)-all represent fertility and abundance. By performing Pūjā, just like by performing a Yajña, despite the fact that the Pūjā does not ask for it, rains would be showered on to the fields, seeds would germinate, there would be plenty on earth. This concept of Śiva and Śakti is further made clearer in the Veda as a union of father and mother who foster the whole world. The Bhagavad Gītā (3.14) denotes that "living entities have evolved from food; food depends on rainfall. Rainfall occurs from the sacrifice (Yajña) unto the supreme Lord. This sacrifice is based on performing actions (Karma) as per Vedic writings."

Cosmic United

The Lord, the life in us, pervades all living beings, be they plants or animals. Hence, they are all regarded as sacred. Human life on earth depends on plants and animals. They give us the vital factors that make life possible on earth: food, oxygen, clothing, shelter, medicines, etc. They lend beauty to our surroundings. They serve man without expectation and sacrifice themselves to sustain us. They epitomise sacrifice. If a stone is thrown on a fruit-laden tree, the tree in turn gives fruit. In fact, the flora and fauna owned the earth before man appeared on it. Presently, the world is seriously threatened by the destruction of forest lands and the extinction of many species of vegetation due to man's callous attitude towards them. We protect only what we value. Hence, in Hinduism, we are taught to regard trees and plants as sacred. Naturally, we will then protect them. That's why the Rīg Vedā explains that nature is protected by different powers with different names."There is one God and the sages give him different names, viz., Indra, Mitra, Varuṇa, Agni, the divine winged Garuḍa, Agni, Yama and Mātariśāvan (the wind)" (RV 1.164.46). "God is one; He created heaven and earth. His eyes are everywhere; His mouth is in all directions. His arms and feet are every where. He pervades the whole universe by his stretched arms and wings" (RV 10.81.3).

Human and God

In the first creation of this earth the process of Ardha showed the merge of Śiva and Śakti. Ardha is the ultimate reality conceived as the divine unity of Śakti (the divine feminine) and Śiva (the divine masculine). Śiva-Śakti is One, All and God. This merging process happens in human being. We call this process of render (the female gamete) capable of development by uniting it with the male gamete: the fertilisation process or Garbha, instead of Hiraṇyāgarbha. The energy mix of this process animates as its vital soul or divine principle. Thus we are a link in the forth-going process from heaven and are gods on earth in microform. So, humans are truly gods. The goal of life is to increase the density of our soul by our status from a micro in a macro cosmos (Bṛhatātmā). This means to grow and to unit with Brahmā or God and to achieve the ultimate reality.

The Oblation

The highest chain in the hierarchy needs explanation in short terms. In the same manner we offer a lot of food to the gods and they achieve just a few drops as essence of the devotional sacrifice. Compared in the line of violence to non-violence, we speak here of the way around. As mentioned before, the carnivore needs a hundred kilo food for one kilo essence. The oblation is comparable with the butter of the milk, which is left after hours of cooking (ceremony) (RV 1.96.1). We find this proportion as soon as we try to find the deeper essence of a product, viz., the Ghī of the butter, or the honey of the flowers. Colour doesn't make any difference. Honey or Madhu has only one colour among all flowers. God is only interested in the essence of the essence. "Who-so-ever learns the holy verses of the Vedas, which contain the essence of the learning of the sages. The Goddess of learning (i.e. Sarasvatī) confers upon them milk, clarified butter, honey and Soma juice" (RV 9.67.32). In meditation, spirituality becomes ripe as soon we can find the essence of wisdom. This is honey or love. Enjoying spirituality is enjoying life and the search of our final destination.

Worship

Pūjā is the core of worshipping God and an aspect of Karma Yoga. Its purpose, in essence, is to propitiate the eternal and boundless God in any of its manifestations. The act is performed by giving a general royal reception through various oblations and offerings (clothes, decorations, feast etc.), accompanied by chanting of hymns or mantras. The sacrifice which is extended on every side by the threads (of created things) spread out by the worship of the gods for a hundred and one (years), these our progenitors, who have preceded us, weave it, weaving forwards, weaving backwards-by combining the superior and inferior weaving, that is, the intellectual and un-intellectual, the enjoyer and the enjoyable, animate and inanimate existence. They worship (Prajāpati) when (the world) is woven.

This first man spreads out this (web), the first man rolls it up, he spread it above in this heaven; his rays have sat down on the seat (of sacrifice), they have made the prayers serve as shuttles for weaving (RV 10.130.1-2). When Prajāpati Brahmā created mankind, he said: "May you evolve by the performance of the sacrifice, and may this yield all that is desirable to you" (Bh.G. 3.10). This performance is a ritual in which a consecrated offering is made to a god or other spiritual being in order to establish, perpetuate, or restore a sacred bond between humanity and the divine. The Atharva Veda gives a comparison with the sacred bond between husband and wife. "Then let thy soul and mind be knit together. Embrace thy consort as her loving husband" (AV 18.1.3: 4241). This bond is also comparable with the relationship between Viṣṇu and Lakṣmī: "Lakṣmī, the spouse of Viṣṇu, is eternal and imperishable. In the manner as He is all pervading and omnipresent, so also is She. Viṣṇu is meaning, She is speech; He is policy, She prudence; He is understanding, She is the intellect; He is the dharma, She is good action. He, is the creator, she is the creation. Lakṣmī is the earth. Viṣṇu is the support of extended space. Viṣṇu is the sun, the lotus-seated goddess its radiance. Lakṣmī is prosperity, Viṣṇu the lord of riches. Lakṣmī is the light, Viṣṇu the lamp. She is the night, He is the day. He is the standard, She is the banner. He is One with all that is male, She with all that is female."

Another method of worship is to reach a spontaneous devotional service as a naturally developed aspect in a person. The nine processes of worship as pure devotional service are: Hearing and chanting about the transcendental holy name, form, qualities, personal belongings and pastimes of the Lord, remembering them, serving the lotus feet of the Lord, offering the Lord respectful worship with sixteen types of His personal belongings, offering prayers to the Lord, becoming His servant, considering the Lord one's best friend, and surrendering everything unto Him (in other words, serving Him with body, mind and words) (Bh.T. 7.5.23-24).

Mental Worship

Purification is a product of pūjā and or meditation. The general oblation is a ritual act in which a consecrated offering is made to a god or other spiritual being in order to establish, perpetuate, or restore a sacred bond between humanity and the divine. The seers perform their sacrifices with oblations in the form of sacred songs and divine mantras. Worship regulates the processes of the subtle body. Everything within this cosmic manifestation is under the control of the Lord. To be enlightened by this perfect knowledge, one should always engage himself in the devotional service of the Lord to return to Siddhaloka or the Ultimate Source (Bh.T. 4.1.80). This is the first oblation or mental worship (RV 4.42.6), also the Adhyātmika form of prayer. This form can not be measured just like wisdom, the so-called son of a matchless man (RV 10.10.13). A matchless is also someone who is prepared to sacrifice his own life for his convictions. The seer merges his prayer in all his efforts and interests, families, states, or organisations. He is skilled in worship, has a firm mind and is pure among mankind (RV 7.3.1-3). A skilled person consists of a human body and a human mind causally interacting with one another. He knows that the intentions of a human being may cause that person's limbs to move. In this way, the mind can also affect the body. In addition, the sense organs of a human being may be affected by light, pressure, or sound, external sources, which in turn affect the brain further affecting mental states. This interaction of mind and body is peculiarly intimate. Unlike the interaction between a pilot and his ship, the connection between mind and body more closely resembles two substances that have been thoroughly mixed together. A businessman would say that the final technique for coming up with new business ideas is to maximise one's strategic degrees of mind freedom. To break out of a market-share stalemate, the strategic thinker must sometimes have the courage to burst these restrictions. The essential nature of individuality lies in the universal element of mind. The force of mind is only as great as its expression; its depth only as deep as its power to expand and lose itself. Looked from the side of universal mind with general spiritual substance, culture means nothing but that this substance gives itself its own self-consciousness, brings about its own inherent process and its own reflection into self.

Astral Sacrifice

The second form is brought into relation with priests, fires, the holy flame and basic characteristics of the sacrifice. This is the fire prayer in the shape of Agni, the Adhidaivika or astral sacrifice (SV 1219). Philosophers use the characteristics of inward obtainable, internal reality, representation in the mind, goal-directedness, creativity and freedom, and consciousness to distinguish mental sacrifice from the physical. Religions, which condemn the pleasures of sense, drive men to seek the pleasures of sacrificial power. Power is the grim idol that the world adores and that can lead someone into destruction. The Spanish novelist and playwright, Benito Pirez Galdus (1843-1920) said in his play Doña Perfecta "Fine pictures, fine statues, beautiful music; pleasure for the senses, and let the devil take the soul!"

The power or fire of destruction dazzles the senses, haunts the imagination, confounds the understanding, and tames the will, by the vastness of its pretensions, and the very hopelessness of resistance. The sacrificial power is comparable with the firepower of the ascetic. An ascetic keeps the fire burning by moral conduct, learning, tranquillity, self-discipline, and mind control. Fire is the great purifier. It purifies the dust and dirt of passions, such as greed, hate, delusion, impatience, anger, self-intoxication and conceit. The British philosopher, Bertrand Russell (1872-1970) indicates that 'pleasure, feeling of happiness, delight, or satisfaction, are only the gratifications of the senses'. This refers to people without sacrificial powers.

Fire as divine power is also compared with the kings on earth. They are justly called Gods, because they exercise a manner or resemblance of divine power upon earth. "O God, may we cross un-surmountable poverty by acquiring cows. May we win our hunger by possessing food-grains like barley. May we obtain wealth from the kings and attain success with our efforts" (RV 10.42.10). For, if you will consider the attributes to God, you'll see how they agree in person of a king. "The ocean is the lord of the rivers. Fire is the lord of the earth. Moon is the lord of the stars. May you excel all in the world" (AV 6.86.2). God has the power to create, to destroy, to make or unmake at his pleasure, to give life or send death, to judge all, and to be neither judged nor accountable to none. To raise low things, and to make high things low at his pleasure and to God are both soul and body due. And the same powers have Kings. "I, the destroyer of the enemies, have become victorious in the world, so that I may gain sovereignty over the masses. Excel All in the world" (RV 10.174.5). They make and unmake their subjects: they have power of rising, and casting down: of life and of death: judges over all their subjects, and in all causes, and yet accountable to none but God only. They have power to exalt low things, and abase high things, and make of their subjects like men at the chess. And to the king is due both the affection of the soul, and the service of the body of his subjects.

Nature Sacrifice

The third form is using the ingredients of nature, bearing the forces of the climates, co-operating for specific purposes and giving consumption provisions. This oblation is called nature sacrifice, the Adhibhautika form of prayer (RV 10.90.6). In general, a climate is the long-term effect of the sun's radiation on the rotating earth's varied surface and atmosphere. It can be understood most easily in terms of annual or seasonal averages of temperature and precipitation. It refers to the inclination of the sun. Besides the effects of solar radiation and its variations, however, climate is also influenced by the complex structure and composition of the atmosphere and by the ways in which it and the ocean transport heat.

Thus, for any given area on earth, not only the latitude (the sun's inclination) must be considered but also the elevation, terrain, distance from the ocean, relation to mountain systems and lakes, and other such influences. Another consideration is scale: A macroclimate refers to a broad region, a meso-climate to a small district, and a microclimate to a minute area. A microclimate, for example, can be specified that is good for growing plants underneath large shade trees. Climate has profound effects on vegetation and animal life, including humans. It plays statistically significant roles in many physiological processes, from conception and growth to health and disease.

The aim of three sorts of oblation is rising the mental force upward (to heaven) and firming the physically force like a newly born bull (SV 1221). Perhaps the most important characteristic of mental phenomena (such as sensation, emotion, imagination, etc.) is that they are inwardly accessible or available to us through introspection. We each know our own minds-our sensation, thoughts, memories, desires, and fantasies-in a direct sense, by internal reflection. Another important characteristic of mind, especially of human minds, is the capacity for choice and imagination. Rather than automatically converting past influences into future actions, individual minds are capable of exhibiting creativity and freedom. In the daily practice of prayer the morning starts with a fit body and a bright mind (bread and butter), onward to working energy and an organised mind in midday (full oily), and ends in midnight with a balanced, harmonised (oblation) and peaceful mind (YV 3114). This should be the rhythm of life because the mind can be driven from all other sources of pride or pleasure. It can fall in love with misery, and grows enamoured of oppression. It gazes after liberty, happiness, comfort, knowledge, which have been torn from it by the unfeeling gripe of wealth and power.

Pūjā and Singing

During the course of a Pūjā, it is customary to chant Mantras, sing Bhajans and make offerings of fruits, flowers and incense to God. Mantras are sacred verses that praise God and seek his blessings. In the more traditional Pūjās, the priest performing it recites the Mantras. A Bhajan is a devotional hymn that is sung by all attendees and may have musical accompaniment. Both Mantras and Bhajans have intense meaning and have a greater effect on those that understand them but it also has a soothing and peaceful effect on those that don't. A Pūjā ends with the Ārati in which fire or incense is moved in a circular motion before God. After the Ārati, all the attendees of the Pūjā partake of the blessings by feeling the warmth of the fire. Hinduism is extremely scientific when it comes to the performing of rituals. Astrologers are consulted before performing rituals and they provide us with the right day and time of day to perform a ritual.

One could go on ad infinitum about all Pūjā rituals and customs but the most important thing to know is their significance. One cannot know of all the rituals and customs that exist but if an effort is made to learn about as many of them as is possible and also to learn of their significance, the quality of one's life as a whole improves and it takes us one step closer to salvation. Performing and knowing about rituals causes us to improve as human beings and most important of all makes us help others do the same. If we know what a certain ritual or custom signifies, then we can help others understand it and prevent them from assuming it to be meaningless and boring. This cycle will surely carry on because learning is contagious and it will pass from one person to another. In conclusion, it is important for us to know about our rituals and customs for they were meant to help us lead a fulfilling and meaningful life. Performing our rituals and customs and speaking our language are probably the only ways by which we can remember our roots.

Small Pūjā Performances

The Lord is the owner of the entire creation. He is therefore the true owner of the house we live in too. Because everything and everybody in this cosmos is a unique identity we need variations, also in the field of daily practices. Nature copies nothing, the reason that we find several entities of Energy, called god. Once a superpower or "god" is produced through the secret power of Pūjā or meditation, the identity remains latent in the cosmos. We can recall this source as god to increase our cosmic power. These entities disappear by dissolving creation. That's why we have 'gods', parts of the One. For example, when you make a clone, you cannot destroy this entity when life is in process. The cloning process is from the beginning of the green stick grasshopper in Malaysia. Once the copy is made she carries it on the back. Everybody has an own identity (thumb), own desires perception and requirements. The Hindu way accesses the facilities with a lot of energy form in stock. Everybody can find an idol that brings us to the primal source. We give, an idea of icons for worship, the choice is yours! The smallest pūjā of a couple of seconds can be performed by greeting the morning Sun. Praying can be done in the car while stepping inside or when you are in a traffic jam. The most effective and easiest is the name of Lord Rāma, Hé Rāma orOṃŚrī Rāmāya Namāh. You can use this word everywhere, in any position, in any working place as a daily mantra. Even in a toilet, or waiting at a bus stop, etc., because this name is par excellence: Rāma se baṛā Rāma ka nāma!

A mantra is a merge of faculties of energies; a word is a combination of characters. As we can see, every mantra is charging our battery or power for the inner self. You are on the road, so you need 'petrol'. It doesn't matter which entity you like, please recall the right person on the right time and on the right place. Don't call the fire God for the job of a fireman!

We give other mantras that can be used in life:

Om Śrīmad Mahā Gaṇādi Pataye Namaḥ.

The mantra of elephant headed God (Gaṇeṣa). Gaṇeṣa opens the door of devotion, as the door of a house. He is like the key of your own home. Open the door first! The mantra removes obstacles and is the bestowal of success.

Om Namo Bhagavate Vāsudevāya

This is the mantra of Lord Viṣṇu. Lord Viṣṇu, who sustains life in the world. Enchanting this mantra saves a devotee from many troubles. It bestows the devotee with prosperity, peace, wealth etc.

Om Śrī Mahā Lakṣmyai Namaḥ

The mantra of Goddess Lakṣmī, goddess of all wealth and prosperity in the world.

Om Namaḥ Śivāya

It is the mantra of Lord Śiva. Many people have become rich from virtually state of starvation by enchanting this mantra. Lord Śiva (Bhole Śankara) is very innocent (Bhole) and bestows his blessings immediately on the devotee.

We explain this mantra etymological as follows:

Om Namaḥ Śivaya: (Sanskrit) "Adoration (or homage) to Śiva". The supreme mantra of Saivism, known as the Pañcākṣara or five syllables.Oṃis the Big Bang. Na is the Lord's veiling grace; Ma is the world; Śi is Śiva; Va is His revealing grace; Ya is the soul. The letters also represent the physical body: Na the legs, Ma the stomach, Śi the shoulders, Va the mouth and Ya the eyes.

Oṃ Śrī Rāmāya Namaḥ

The description of word "Rāma" is unlimited. Lord Rāma is the incarnation of Viṣṇu. Ra stands for knowledge and Mā for Purūṣa or God. The meaning is Science of God. Upside down is Marā, which means go to God or death A devotee can gain overall benefits in all fields of his or her life by enchanting this mantra.

Oṃ Śrī Kṛṣṇāya Namaḥ

This is the mantra of Lord Kṛṣṇa, the incarnation of Lord Viṣṇu. It solves all the problems of a devotee and bestows him with wealth and prosperity.

Oṃ Aiṁ Hriṁ Kliṁ Cāmuṇḍāye Vicaye Namaḥ (Śakti Durgā). This mantra is of Goddess Durgā the combined form of the powers of Lakṣmī, Sarasvatī and Kālī. By enchanting this mantra all the physical, mental, economic problems are solved. Mother protects and blesses with all comforts.

The smallest Gāyatrī mantra:

Oṃ Bhūr Bhuvah Svah

Tat Savitur Vareṇyam Bhargo Devasya Dhīmahi

Dhi Yo Yonah Pracodayāt

The Gāyatrī Mantra may be translated as follows:

"Oṃ (O, Cosmos)-we meditate (dhīmahi) upon the spiritual effulgence (bhargo) of that adorable supreme divine reality (vareṇyam devasya), the source (savitur or Sun) of the physical (bhūr), the astral (bhuvaḥ), and the heavenly (svāhaḥ) spheres of existence. May that (tat) supreme divine being enlighten (pracodayāt) our (nah) intellect (dhiyo) so that we may realise the supreme truth (Oṃ)".

Another alternative for a small pūjā is touching the feet of the elderly, (parent, Master, image of God (Mūrti (sculpture, picture). Man stands on his feet. Touching the feet in prostration is a sign of respect for the age, maturity, nobility and divinity that our elders personify. It symbolises recognition of their selfless love, and access to society. Good wishes (Saṁkalpa) and blessings (Aśīrvāda) of elders are highly valued. We prostrate to seek them. Good thoughts and acts create positive vibrations. Therefore a good heart is necessary. This is why the posture assumed whether it is in the standing or prone position enables the entire body to receive the energy. Posture or sculpture is a symbol of positive energy, viz., characters or digits. A combining word recalls the meaning or secret behind it in our mind. This is a mental healing of growth. Without acceptation we have no perception, no idea and no experience. There is no teaching without a sample or model. Academics say "without sample we speak of verbalism". The master today was a teacher before. Don't touch the sentence of the criminal world. Hinduism avoids verbalism, and that is to touch. In other words: A Hindu doesn't use words considered as predominating over or obscuring ideas or reality.

Table 10: Pūjā in Time Schedule (Good Fortune)

Deity	**Mantra**	**Time limit**	**Results in Vedas**
Lord Rāma	Hé Rāma	in all life circum-stances	rest, peace, harmony, balance, no fear in life (AV 3043)
Lord Gaṇeṣa	Om Śrīmad Mahā Gaṇādi Pataye Namaḥ	10 seconds	remove all pain, miseries and obstacles in life (AV 1026)
Lord Sūrya: Greeting the Sun outside	Om Ghrini Sūryāya Namaḥ	15 seconds	strengthening the mind and brain, beauty, strength (AV 1440)
Goddess Durgā	Om Aiṁ Hriṁ Kliṁ Cāmuṇḍāye Vicaye Namaḥ	30 seconds	love, peace, solving of mental enemies (RV 1.92.1)
Goddess Gāyatrī	Om Bhūr-bhuvaḥ Svāhaḥ Tat Savitur Vareṇyam Bhargo Devasya Dhīmahi Dhi Yo Yonah Pracodayāt	45 seconds	liberation, enlightenment, mindforce (YV 1566) Third Eye
Śrī Yantra-Lakṣmī Yantra	Om Sriṁ Hriṁ ŚrīṁKamle KamlālayePrasida PrasidaOm Sriṁ HriṁŚrī Mahā Lakṣmyai Namaḥ	50 seconds	wisdom, beauty, honour, happiness, wealth (RV 1.125.3) Third Eye

Deity	Mantra	Time limit	Results in Vedas
Goddess Lakṣmī (lightning a Dīya or lamp and incense)	Oṃ Sriṁ Hriṁ Śrī Mahā Lakṣmyai Namaḥ	3 minutes	money, beauty, youthful appearance, good marriage, motherhood (SV 306)

Deity	Mantra	Time limit	Results in Vedas
The Guru Prāṇāyāma Lord Viṣṇu and Lakṣmī	1.Gurur Brahmā Gurur Viṣṇu Gurur Devo Maheśvarah Gurur Sākṣāt Pārabrahma Tasmai Śrī Gurāve Namaḥ 2.Om Namaḥ Sivāya (1:4:2) 3.Śāntākāraṁ Bhujaga-Śayanaṁ Padmanābhaṁ Sureśaṁ Viśvādhāraṁ Gagana-sadṛśaṁ Meghavarṇaṁ Śubhāṅgaṁ Lakṣmīkāntaṁ Kamalanayanaṁ Yogibhir-dhyānagamyaṁ Vaṅde Viṣṇuṁ Bhavabhayaharaṁ Sarvalokaikanāthaṁ	10 minutes	dedication, devotion, love, peace, harmony, knowledge, wisdom, breath control, good concentration, study improvement (AV 1779, 2476) All in One

Results of Pūjā or meditation, according to the Vedas.

"O men, in this world, the Immortal God, All-pervading like space, beyond the light of day, early in the morning before dawn, grants to the learned and immortal soul, happiness that removes miseries and is most excellent. Know and realise Him following the instructions of the Vedas! Those who say their prayer and remember God early in the morning before sunrise, attain to happiness and get freedom from misery" (AV 1026).

"This sweetest Soma juice has been expressed for you at morning rites" (SV 306).

"May the morning prayer realise God's two powers of Pervasion and Excellence, which govern the universe unrestricted through might. Through these two powers, different planets are established, which are strongest and most heroic in their vigour" (AV 1797). "For the householder, who knows how to honour a guest, the rising Sun brings the message of joy, the early morning Sun filled with rays sings praise, the mid-day Sun chants his virtues, the afternoon Sun grants nourishment, the setting Sun grants shelter. He becomes the abiding place of welfare, of progeny, and of cattle" (AV 2476). "The preceptor should say to the seeker after truth, "If thou will try to realise God with eyes different from those of the ancient sages, thou wilt be blind" verily have I now realised God, Who exists after the dissolution of the universe, is far from the ignorant, and near the learned. Like the ancient sages with divine eyes of the Sun and Moon, have I perceived God and acquired Him. Verily this God is Resourceful, Nourishing, and Serviceable. He who thus knows God, becomes resourceful, nourishing, and serviceable" (AV 3043).

"O God, mortal man cannot comprehend the immensity and virility of Thy power. Thou makest every one tremble with Thy fear. Thou destroyest sin, as a cow eats her secundines. God is subtle in contemplation, and grand, expanded in nature to the naked eye, just as the sun contracts in the morning and evening when it sets, and expands and grows warmer in daytime. Just as the jaws of a man press and chew food, so the destructive powers of God devour the universe at the time of dissolution" (AV 1440).

"These divinities of the morning have spread light (over the world); they manifest light in the eastern portion of the firmament, brightening all things, like warriors burnishing their weapons; the radiant and progressing mothers (of the earth), they travel daily (on their course)" (RV 1.92.1).

"Morning and Night, divine Ones, have strengthened bright Indra, strength-giver, the Goddesses advanced the God, With the Anustup laying power in Indra, strength and vital force. For gain of wealth, let them enjoy. Pay sacrifice" (YV 1566).

"Desirous (of again beholding you), I have this day obtained you, who have done in the morning a good deed; the performer of a sacrifice with a wealth-laden car, refresh yourself with the effused juice of the exhilarating (Soma) creeper, and augment with sincere prayers (the prosperity) of the chief of flourishing race" (RV 1.125.3).

God is Light

Performing Pūjā everyday at least for a few minutes, leads one to develop inner purity and peace. Another simpler method is to perform pūjā for a Mūrti as a picture or to a Dīpa as lamp. Both the above methods are of equal value.

All auspicious functions and moments like daily worship, rituals and festivals and even many social occasions like inaugurations commence with the lighting of the lamp, which is often maintained right through the occasion. Light symbolises knowledge, and darkness ignorance. The Lord is the principle knowledge or Caitanya who is the source, the enlivener and the illuminator of all knowledge. Knowledge removes ignorance just as light removes darkness. Also knowledge is a lasting inner wealth by which all outer achievements can be accomplished. Hence we light the lamp to bow down to knowledge as the greatest of all forms of wealth. Knowledge backs all our actions whether good or bad. We therefore keep a lamp lit during all auspicious occasions as a witness to our thoughts and actions. The butter or Ghī in the lamp symbolises our negative tendencies or Vāsanās and the wick, the ego. When lit by spiritual knowledge, those tendencies get slowly exhausted and the ego too finally perishes. The term Namaḥ is also literally interpreted as "na ma" (not mine). It has a spiritual significance of negating or reducing one's ego in the presence of another. We bow is Namaḥ .

The flame of a lamp always burns upwards. Similarly, we should acquire such knowledge as to take us towards higher ideals.

Lighting of the candles has been accepted throughout the world to illuminate and to provide knowledge. Knowledge is something like a candle burning inside an earthen pot having infinite number of holes. Each hole has a shutter. We describe the shutter here as a sample of energy sources. When a shutter is open, a ray of light emerging out of the pot illuminates the thing in its way and provides us with its knowledge. The shutter named ear provides us the sense of sound. The shutter tongue provides us the sense of taste. The shutter eye provides us the sense of sight. The shutter nose provides us the sense of smell. The shutter skin provides us the sense of touch. The shutter mind, if open, provides us righteousness. The more shutters that are open, the more will be the knowledge. If the shutters are closed, it will be a darkness of ignorance. If all the shutters are open, there will be nothing but knowledge. When the number of open shutters tend to infinity, the pot disappears. There will be nothing but light, means knowledge.

Knowledge is Light in Our Life

Academics declare that light is everywhere in our world. We need enough light to see, because it carries information from the world to our eyes and brains. Seeing colours and shapes is a second nature to us. Colour is more than decoration, and perceiving colour is tricky. Our brains and eyes act together, to make extraordinary things happen in perception. Light acts like particles, little light bullets that stream from the source. Light also acts like waves. Scientists have spent lifetimes developing consistent physical, biological, chemical, and mathematical explanations for these principles.

The knowledge we use for people in speeches to open the light or mind. The speaker bridges the audience with knowledge. Before starting a speech we need to concentrate on the latent knowledge in the cosmos. The Hindu in practical life uses mantras before holding a speech or at the commencement and closing of a ceremony. Some of these mantras we mention below. Therefore we focus on the energy or light regarding the faculties.

Gaṇeṣa, the Big Opener

Gajānanaṁ Bhūta Gaṇādi Sevitaṁ
Kapitha Jambū Phalacāra Bhakṣaṇaṁ
Umāsutaṁ Śoka Vināśakārakaṁ
Namāmi Vighneśvara Pāda Pañkajaṁ

"For Him, who has the face of an elephant and is worshipped by the deities of nature; for Him, who eats the essence of kapitha and Jambu fruits; for Him, who is the son of Umā Devī and who destroys all grieves and ill feelings in us; O, Lord Vighneśvara, I offer my homage at your Divine feet".

The Guru, the Eye Opener

Gurur Brahmā Gurur Viṣṇu
Gurur Devo Maheśvarah

Gurur Sākśāt Pārabrahma
Tasmai Śrī Guruve Namaḥ

"Know the Guru to be Brahmā himself. He is Viṣṇu. He is also Śiva. Know him to be the Supreme Brahmā, and offer thy adorations unto that peerless Guru".

The Creators Viṣṇu and Lakṣmī

Śāntākāraṁ Bhujaṁgā-Śayanaṁ Padmanābhaṁ Sureśaṁ
Viśvadhāraṁ Gagana-sadriśaṁ Meghavaraṇaṁ Śubhāngaṁ
Lakṣmīkāntaṁ Kamalanayanaṁ Yogibhirdhyānagamyaṁ
Vande Viṣṇuṁ Bhavabhayaharaṁ Sarvalokaikanathaṁ

"He is of blissful form and lies on a serpent bed. He sports a lotus on his navel and is the Lord of the celestials. He supports the whole cosmos, his limbs are exquisite, and his complexion is blue like that of the sky and the rain cloud. He is the consort of Lakṣmī and has eyes rivalling the lotus. All the yogis meditate on Him in their innermost heart. I bow down before Viṣṇu, the Lord of all worlds and the remover of all causes of fear".

Pūjā Customs

The sacrificer repeats the following six formulas in accordance to the six oblations, one for each season belonging to Prajāpati as Lord of the Year. In this context, word sacrifice means the Vājapeya now in course of performance. The Yajur Veda gives the importance of sacrifice with the following prayer: "May life succeed through sacrifice? May life-breath thrive by sacrifice? May the eye thrive by sacrifice? May the ear thrive by sacrifice? May the back thrive by sacrifice? May sacrifice thrive by sacrifice? We have become the children of Prajāpati. Gods, we have gone to heaven. We have become immortal (YV 9.12: 377). We sincerely pray to the Lord that at least while we undertake special tasks or even in our daily lives, there are no problems or that, problems are minimised.

Tilaka and Kumkuma

The Lord Viṣṇu worshipers apply a Candan Tilaka of the shape of "U", Lord Śiva worshipers apply a Tripundra Bhasma, Devi worshippers apply red dot of Kumkuma. The Chandana, Kumkuma or Bhasma which is offered to the Lord is taken back as Prasāda and applied on foreheads. The Tilaka covers the spot between the eye brows, which is the seat of memory and thinking. It is known as the Ājñā cakra in the language of yoga. The Tilaka is applied with the prayer - "May I remember the Lord. May this pious feeling pervade all my activities. May I be righteous in my deeds". Even when we temporarily forget this prayerful attitude, the mark on another reminds us of our resolve. The Tilaka is thus a blessing of the Lord and protection against wrong tendencies and forces. The entire body emanates energy in the form of electro-magnetic waves-the forehead and the subtle spot between the eye brows especially so. That is why worry generates heat and causes a headache. The Tilaka cools the forehead, protects us and prevents energy loss.

Bhasma

Bhasma (the holy ash) is the ash from the sacrificial fire where special wood along with ghee and other herbs is offered by pouring ash and is then distributed as Bhasma. It is generally applied on the forehead. Some apply it on certain parts of the body, like the upper arms, chest etc. Some ascetics rub it all over the body. Many consume a pinch of it each time they receive it. The word Bhasma means that by which our sins are destroyed and the Lord is remembered. Bha implies Bhartsanam or to destroy, and Sma implies Smaranam or to remember. The application of Bhasma therefore signifies destruction of the evil and remembrance of the divine. Bhasma is also called Vibhūti which means glory as it gives glory to one who applies. It has also a source of protection as it protects the wearer from ill health and evil, by purifying him or her. In the Bible is mentioned: Thy are dust and to dust you shall return (Gen. 3:19).

Bhasma is specially associated with Lord Śiva who applies it all over his body. lord Śiva, devotees apply Bhasma as a Tripuṇḍra. When applied with a red spot in the centre, the mark symbolises Śiva-Śakti or Androgyne: the unity of energy and matter that creates the entire seen and un-seen universe. Ash is what remains when all the wood is burnt away and it does not decay. Similarly, the Lord is the imperishable Truth that remains when the entire creation of innumerable names and forms is dissolved. Bhasma has medicinal value and is used in many āyurvedic medicines. It absorbs excess moisture from the body and prevents colds and headaches. The Upaniṣads say that the famous Mṛtyuñjaya mantra should be chanted while applying ash on the forehead.

Prasāda

In western tradition food is partaken after a thanks giving prayer-grace. Indians make an offering of it to the Lord and later partake of it as Prasāda - a holy gift from the Lord. In temples and in many homes, the cooked food is first offered to the Lord each day. The offered food is mixed with the rest of the food and then served as Prasāda. In our daily ritualistic worship (pūjā) too we offer Naivedyam (food to the Lord). This is done because: The Lord is omnipotent and omniscient. Man is a part, while the Lord is the totality. All that we do, is by his strength and knowledge alone. Hence what we receive in life as a result of our actions is really his alone. We acknowledge this thru the act of offering food to him: "I offer what is yours to you. Thereafter it is akin to his gift to us, graced by his divine touch". The food offered will naturally be pure and the best. We share what we get with others before consuming it. We do not demand, complain or criticise the quality of the food we get. We do not waste or reject it. We eat it with cheerful acceptance (Prasāda Buddhi). When we become established in this attitude, this goes beyond the pre-view of food and pervades our entire life. We are then able to cheerfully accept all we get in life as his.

Before we eat daily meals, we first sprinkle water around the plate as an act of purification. There after the Lord, the life force, who is also within us as the five life-giving physiological functions, is offered the food. The five life-giving functions are prāṇāya (respiratory), apānāya (extretory), vyānāya (circulatory), udānāya (reversal) and samānāya (digestive). After offering the food thus, it is eaten as Prasāda -blessed food.

Kamala

The Kamala or lotus is India's national flower and rightly so. Not long ago, the lakes and ponds of India were full of many hued lotuses. The lotus is the symbol of truth, auspiciousness and beauty (Satyam, Śivam, Sundaram). The Lord is also of that nature and therefore, His various aspects are compared to a lotus (i.e. lotus eyes, lotus feet, lotus hands, the lotus of heart etc.). Our scriptures and ancient literature extol the beauty of the lotus. Art and architecture also portray the lotus in various decorative motifs and paintings. Many people have names of or related to the lotus: Padma, Paṅkaja, Kamalā, Kamalā, Kāmalakṣmī etc. The Goddess of wealth, Lakṣmī, sits on a lotus and carries one in Her hand.

The lotus blooms with the rising sun and closes at night. Similarly, our minds open up and expand with the light of knowledge. The lotus grows even in slushy areas. It remains beautiful and untainted despite its surroundings, reminding us that we too can and should strive to remain pure and beautiful within, under all circumstances. The lotus leaf never gets wet although it is always in water. It symbolises the man of wisdom who remains ever joyous, unaffected by the world of sorrow and change. The lotus posture, Padmāsana is recommended when one sits for meditation.

A lotus emerged from the navel of Lord Viṣṇu. Lord Brahmā originated from it to create the world. Hence, the lotus symbolises the link between the creator and the supreme Cause. It also symbolises Brahmloka, the abode of Lord Brahmā.

The auspicious sign of the Svastika is said to have evolved from the lotus. From the above, we can well appreciate why the lotus is, India's national flower and so special to Hindus.

Śānti

Śānti, meaning peace, is a natural state of being. Others or we create either disturbance. For example, peace already exists in a place until someone makes noise. Therefore, peace underlies all our agitations. When agitations end, peace is naturally experienced since it is already there. Where there is peace, there is happiness. Therefore, everyone without exception desires peace in his/her life. However, peace within or without seems very hard to attain because it is covered by our own agitations. A rare few manage to remain peaceful within even in the midst of external agitation and troubles. To invoke peace, we chant prayers. By chanting prayers, troubles end and peace is experienced internally, irrespective of the external disturbances. All such prayers end by the chanting Śānti thrice. It is believed that Trivaram Satyam-that which is said thrice comes true. For emphasising a point we repeat a thing thrice. In the court of law also, one who takes the witness stand says, "I shall speak the truth, the whole truth and nothing but the truth". We chant Śanti thrice to emphasise our intense desire for peace. All obstacles, problems and sorrows originate three sources:

- Adhidaivic: The unseen divine forces over which we have little or no control like earthquakes, floods, volcanic eruptions etc.
- Adhibhautic: the known factors around us like accidents, human contacts, pollution, crime etc.
- Adhyātmic: Problems of our bodies and minds like diseases, anger, frustrations etc.

May peace alone prevail. Hence Śānti is chanted thrice. It is chanted aloud the first time, addressing the unseen forces. It is chanted softer the second time, directed to our immediate surroundings and those around, and softest the last time as it is addressed to oneself.

Amṛita Phala

In the traditional, Abhiṣekha ritual done in all temples and many homes, several materials are poured over the deity like milk, curd, honey, tender coconut water, sandal paste, holy ash etc. Each material has a specific significance of bestowing certain benefits on worshippers. Tender coconut water is used since it is believed to bestow spiritual growth on the seeker.

The marks on the coconut make it look like the head of a human being. The coconut is broken, symbolising the breaking of the ego. The juice within representing the inner tendencies (Vāsanās) if offered along with the white kernel-the mind, to the Lord. A mind thus purified by the touch of the Lord is used as Prasāda (a holy offering). The coconut also symbolises selfless service. Every part of the coconut tree-the truck, leaves, fruit, coir etc. is used in innumerable ways like thatches, mats, tasty dishes, oil etc. It takes in salty water and converts it into sweet nutritive water that is especially beneficial to the sick. It is also used in the preparation of many Āyurvedic medicines and applications. The marks on the coconut are even thought to represent the three-eyed Lord Śiva and therefore it is considered to be a means to fulfil our desires.

Śaṅkha

The conch sound served to briefly elevate people's minds to a prayerful attitude even in the middle of their busy daily routine. When the conch is blown, the primordial sound of Om emanates.Oṃis an auspicious sound that was chanted by the Lord before creating the world. It represents the world and the truth behind it. In temples or at homes, the conch is blown once or several times before ritualistic worship. It is sometimes blown whilst during Ārati or to mark an auspicious occasion. Towards the end of every ritualistic worship (Pūjā or Bhajan) of the Lord or to welcome an honoured guest or saint, we perform the Ārati. This is always accompanied by the ringing of the bell and sometimes by singing, playing of musical instruments and clapping. The conch is also blown before a battle starts or to announce the victory of an army. The battle of Mahābhārata started with this act. The conch is also placed at the altar in temples and homes next to the Lord as a symbol of Nāda Brahm (Divine Sound), the Vedas, Om, Dharma, victory and auspiciousness. It is often used to offer devotees Tīrtha (sanctified water) to raise their minds to the highest truth.

Kalaśa

A kalaśa is a brass, mud or copper pot filled with water. Mango leaves are placed in the mouth of the pot and a coconut is placed over it. A red or white thread is tied around its neck or sometimes all around it in an intricate diamond-shaped pattern. The pot may be decorated with designs. When the pot is filled with water or rice, it is known as Pūrṇakumbha representing the inert body which when filled with divine life force gains power to do all the wonderful things that makes life what it is.

A Kalaśa is placed with due rituals on all important occasions like the traditional house warming (Gṛhapraveśa), wedding, daily worship etc. It is placed near the entrance as a sign of welcome. It is also used in a traditional manner while receiving holy personages.

Before creation came into being, Lord Viṣṇu was reclining on His snake-bed in the milky ocean. From His navel emerged a lotus from which appeared Lord Brahmā, the Creator, who thereafter created this world. The water in the Kalaśa symbolises the primordial water from which the entire creation emerged. It is the giver of life to all and has the potential of creating innumerable names and forms, the inert objects and the sentient beings and all that is auspicious in the world from the energy behind the universe. The leaves and coconut represent creation. The thread represents the love that 'binds' all in creation. The Kalaśa is therefore considered auspicious and worshipped.

The waters from all the holy rivers, the knowledge of all the Vedas and the blessings of all the deities are invoked in the Kalaśa and its water is thereafter used for all the rituals, including the Abhiṣeka. The consecration (Kumbha-abhiṣeka) of a temple is done in a grand manner with elaborate rituals including the pouring of one or more Kalaśa of holy water on the top of the temple.

When the demons and the demigods churned the milky ocean, the Lord appeared bearing the pot of nectar which blessed one with everlasting life. Thus the Kalaśa also symbolises immortality. Men of wisdom are full and complete as they identify the infinite truth (Pūrṇatvam). They brim with joy and love and represent all that is auspicious. We greet them with a Pūrṇakumbha (full pot) acknowledging their greatness and as a sign of respectful reverential welcome, with a full heart.

Navagraha (Nine Planets) Pūjā

Navagrahas are the secondary deities and usually in Śiva temples. Here, the Sun is the main deity and the other eight planets have their separate Shrines around the Sun. The antiquity of this holy place can be traced to the days of Mahā Bhārata. The Purāṇas subscribe to the same view that all sorts of physical and mental ailments will be mitigated when people worship this temple. It is customary to light Ghiī Dīpams to Navagrahas separately. The Sun is the main deity and Saturn etc., are the Parivāra Devas, and so the sun annuls the influence of Saturn. The Sun, the restorer of the world from darkness to light is also the restorer of mankind from adversity to prosperity. By prayers and Pūjās done to all the nine Graha Devtās (Nine planet's Gods) devotees cast off their physical and mental agonies and derive inward harmony, equanimity, and adjustment.

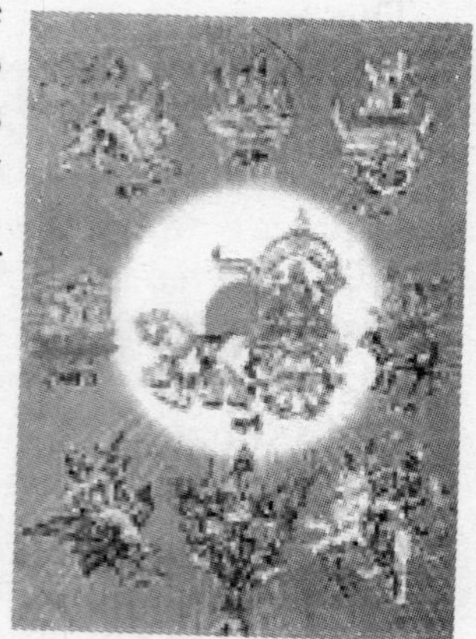

"The moon was born from His mind; the sun was born from His eye; Indra and Agni were born from His mouth, Vāyu from His breath" (RV 10.90.12). There is an ideal world in which a world of ideas exists and in which the mind is the boss. In each activity, thus also at concentration, we must call the idea or the mind at first. This is a cosmic principle. This is the reason why we first light the fire or fire lamp (a) and afterwards the incense at the pray. The woman is related with the moon and in daily costume we say: 'ladies first'.

Sūrya (Sun)

The physically body of God in the cosmos is the Sun. Those who aspire for sound health, prosperity, good eyesight, strength and courage, success, cure of chronic diseases like leprosy, heart ailment, nervous weakness, asthma etc., should worship the Sun. This planet is known for his Power, strength and glory.

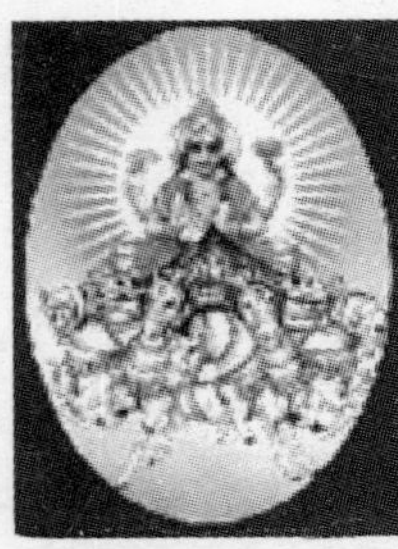

Mantra of the Sun:
Om Jabakusuma Sankāśam Kaśyapayam Mahādyutim Tamorim Sarvapāpaghnam Praṇato-Smi Divākaram OṃSūryāya Namaḥ.
"Om, I bow down with devotion to the shining light that is shining red like a hibiscus flower, shining onto the earth, removing all the darkness and removing sin. Om, I bow to the Sun".

The prayer of the God of Sun is a dynamic exercise, which exists from a consecution of 12 attitudes. She brings all muscles in action and warms these as preparation for the *Āsanas.* For this reason this greeting forms already is a complete exercise on itself. The general twelve mantras of the Sūrya Namaskār are as following [cf. Asana Pranayama Mudra Bandha, Swami Satyananda Saraswati, Bihar Yoga Bharati, India, 1997].

Oṃ Mitrāya Namaḥ, OṃRavaye Namaḥ, OṃSūryāya Namaḥ, OṃBhānave Namaḥ, OṃKhagāya Namaḥ, OṃPuṣane Namaḥ, OṃHiranyagarbhāya Namaḥ, OṃMarīcaye Namaḥ, OṃĀdityāya Namaḥ, OṃSavitre Namaḥ, OṃArkāya Namaḥ, OṃBhāskarāya Namaḥ.

Candra or Moon

The moon stands for the spirit that reacts on the impulses of the eyes as soon as they behold something. One sees in the light and that is one aspect of the sun. In this manner sun and moon have something with each other the same manner that man and wife in the family can be regarded as incense.

The moon regulates the cycle of the fertilisation process and the termination of the germination process. For concentration, mental peace, pleasing personality, control of emotions and to get rid of mental depression one should worship the moon god.

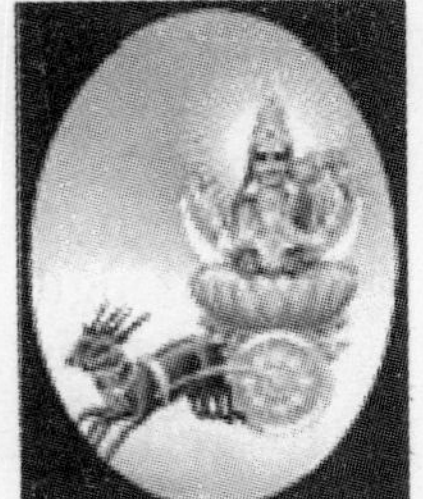

The mantra of the Moon:
Dadhi Śankha Tushārabham Kṣīrodārnasambhavam ˇNamāmi Śaśinām Somam Śambhormukuta Bhuśanam
Om Candrāya Namaḥ
"I bow down to the Moon, who is creamy white like a container of yogurt (dahī) and

most pleasing, born from the churning ocean of milk, the effulgent emblem of devotion, which adorns the head of Lord Śiva. Om, I bow to the Moon".

Maṅgala (Mars) Pūjā

If giving bad results, needs to be propitiated well. It is one of those planets that give very visible positive or negative results. The brain power, willpower and guts, healing power, etc., are provided by the Viśuddhacakra in our body by the Mars (Maṅgala) in the form of cosmic energy.

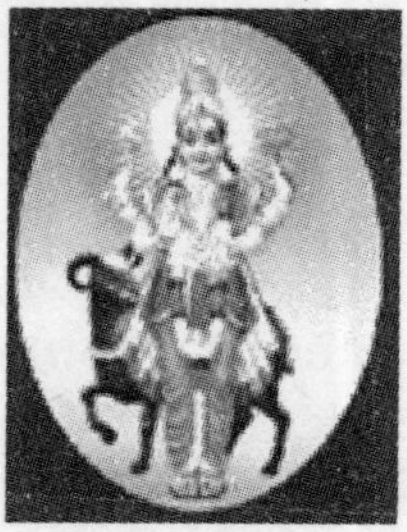

The mantra of Mars:

Dharaṇīgarbhasambhūtam Vidyutkānti Samaprabham ˇKumāram Śaktihastam Ca Tam Maṅgalam Praṇamāmyaham OṃMaṅgalāya Namaḥ

"I bow down to Mars, the auspicious one, who supports the womb of all creation, shines forth with the radiance of beauty enhanced by love, and wields power in his hand. Om, I bow down to Mars".

Budha (Mercury) Pūjā

Those who are weak at studies, lack concentration and suffer from blood pressure and sugar problem etc., should worship Budha. A prayer to Budha, on Wednesdays, brings in manifold benefits like removing obstacles, progeny, possession of fertile lands, etc.

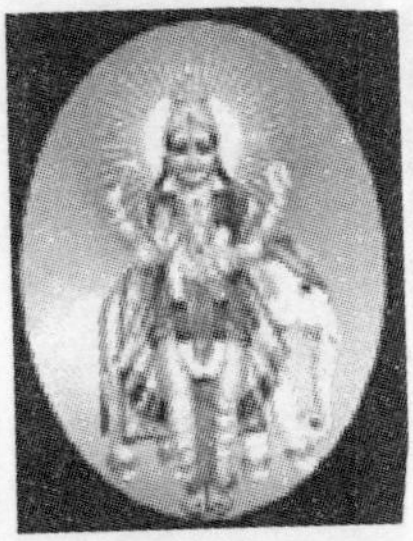

The mantra of Mercury:

Priyaṅgukalikaśyamam Rupenā-Pratimam Budham Saumyam Saumyamguṇopetam Tam Budham Praṇamāmyaham Oṃ Budhāya Namaḥ

"I bow down to Mercury, whose beloved body is dark like the night, the symbol of intelligence, and whose qualities are most beautiful. Oṃ, I bow down to Mercury".

Guru (Jupiter) Pūjā

It is reputed as the father of every living thing. The worship

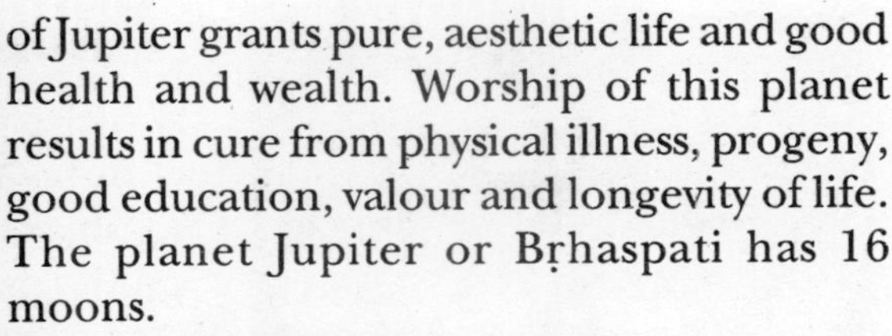

of Jupiter grants pure, aesthetic life and good health and wealth. Worship of this planet results in cure from physical illness, progeny, good education, valour and longevity of life. The planet Jupiter or Bṛhaspati has 16 moons.

The mantra of Jupiter:

Devānānca Rṣanca Gurum Kāncana Sannibham Buddhi Bhūtam Trilokeśam Tam Namāmi Bṛhaspatim Oṃ Gurave Namaḥ

"I bow down to Jupiter, teacher of gods and sages, the greatest treasure, and the most intelligent of all creation. Oṃ, I bow down to Jupiter."

Śukra (Venus) Pūjā

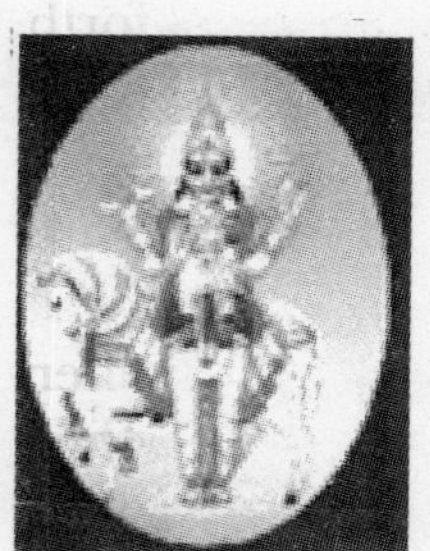

The planet Venus (Śukra) is the most benevolent of all the planets. To have a happy married life, one should worship this planet. In the embryo development (the seventh month) the foetus possesses its complete physical structure through the production of *Ojas* or life power, the essence of Śukra or Venus.

The mantra of Venus:

Hima Kuṇḍa Mrinalabham Daityanām Paramam Gurumāram Bhārgavam Praṇamāmyaham Oṃ Śukrāya Namaḥ

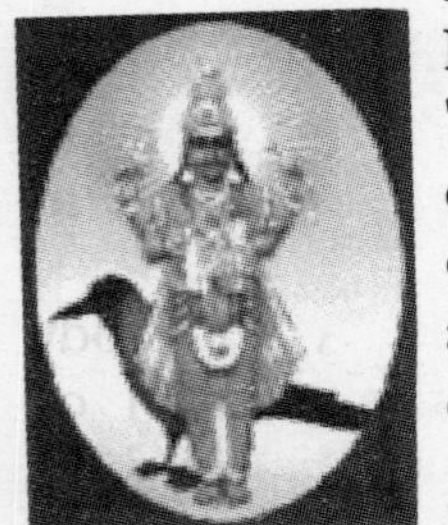

"I bow down to Venus, who is fragrant like crushed sandal and jasmine, the great guru of the demons, expounding all scriptures, and the descendant of sage Bhṛgu. Om, I bow down to Venus".

Śani (Saturn) Pūjā

Saturn or Śani, the sun of Sūrya and Chāyā is also known as 'Īśvara' (The Supreme). It can make a person a king or a beggar according to the native's karmas. This deity is the most sought out among all the planets.

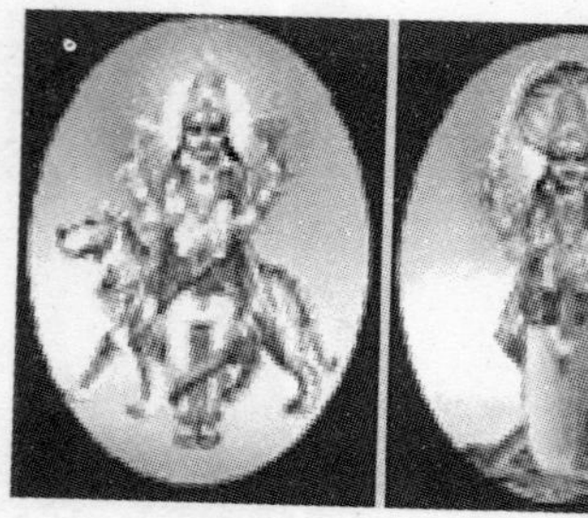

The mantra of Saturn:

Nīlāmbujasamabhāsam Raviputram Yamagrajam Chāyāmar-tandasāmbhūtam Namāmi Śanaśācaram Oṃ Śanaiccarāya Namaḥ

"I bow down to Saturn, who is blue like a storm cloud, the son of the Sun and the brother of Death, who can cast his shadow even over the Sun. Oṃ, I bow down to Saturn".

Rāhu (Dragon Head) Ketu (Dragon Tail) Pūjā

Rāhu and Ketu are shadow planets and have the powers of Saturn and mars respectively. The proper worship of both the planets blesses all those who suffer from sudden illness, loss of money and delay in marriage. Rāhu is instrumental is strengthening one's power and converting an enemy into a friend. The effect of snake bite is removed by His grace.

The mantras of Rāhu and Ketu:

Ardhakāyam Mahāvīryam Candradityavimardanam
Simhikagarbha Sambhūtam Tam Rāhu Praṇamāmyaham
Oṃ Rāhave Namaḥ

"I bow down to Rāhu, the great warrior who divides even the Sun and Moon in half, born from the womb of Simhika. Oṃ, I bow down to Rāhu".

Palaśapuśpa Sankaśam Tārakagrahamaṣṭakam
Raudram Raudrātmakam Ghorām Tam Ketu Praṇamām-yahamOṃKetave Namaḥ

"I bow down to Ketu, who is red like a palāsha flower, who makes the star-eyed constellation to set, terrible and awesome to behold. Om, I bow down to Ketu."

Janam Divas (Birthday) Pūjā

Birthday is one of the most important day in ones life. Birthday pūjā is done on the date of birth and recommended for everyone for a happy long life. This is done once in a lifetime. Every person should do a birthday pūjā.

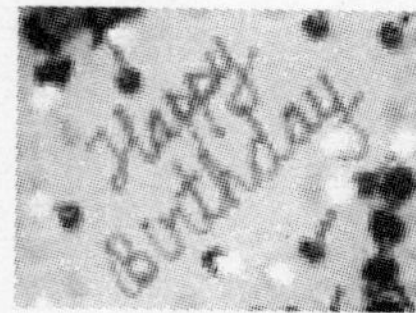

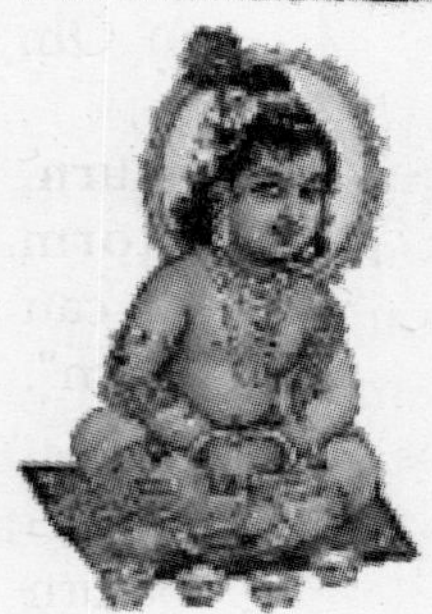

Children are nature's gift for the happiness of a family. When a native is devoid of a child, life becomes hell. Peace of mind is destroyed in spite of having all comforts of life if there is no child or any issue out of the couple. If there are obstacles or delay in progeny and some complications/ obstacles arises during pregnancy Santāna Gopālana Homa is performed for childless couple, who wish to have a child. This pūjā is performed on your behalf, to beget a child. Those who are expecting, shall also perform this pūjā for a healthy and intelligent child. After performing this homam one will be blessed with a child, wealth, property, gain, and prosperity. Those who wish progeny, success in endeavours, worldly enjoyment and final emancipation shall attain it by performing this homam.

Lord Gaṇeṣa Pūjā

Gaṇapati or Gaṇeṣa, the Lord of Gaṇas, the elephant faced God, represents the power of the Supreme Being that removes obstacles and ensures success in human endeavors. Gaṇeṣa is revered as the son of the Śiva and Pārvati, and is always honored first in most worship services and rituals. Gaṇeṣa is also known as Gaṇapati, Vighneśvara, Vināyaka, Gajamukha and so forth. He is worshipped for siddhi, success in undertakings, and buddhi, intelligence. He is worshipped before any venture is started. He is also the God of education, knowledge and wisdom, literature, and the fine arts. Gaṇeṣa is also one of the five Gods the worship of whom was popularised by Ādi Shankarāchārya; the other four are Viṣṇu, Śiva, Devi and Sūrya. The worship of these five deities is called the Pañcāyatana Pūjā. In some cases, a sixth God, Skanda is also worshipped.

The large head of an elephant symbolises wisdom, understanding, and a discriminating intellect that one must possess to attain perfection in life. The wide mouth represents the natural human desire to enjoy life in the world. The large ears signify that a perfect person is the one who possesses a great capacity to listen to others and assimilate ideas. The trunk relates to the power of human mind, which must be strong enough to face the ups and downs of the external world and yet delicate enough to explore the subtle realms of the inner world. The two tusks denote the two aspects of the human personality, wisdom and emotion. The right tusk represents wisdom left tusk represents emotion. A broken left tusk conveys the idea that one must conquer emotions with wisdom to attain perfection. The eyes: the elephant eyes are said to possess natural deceptiveness that allows them to perceive objects to be bigger than what they really are. Thus one's pride and attain humility.

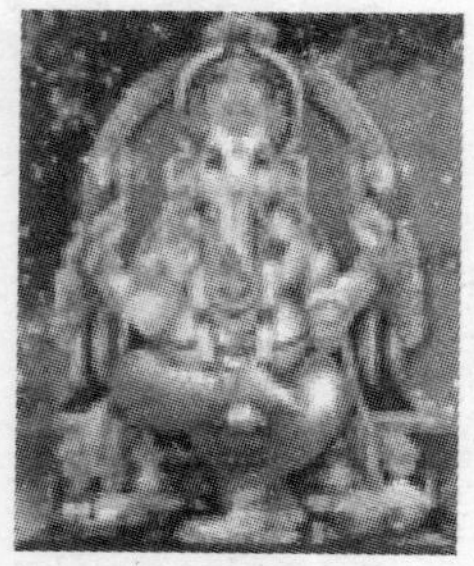

The four arms and various objects in the four hands: the four arms indicate that the Lord is omnipresent and omnipotent. The left side of the body symbolises emotion and the right side symbolises reason. An axe in the upper left hand and a lotus in the upper right hand signify that in order to attain spiritual perfection, one should cut worldly attachments and conquer emotions. This enables one to live in the world without being affected by earthly temptations, just as a lotus remains in water but is not affected by it.

A tray of Laḍḍus near the Lord denotes that He bestows wealth and prosperity upon His devotees. The lower right hand is shown in a blessing pose, which signifies that gaṇeṣa always blesses his devotees.

A body with a big belly: the human body possesses a human heart, which is a symbol of kindness and compassion toward all. Gaṇeṣa's body is usually portrayed wearing red and yellow clothes. Yellow symbolizes purity, peace and truthfulness. Red symbolises the activity in the world.

A mouse sitting near the feet of Gaṇeṣa and gazing at the tray of Laḍḍus: a mouse symbolises the ego that can nibble all that is good and noble in a person. A mouse sitting near the feet of Gaṇeṣa indicates that a perfect person is one who has conquered his (or her) ego. Right foot dangling over the left foot illustrates that in order to live a successful life one should utilise knowledge and reason to overcome emotions.

Hanumāna Pūjā

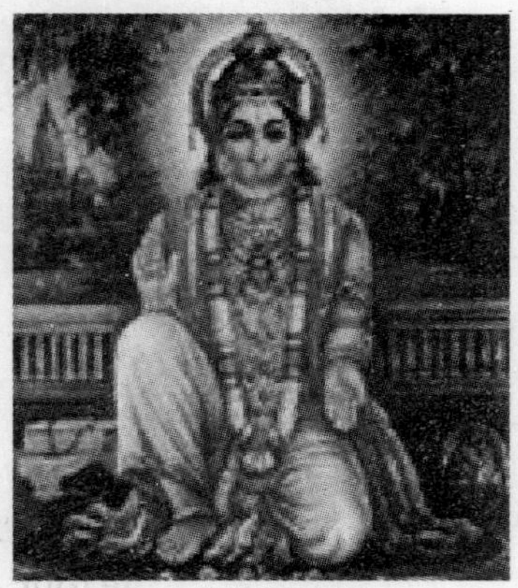

Śrī Hanumānajī is known to be the incarnation of Lord Śiva. It is believed that when Lord Viṣṇu took birth, in the form of Rāma to vanish, the greatest demon king Rāvaṇa, the other Gods also were born in monkey and bear races to help him. God Śeṣanāga and Lord Śiva incarnated as Lakṣmaṇa and Hanumāna respectively. He was born on the full moon day (Pūrṇimā) of the month Caitra (March) on Tuesday. That is why, every year when Caitra month's full moon day arrives, his birthday is celebrated, which is called Śrī Hanumāna Jayanti and Tuesday is considered very auspicious day to worship Hanumānajī. Its pūjā cures all illness and gives a person courage to fight the illness and gives peace of mind.

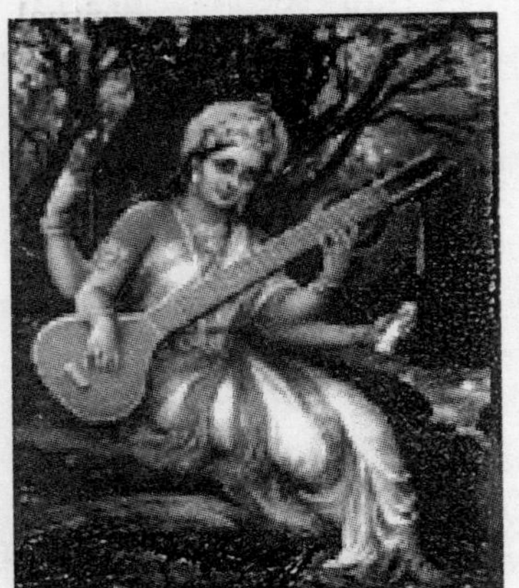

Sarasvatī Pūjā

Goddess Sarasvatī is the wife (consort) of Lord Brahmā and possesses the powers of speech, wisdom and learning. She has four hands representing four aspects of human personality in learning; mind, intellect, alertness and ego. Sarasvatī Devī is controller of education, intelligence and speech. In case a man stammers, his stammering will be controlled by this pūjā. By performing this pūjā one will be blessed with success in the examinations, will have concentration in education, will not forget but retain and remember whatever he or she reads.

Mahāmṛtyuñjaya Homm

This powerful mantra of Śiva the Rudra removes physical, mental, and celestial ailments. Like Gāyatrī, this is an all-purpose mantra and is commonly prescribed by astrologers, Vaidyas (medicine men), and Tantrics. Recitation or Japa of 125,000 times removes the fear of death, even if the condition of the ailing person is so severe that the doctors become helpless and no medicine works.

After the Japa, Homa or fire sacrifice should be done with 12,500 repetitions of the mantra and an offering of black sesame seeds with each. Mahāmṛtyuñjaya is a name of Śiva, the Lord of Destruction. As Mahākāla He is Lord of Death.

Meditation on Śiva with four arms is necessary. In his Mahāmṛtyuñjaya form, Śiva is sitting in a pond. Two of his arms are holding water pots, from which he is pouring water over his head. His third hand on the right side is doing a mala, and in his fourth hand on the left side he has another water pot, from which water is constantly issuing. Sometimes one of his right hands is shown in a blessing Mudra (gesture). Mahāmṛtyuñjaya Mantra also known as the Śiva-Gāyatrī, due to the three parts in this mantra starting with Bhūr-bhuvah Svah. This mantra is supposed to give victory over death, suffering, and disease. It removes obstacles, creates a suitable environment, and brings happiness to life.

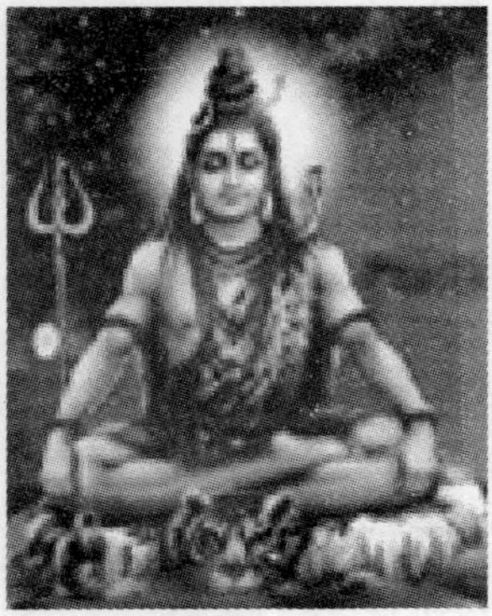

Mahāmṛtyuñjaya Homam is dedicated to Lord Śiva to avoid untimely death. This Homa is performed to achieve Jaya or victory over Mṛtyu or death. It is performed for longevity, on birthdays. It is also done for extending life time and performed for cure for chronic illness and healthy life.

The mantra of Mahāmṛtyuñjaya is as follows:
Oṃ Hraum Jūm Sah.Oṃ Bhūrbhuvah Svaḥ
Oṃ Trayambakam Yajāmahe, Sugandhim Puṣṭivar-

dhanam. Urvārukamiva Bandhanān Mṛtyormukśiya Māmṛtāt. Oṃ Svaḥ bhuvah Bhūh Oṃ Sah Jūm Hraum Oṃ.

Abhiśeka is a part of the worship of Lord Śiva. Without it, the worship is incomplete. It is the ceremonial bathing of the Śiva Liṅgam in Śiva temples. A pot made of copper or brass, with a tiny hole in the centre, is kept hanging over the image or Liṅgam of Śiva. Water drips (falls) on the image throughout the day and night. Pouring water, milk, ghee (clarified butter), curd, and honey, or coconut water over the Lingam is also Abhiṣeka. Whilst this is done, the Rudram is chanted loudly with devotion and love. Lord Śiva is invoked by performing this Abhiśeka.

Monday is a very important day for worshipping Lord Śiva. The thirteenth day (Pradośa) of the bright and dark fortnights is also considered sacred. On these days, devotees of Lord Śiva offer special worship with plenty of Prasāda.

The water of the Abhiśeka is considered very sacred. It is known to grant great benefits on the devotees who take it as the Lord's Prasāda. It purifies the heart and destroys countless sins. You should take it with intense faith and devotion.

When you perform Abhiśeka with devotion, your mind is concentrated. Your heart is filled with divine thoughts and with the image of the Lord. You forget your body and your surroundings. Egoism vanishes. When the body is forgotten, you begin to enjoy and taste the eternal bliss of Lord Siva. The recitation of Mantras during the Abhiśeka purifies the mind. The greatest and the highest Abhiśeka is to pour the waters of pure love on the Lingam in the lotus of the heart. The external Abhiśeka with objects is intended to lead to this internal Abhiśeka, wherein there is a flow of pure love.

The sacred Prasāda of the Lord and the holy water of the Abhiśeka purifies the heart if taken with faith and devotion. They can bring peace and prosperity. Incurable diseases are cured by performing Abhiśeka. It bestows health, wealth, and prosperity, peace of mind and purity of heart. It expands the heart. It calls for self-sacrifice and self-surrender. There must be a natural feeling in the heart. "I am Thine, my Lord. All is Thine, my Lord."

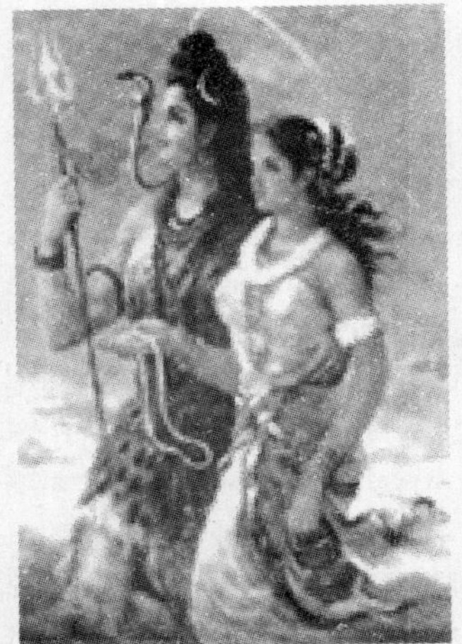

Umā Maheśvarī Pūjā

'Marriages are made in heaven', goes the proverb. Two people start a new journey towards the future, hand in hand, sharing at each step new outlooks, responsibilities and love. Marriage is an auspicious occasion among us. Arranged marriage is still a common practice while love marriages (Gandharva Vivāha), where partners choose each other without the intervention of their family members, are more prevalent in recent times. Arranged marriages are still a widely practiced form of forming an eternal partnership where two completely unknown people tie the knot for life with the initial introduction done by the help of both the families. These relationships are more based upon the foundation of adjustments, compromises, and sacrifices and a liking for each other which blossoms into love.

Uma Maheśvari pūjā is for long and happy married life. Umā (Goddess Pārvatī the wife of Lord Śiva) and Lord Śiva pūjā is performed as they are considered to be the perfect match i.e., Śiva and Śakti. This pūjā is considered to be best for marital happiness if there is any discord in the relationship, all will be resolved. One should conduct this pūjā at least once a year for a happy married life.

Viṣṇu Pūjā

Lord Viṣṇu represents the aspect of the Supreme Reality-is the Lord of protection and maintenance. His consort Lakṣmī is the possessor of wealth, which is a necessity for maintenance. Goddess Lakṣmī represents not only material wealth, but also the wealth of grains, courage, valour, offsprings, success, luxurious life, eternal bliss. Viṣṇu symbolises the all-pervading protective aspect of the Supreme God, Brahmā. However, according to Hindu mythology, Viṣṇu is reincarnated on earth from time to time, to destroy evil in the world. The four arms indicate the Lord's omnipresence and omnipotence. The right side of the body represents the creative activities of the mind and the intellect. The left side symbolises the activities of the heart; that is, love, kindness, and compassion.

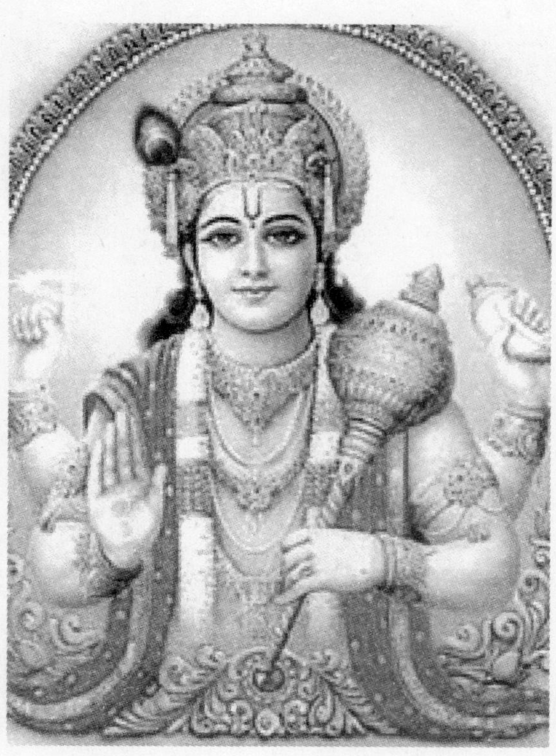

BIBLIOGRAPHY

- ***All About Hinduism;*** Sri Swami Sivananda; The Divine Life Society; Himalayas; India; 1993.
- ***An integrated theory of the earth;*** Murthy, S.R.N.; Kalpatharu Research Academy; Bangalore; 1987.
- ***Ancient Indian Rituals and their Social Contents;*** N. N. Bhattacharyya; Manohar Publishers & Distributors; New Delhi; 1996.
- ***Asana Pranayama Mudra Bandha;*** Swami Satyananda Saraswati; Bihar Yoga Bharati; India; 1997.
- ***Aspects of Hindu Morality;*** Jhingran, Saral; Motilal Banarsidass Publishers Pvt. Ltd.; Delhi; 1999.
- ***Aspects of Yoga;*** Kaul, H. Kumar; B.R. Publishing Corporation; Delhi; 1994.
- ***Beginnings of Life, Culture and History (vol I);*** Kulkarni, S.D., Vedavyasa, Shri Bhagavan; Itihasa Samshodhana Mandira (BHISMA); Bombay; 1988.
- ***Breath, Mind and Consciousness;*** Harish Johari, Rochester; Vermont; Destiny Books; U.S.A.; 1989 (page 15).
- ***Chakras; Energy Centers of transformation;*** Harish Johari; Destiny Books; U.S.A; 1994.
- ***Classical Indian Ethical Thought;*** Tiwari, Kedar Nath; Motilal Banarsidass Publishers Pvt. Ltd.; Delhi; 1998.
- ***Comparative Ethics in Hindu and Buddhist Traditions;*** Hindery, Roderick; Motilal Banarsidass Publishers Pvt. Ltd.; Delhi; 1978.

- ***Concentration and Meditation;*** Sri Swami Sivananda; The Divine Life Society, U.P., India, 1994.
- ***Cyclic Universe, Creation, Evolution, Involution and Dissolution of the Universe, vol. 1 The Unsolved Riddle;*** Panda, N.C.; D.K. Printworld (P) Ltd.; Delhi; 2002.
- ***Dancing with Siva; Hinduism's Contemporary Catechism;*** Satguru Sivaya Subramuniyaswami; Himalayan Academy India; USA; 1993.
- ***Dead and Eternal life;*** John Hick; The Dutch version was published in by Helmond and Helmond, Deventer; 1976 (p.34).
- ***First steps to Higher Yoga;*** Shri Yogeshwarananda Parmahans; Yoga Niketan Trust; New Delhi; 1987.
- ***Hatha Yoga Pradipika;*** Swami Visnu-Devananda; Om lotus Publications, Motilal Banarsidass Publishers Pvt. Ltd., New Delhi, 1987.
- ***Hatha Yoga, The hidden language;*** Symbols, Secrets, and Metaphor, Swami Sivananda Radha, Jaico publishing house, Bombay, 1998.
- ***Hindu Samskaras, Socio-Religious Study of the Hindu Sacraments;*** Pandey, Rajbali; Motilal Banarsidass Publishers Pvt. Ltd.; Delhi; 1993.
- ***Hindu Spirituality. Vedas through Vedanta;*** Sivaraman, Krishna (ed.); Motilal Banarsidass Publishers Pvt. Ltd.; Delhi; 1989.
- ***Hindu World (volume 1-2);*** An encyclopaedic survey of Hinduism, Benjamin Walker; HarperCollins Publishers India; New Delhi, 1995.
- ***Hinduism and Scientific Quest;*** Iyengar, T.R.R.; D.K. Printworld (P) Ltd.; Delhi; 1997.

- ***Hinduism: The Anthropology of a Civilization;*** Biardeau, Madeleine; Calcutta, Chennai, Mumbai; Oxford University Press; 1997.
- ***History of Civilizations of central Asia volume I to III;*** Dani, A.H., Masson, V.M.; Motilal Banarsidass Publishers Pvt. Ltd.; Delhi; 1999.
- ***Indian Music in Professional and Academic Institutions;*** Dr. (Mrs.) Manjusree Chaudhuri; Sanjay Prakashan; Delhi 1999.
- ***Introduction to Buddhism;*** Kelsang Gyatso, Geshe; Motilal Banarsidass Publishers Pvt. Ltd.; Delhi; 1992.
- ***Introduction to Religious Philosophy;*** Masih, Y.; Motilal Banarsidass Publishers Pvt. Ltd.; Delhi; 2002.
- ***Introduction to Tantra Śastra;*** Sir John Woodroffe; Ganesh & Company; Madras; 1997 (page 127).
- ***Kuṇḍalini Yoga;*** Swami Sivananda Radhas; Motilal Banarsidass Publishers Pvt. Ltd., New Delhi, 1992.
- ***Kundalini Yoga;*** Swami Sivananda; The Devine Life Society, U.P., India, 1994.
- ***Kundalini, An Occult Experience***; Arundale, G.S., Adyar; Madras, 1947.
- ***Light on Pranayam;*** Pranayam Dipika; B.K.S. Iyengar; HarperCollins Publishers India Pvt Ltd, New Delhi, 1993.
- ***Mantra-Yoga Samhita;*** Dr. Ramkumar Rai; Chaukhambha Orientalia; A house of Oriental and Antiquarian Books; Delhi; 1982 (pag.71).
- ***Meditation and Mantra's;*** Swami Visnu-Devananda; Om lotus publications, Motilal Banarsidass Publishers Pvt. Ltd., New Delhi, 1978.

- ***Meditation on OM and Mandukya Upanishad;*** Sri Swami Sivananda; The Devine Life Society, U.P., India, 1997.
- ***Music and Musical Thought in Early India;*** Lewis Rowell; Munshiram Manoharlal Publishers Pvt. Ltd.; New Delhi 1998.
- ***Patanjali's Yoga Sustras, with the commentary of Vyasa and the gloss of Vachaspati Misra;*** Munshiram Manoharlal Publishers Pvt. Ltd., New Delhi, India, 1998.
- ***Practicals of Yantras;*** L.R. Chawdhri; Sagar Publications; New Delhi; 1990.
- ***Pure Yoga;*** Yogi Pranavananda; Motilal Banarsidass Publishers Pvt. Ltd., New Delhi, India, 1997.
- ***Ritual and Mantras: Rules Without Meaning;*** Staal, Frits; Motilal Banarsidass Publishers Pvt. Ltd.; Delhi; 1996.
- ***Science and Mysticism, The essence of Vedic Philosophy;*** Kesavan H.K.; New Age International Publishers; Delhi; 1997.
- ***Secret Power of Tantrik Breathing;*** Swami Sivapriyananda; Abhinav Publications; Delhi; 1996.
- ***Sivasvarodaya;*** Ram Kumar Rai, Prachya Prakashan Varanasi; Second Edition 1987.
- ***Spiritual Experiences;*** Shri Swami Sivananda; A Divine Life Society Publication; Delhi; 1995.
- ***Ten Upanishads;*** Swami Sivananda; A Divine Life Society Publication; Tehri-Garhwal; U.P. Himalaya's; 1993 (page 34).
- ***The Art of Yoga;*** BKS Iyengar; Harper Collins Publishers India Pvt Ltd; New Delhi; 1985.
- ***The Concept of Man, A study in comparative philosophy;*** Radhakrishnan, S., Raju, P.T.; HarperCollins Publishers; Delhi; 1997.

- ***The cosmic vibration AUM, OM;*** Ashima Kaul Bhatia, Aravali Books International, New Delhi, 1998.
- ***The Hindu quest for the perfection of man;*** Organ, Troy Wilson; Munshiram Manoharlal Publishers Pvt. Ltd.; Delhi; 1994.
- ***The Hinduism Rimer;*** Gopsons Paper Ltd. Noida; India; 1993.
- ***The Holistic Way to Health, Happiness and Harmony;*** V.K. Subramanian; Shakti Malik Abhinav Publications; New Delhi; 1996.
- ***The illustrated guide to Astronomy;*** Bill Yenne, Ars Scribendi BV, Harmelen; Belgium; 1995 (page 181).
- ***The Naradiya Purana;*** Dr. S.S. Upadhyaya, Srimati Kumud Kumari Upadhyaya; Muzaffarpur, Bihar; 1983.
- ***The Primal Power of Man or Kundalini Sakti;*** Narayananda, Swami; Rishikesh, India, 1950.
- ***The Religions hidden Cults of India;*** Macmunn, Sir Goerge; Neeraj Publishing House; Delhi; 1982.
- ***The science of Pranayama;*** Swami Sivananda; The Divine Life Society, U.P., India, 1997.
- ***The Secret Serpent;*** Datta, M.R.; Motilal Banarsidass Publishers Pvt. Ltd., New Delhi, India, 1994.
- ***The Serpent Power;*** Sir John Woodroffe; Ganesh & Company; Madras; 1997.
- ***The Spectrum of Consciousness;*** Wilber, Ken; Motilal Banarsidass Publishers Pvt. Ltd.; Delhi; 2002.
- ***The Tantric Way;*** Ajit Mookerjee and Madhu Khanna; Thames and Hudson; London; 1977.
- ***The Textbook of Yoga;*** George Feuerstein, Ank-Hermes bv; Deventer; 1978.

- ***The Tree of Yoga;*** B.K.S. Iyengar; Harper Collins Publishers India Pvt Ltd.; New Delhi; 2000.
- ***The World's Great Religions;*** Hutchinson, Paul; Golden Press, Inc.; New York; 1958.
- ***Theories of the Chakras,*** Bridge to Higher Consiousness, Hiroshi Motoyama; Uitgeverij Ank-Hermes bv, Deventer, 1990.
- ***Tools for Tantra;*** Harish Johari; Destiny Books; Rochester; Vermont; 1986
- ***The Hindu Connection, Roots of the New Age;*** Victor Raj, A.R.; Concordia Publishing House; St. Louis; 1995.
- ***What is Yoga: Een inleiding tot universeel denken;*** Hans Wesseling; Uitgeverij Bert Bakker; Amsterdam, 1978.
- ***What becomes of the soul after Death;*** Swami Sivananda; A Divine Life Society Publication; Tehri-Garhwal; U.P.; 1997 (page 14 tm 24).
- ***Wisdom, The Absolute is Adorable;*** Nataraja Guru; D.K. Printworld (P) Ltd.; Delhi; 1995.
- ***Yoga & Ayurveda, Self-Healing and Self-Realization;*** David Frawley; Motilal Banarsidass Publishers Pvt. Ltd., New Delhi, India, 2002.
- ***Yoga & Sex;*** Pandit Shiv Sharma & Kailash Nath Sharma; B.I. Publications PVT Ltd., New Delhi, 1973.
- ***Yoga Darshan: Vision on the Yoga Upanishads;*** Paramhansa Satyananda; Ganga Darshan; India; 1993.
- ***Yoga Philosophy: In relation to other systems of Indian Thought;*** S.N. Dasgupta; Motilal Banarsidass Publishers P ltd., Delhi, 1996.
- ***Yoga Suras, with the commentary of Vyasa and the gloss of***

Vachaspati Misra; translated by Rama Prasada; Munshiram Manoharlal Publishers Pvt. Ltd.; New Delhi; 1998.

- ***Yogacarya Astadala Yogamala;*** B.K.S. Iyengar; Allied Publishers Limited; New Delhi; 2000.

Index of Oral and Practical Science

Below I present a list of the persons and institutions that provided information to make this book possible.

The Netherlands

- Widwad Parishad Nederland (WPN), Den Haag.
- Sanātan Dharm Brahm Widwad Parishad Nederland, Rotterdam.
- Stichting Shri Sanātan Dharm Rotterdam.
- Stichting Lallarookh Nederland, Utrecht.
- Stichting voor Surinamers, Den Haag.
- Sanātan Hindoe Parishad Nederland (SHPN), Den Haag.
- Shrimati S. Lalta, Rotterdam-India.
- Prof. Dr. W.R.W. Donner, Rotterdam.
- Prof. M.K. Gautam, Leiden.
- Shri S. Changoe Āchārya, Den Haag.
- Shri A. Bhageloe Panday Shastrārd Kesari, Rotterdam.
- Shri H. Sardjoe Misier, Den Haag.
- Shri A. Ardjoen Sharma, Hoofddorp.
- Shri V. Mahadew Panday, Rotterdam.
- Drs. D. Shriemisier, Purmerend.
- Shri R. Ramdoelare Panday, Amsterdam.
- Shri P. Tewarie, Den Haag.
- Shri R. Baidjnath Misier, Rotterdam.
- Shri W. Jaipal, Rotterdam.
- Shri Sillivis Smith (Reformed Minister), Rotterdam.

Surinam

- Shri Sanātan Dharm Māhā Sabhā Paramaribo.
- Dr. R.M. Nannan Panday, Paramaribo.
- Shri Haldhar Mathoerapersad Sharma Ācārya, Paramaribo.
- Shri C. Sewpersad, Paramaribo.
- Dr. Rajiv Lochanāchāryaji (International Chaitanya *Kundaliniyoga*-mission, Madhya Pradesh), India.
- Shri B. Jaggoe (Maulāna), Paramaribo.

India

- Vishva Hindu Parishad, New Delhi, Shri Ashok Singhal Ji, Girijraj Kishore Ācārya Ji and Shri Dr. R. Ojha Ji.
- Jayarāma Āshrama Rishikesh, Shree Devindra Svarupa Brahmāchari Shāstri Ji.
- Jayarāma Āshrama Haridwār, Shri Brahmasvarupa Brahmāchariji.
- Dr. Premācārya ji, Vaidic Sahitya Shāstrard Mahā Rathi, New Delhi.
- Shri Shrikant Chaturveda Bhasyakāra Shāstri Ji, New Delhi.
- Professor J.S.L Tripathi, Benares Hindu University of India (BHU).

Pitha Adishvara; provincial research coordinator (Pastor)

- Swāmi Sarvadānanda Sarasvati Naimishvyash Jagatācārya Pithādhisvar, Naymisaranya.
- Shri Bhānupura Pithādhisvar Sankarācārya (Jagatguru), Mansur.

Vedapāthi (Veda-specialists)

- Shri Dinesh Chandra Vedapāthi Ji *(Rig Veda).*
- Dr. Gangadhar Shāstri Ji *(Sāma Veda).*
- Shri Sanjeev Kumar Avasthi Vedapāthi Ji *(Yajur-and Atharva Veda)*.
- Shri Shridhar Vedpathi Ji *(Sāma Veda)*.

Priests and teachers

- Dr. Bhagavadālankar Shukerle Ji Upadhyaya, Khwalipur.
- Dr. Sauvnak Brahmāchary Ji Mahāraj, Kanpur.
- Shri Nathu Ram Pandey Ji, Ācārya, Chitrakoot, Uttar Pradesh.
- Shri Munis Chanda Shāstri Ji, New Delhi.
- Shri Brajesh Shāstri Ji, New Delhi.
- Dr. Sukhratna Upadhiyaya Ji.

Index

P

R

S

BOOKS OF RELATED INTEREST

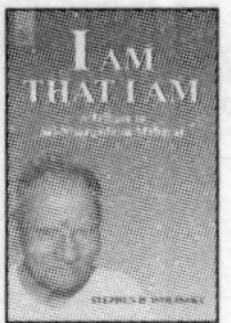

I AM THAT I AM
A Tribute to Sri Nisaradatta Maharaj
Stephen H. Wolinsky
81-7822-262-0

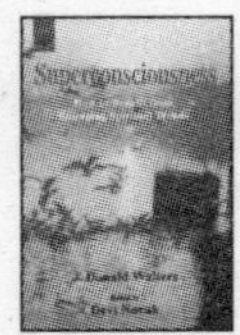

SUPERCONSCIOUSNESS
How to Benefit from Emerging Spiritual Trends
J. Donald Walters
81-7822-026-1

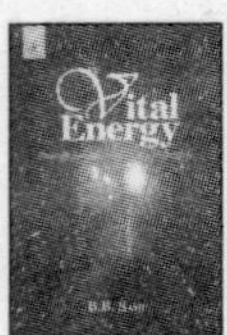

VITAL ENERGY
Energy for Normal Body Function
B.B. Sahi
81-7822-081-4

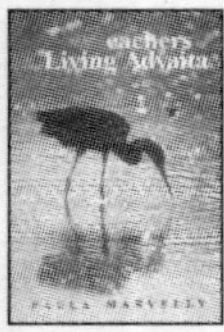

THE TEACHERS OF ONE LIVING ADVAITA
Conversations on the Nature of Non-Duality
Paula Marvelly
81-7822-144-6

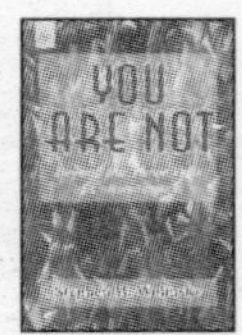

YOU ARE NOT
Beyond the Three Veils of Consciousness
Stephen H. Wolinsky
81-7822-261-2

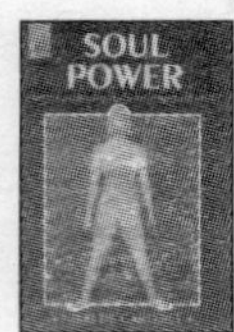

SOUL POWER
The Transformation That Happens When You Know
Nikki De Carteret
81-7822-145-4

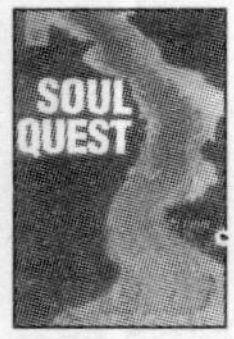

SOUL QUEST
Journey From Death to Immortality
Anand Krishna
81-7822-234-5

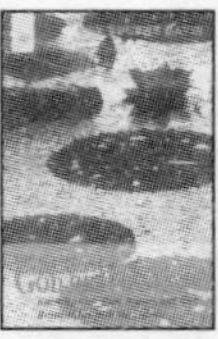

THE SCIENCE OF GOD-REALIZATION
Knowing Our True Nature and Our Relationship With the Infinite
Roy Eugene Davis
81-7822-082-2

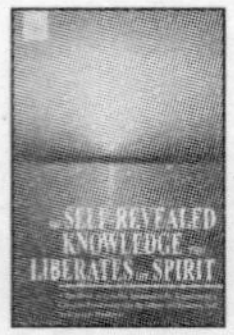

THE SELF-REVEALED KNOWLEDGE THAT LIBERATES THE SPIRIT
A Handbook of Essential Information for Experiencing a Concious Relationship with the Infinite and Restoring Soul Awareness to Wholeness
Roy Eugene Davis
81-7822-050-4